LIFE AND ETHICS IN JAPAN

―in consideration of history, religion and culture―

Norihiko Aoki

Yanagihara Shuppan

Life and Ethics in Japan
— in consideration of history, religion and culture—
by Norihiko Aoki
Copyright © 2008 Norihiko Aoki

Published by Yanagihara Shuppan Ltd.(Publishers Since 1747)
74,Kawashima-Kitaura-cho,Nishikyo-ku,Kyoto,Japan
All rights reserved.Printed in Japan.
ISBN 978-4-8409-7049-5
http://www.yanagihara-pub.com/

LIFE AND ETHICS IN JAPAN

—in consideration of history, religion and culture—

Norihiko Aoki

In memory of my affectionate parents, Tsuya Aoki (1904-1996) and Morishiroh Aoki (1905-1996), who lived long and died in the same year, leaving in me a deep compassion for all living things and an ever-lasting philosophical curiosity about the world.

Preface

Bioethics has only a short history.

It is a new discipline which came into bloom in the late 20th century as a modern subtype of ethics, which has been a field of great concern for humans as having a long history dating back to Confucius of about 2500 years ago and Aristotle in ancient Greece. Bioethics was born mainly because a new area of scientific investigation called life science was born in the late 20th century, when a mechanistic or scientific approach even to life funned out to be possible, with the same methodology as in physics and chemistry, and because this life science needs essentially ethics.

The essence of ethics is learning from practice, unlike science, which is based on the law of causality. Since it is learning from practice, it should have flexibility, that is, adaptability and applicability to actual society. Otherwise, it remains to be a classical ethics or knowledge lacking usefulness in our time. Also, ethics spreads its thick root deep into the ethos (customs and mores). That is, we have to admit that ethics is strongly affected by regional characteristics, ethnicity, national character, religious belief and the course of history, and therefore that it is relative.

Bioethics is rapidly growing in recent years in the Western cultural sphere, especially in the U.S. There are several major reasons for this. One is that the progress in life science such as gene manipulation, cloning technology and organ transplantation has raised unprecedented and entirely new ethical questions, that is, life is not a sanctuary or a mystic area anymore, unlike until the beginning of the 20th century. Secondly, the principles of individual freedom, human rights and equality based on liberal individualism have spread the results of modern science and modern culture to every corner of the free world. Thirdly, the unexpectedly rapid spread and development of communications networks, as symbolized by the IT revolution in the 1990s, has brought about an almost uniform spread of knowledge with associated ethical conflicts throughout the world under the name of globalization.

When this new wave of bioethics propagating from the U.S. reaches countries which are not part of the free world politically or reliziously, some friction is bound to occur with the local traditional ethics, because the globalization is slower in ethics than in science or the economy. In this respect, ethics, understood as learning from practice, differs from science as universal learning, because ethics relies on the spirituality of people to a considerable extent.

This just applies to bioethics in Japan, which is in a sort of dilemma. While life science in Japan has progressed as fast as in Europe and the U.S. along with well-developed natural science basing on general thought of the Western-style liberalism imported after WW II, decisions about ethical issues are not clear-cut because the principle on which Japanese ethics is based is a mixture of the communitarianism prevalent for such a long time until the end of the war and the liberalism hastily adopted after the war. For instance, while we understand well organ transplantation scientifically, we also have a traditional spirituality (culture, customs, ethos) which prevents us from introducing the transplantation freely into Japan. This is easily understandable, considering that ethics has a historical and regional characters, but it may be incomprehensible for Westerners who have not experienced this ethics from inside.

I have considered for a long time that Japanese people need a book on bioethics which attaches importance to the historical and cultural aspects of Japanese ethics while describing life science as a new important field of science, that is, a book on bioethics from the Asian or the Japanese viewpoint. I hope that this book, which offers an entirely new viewpoint, will be of some help in changing Japanese culture and establishing a proper Japanese identity in the future.

Norihiko Aoki

Kinki University
Osaka, Japan

CONTENTS

Preface

Chapter I : *The background of bioethics and environmental ethics*   1

Chapter II : *DNA and Life*   27

Chapter III : *Greek Culture and Its Significance for the Later Development of Science and Ethics*   47

Chapter IV : *Japanese Religion*   71

Chapter V : *Culture and Ethics*   121

Chapter VI : *Science and ethics for their proper orientation*   175

Chapter VII : *Environmental ethics, environmental hormones and various current problems*   219

Afterword   244

Index

Chapter I : *The background of bioethics and environmental ethics*

1. Recollections of the 20th century

Environmental ethics and bioethics are new academic fields which emerged in the U.S. and Europe in the 1960s and 1970s.

The Japan Association for Bioethics was founded on November 13, 1988. The 14th annual meeting of the Association was held in Hiroshima in 2002. People specializing in ethics and philosophy, jurists, attorneys, doctors, etc., conducted lively discussions at the meeting, where there was an air of eagerness and excitement. This tendency was most significant among the ethicists and jurists, both groups belonging to an historically established category that can be said to be classic. It was a scene which vividly illustrated that "bioethics" is a newly created interdisciplinary field which emerged suddenly at the end of the 20th century in response to the demands of the times. The 15th annual meeting of the Association for Bioethics was held at Sophia University of Tokyo in 2003. A new initiative to adopt a religious atmosphere to a large extent was tested at the meeting, and this was a large step toward a new phase in bioethics. Religions faced the task of shedding their older styles in order to contribute to the founding of a new wisdom and overcome the differences between dogmas. In other words, this is an age when specialists in the fields of religion, philosophy, ethics, law, molecular biology, medicine, medical services, etc., are requested to cooperate with each other in breaking down barriers, and the result at that meeting was that the incarnation of a new wisdom emerged.

Environmental ethics is a field that expands the scope of bioethics to include the environment and nature. Up until now, human beings have developed weapons of genocide and ecological mass-destruction: the atomic bomb, the hydrogen bomb, Agent Orange (dioxin defoliant used in Vietnam), the Star Bomb, the Daisy Cutter, depleted-uranium shells, and so forth, and it is undeniable that scientists have participated directly in the development of these weapons. Of course, those scientists experienced personal joy whenever they made discoveries and were able to develop their knowledge into practical applications. However, they were simply expendable and were in many cases ultimately ripped off in the politics and economics of the scientific process. Scientists in the future must abandon this ignorance of worldly matters outside their special field of study. We should consider that environmental ethics has appeared recently based on the fact that scientists are essentially required to maintain definite ethical principles as well as a scientific mind. Indeed, it is a time when scientists must use their wisdom to perform their duty and bring under control the large amount of weapons, chemical drugs, artificial chemical agents, etc., thus far produced in the course of the development of their scientific wisdom.

When thinking back on the rise of environmental ethics and bioethics in Europe and the United States, we could say that it was a like a scream finally given by human beings who at first participated in the development of material civilization from an innocent motivation but finally had to confront its intolerable invasion into human existence. As a result of modernization, or the application of science's results to people's lives, material civilization evolved at an unexpected speed in the latter half of the 20th century. The rise of environmental ethics seems to indicate that human beings have started the process of positive self-control in order to survive on this relatively small planet. If these kinds of self-interest activities are effective, human beings can surely survive while sharing this habitat called "Earth." In this context, human beings can contrive new self-defense measures and adjust themselves in a macroscopic manner to other living things.

This adjustment involves not only human beings but also ecological systems, including plants, animals, microorganisms, and so on. This is very close to the Asian viewpoint. Needless to say, it requires the modification of the traditional European idea originated by Aristotle that "human beings are the rulers of nature" (a mixture of Greek idealism, rational thinking, modern science, etc.), and the establishment of a new paradigm which underlies Asian thought and which states that all living things are equal, each contributing to the formation of a complete world whole.

The acme of Greek civilization (Empedocles: 493-433 B.C., Plato: 427-347 B.C., and Hippocrates: 460-370 B.C.), the age of Buddha or Shakyamuni (566-468 B.C.) and the age of Confucius (551-479 B.C.), who established Confucianism in China, all occurred in approximately the same period in the history of mankind. This is a sort of "synchronization," as each civilization developed along specific lines in its own inherent environment that was geographically distant from those of the others. However, it is interesting to find that there was a transcendental commonness in all civilizations, something like the "collective unconscious" as defined by Carl G. Jung (1875-1961). For instance, they all had religious values or some form of religious feeling as indispensable elements. However, when verifying the various events which subsequently occurred throughout world history, we find that independent and inherent religions, cultures and civilizations have been generated in many quarters of the globe, forging their identities by strictly distinguishing themselves from others. There have been many wars and atrocities waged in order to establish or claim these identities, and these wars and atrocities still persist today. The so-called "modernization," which started in the 17th century, evolved on such rational principles as causality, mechanistic theory and scientism, all derived from Greek thought. This was a phenomenon which began the trend toward the westernization of the whole world. Modernization, at first, was incarnated in the form of the Industrial Revolution (circa 1760), and then caused the world to shift to a material civilization associated with improvements in the standard of living, means of transportation, means of production, circulation, politics, industries, economics, and so on. At the same time, modernization also caused heightened interaction, interference and collision among civilizations.

In the 20th century, science was split into new specialties (quantum theory, electronic engineering, synthetic organic chemistry, physical chemistry, molecular genetics, molecular biology, eugenics, microbial engineering, immunology, zootechny, the science of breeding, information engineering, life science, many splintered fields of medical science, etc.). It is possible to say that the 20th century was the era when the principles of nature were elucidated in each field. This process was largely promoted by western ideas backed by physics, natural science and monotheistic Christianity. The discovery of the principles governing the world immediately generated a number of related applied sciences, including petrochemistry, computer information science, gene recombination and the industrialization of cloned species production. As a result, a considerable amount of artificial materials (e.g. freon gas and industrial waste) started to accumulate around the globe. There were changes in the global environment, such as global warming, the disturbance of the ecosystem, the degradation of human living conditions, and specific cultures were transformed worldwide on a massive scale. People began labeling these changes with a new universal word, "globalization" in the 1990s.

Under such circumstances, environmental ethics and bioethics arose out of necessity. It was a normal reaction of the spirit of those human beings who noticed that natural science, which is rational and positivistic, has progressed very rapidly, so much so that it has become automatized and uncontrollable. These branches of ethics appeared because human beings saw them as a necessity in the course of modernization, or the development of a scientific civilization.

We now stand at the dawn of a new millennium. As we reflect on the passage of the 20th century, we can say that it was "a century of wars," "a century of material civilization," "a century of the clash of civilizations" or "a century of ideology," "an era of bipolar conflict" or "an era when the principles of natural science were elucidated." However, regrettably, we cannot help but say that these are all superficial or one-sided ways of looking at things, even though they are seemingly to the point. That is to say that the present is huge and has become a "complicated system." It may be inevitable for us to define contemporary humans in a negative light. For instance, as a result of the accelerated and hypertrophied development of natural science, the induced material civilization ("things") has begun to invade the psyche, or the inherent primary region of human existence emphasized since the days of Socrates. Human beings are on the verge of losing their identity as a "mind-body unity." Such is the present age. I call it "scientific anarchism." If human beings cannot wisely monitor the progression of science, which is what we should have been doing all along, it will be like the future of an atomic reactor which has lost its control rods. A phenomenon like this occurred in a burst in the 1990s, when the synergistic effects of the information technology revolution and the genomic analysis of major living organisms were substantially completed. This is akin to a child who is given free reign over a toy box. He is allowed to use the toys freely, takes out the toys one after another for fun, playing with them in his room. He does not, however, put away the toys which he has been playing with and starts playing with other toys self-indulgently. Ultimately, his room is full of these toys which he has never mastered, and therefore does not know how to put away.

When we sum up the 20th century, our responsibility in the 21st century is obvious. It is to harmonize the individual sciences that have become splintered and never cease to become increasingly so, to bring them under the control of humans so that these sciences can regain their integrity. The mind (spirit) of men must accomplish this. From the academic viewpoint, it is the business of philosophy and ethics, and, at the present day, the emerging field of bioethics should have the responsibility for this process of reintegration by developing and systematizing itself.

This notion is based on the idea that what controls the sciences is the mind (spirit, psyche, contemplation) and human beings, and this is obviously different from the stance according to which science controls all human behavior, including our minds, thoughts and creativity. Otherwise, the sciences, which are always intrinsically self-propagating, will run out of control because they naturally lack an integrated or philosophical perspective on the world.

Today, the idea that reductionism based on scientism will finally elucidate even the processes of the mind is only a deduction engendered by the pomposity of science. It is predicted that natural science will be able to explain more psychological phenomena, in particular pathological ones, than it does now. However, a "complex system" produces human behaviors related to the spirit, such as music, religion and a variety of other creative endeavors. This is a standpoint that relies on the long history of idealism, beginning with Socrates and Plato, and the massive amount of human creative activities. This is explained away using a caricatural understanding. As animals cannot survive long by eating their own tails or one of their four limbs, so the human mind and spirit have a core of existence that cannot be invaded by scientific reductionism.

Table 1 shows the background of environmental ethics and bioethics through the 100 years of the 20th century.

Aldo Leopold (author of "A Sand County Almanac," translated into Japanese by Yoshiaki Nihjima, Kodansha Publishers, Ltd.), who warned against global environmental destruction at an early date, died in 1948. Hiroshima suffered the atomic bomb in 1945. The spiral structure of the DNA was discovered in 1953. Karl Jaspers, who admitted that science, however capable it may be, has its limits and there is a communication channel between "*Transzendenz*" and "*Existenz*," died in 1956.

Table 1

Chronological table for environmental ethics and bioethics through the 20th century

1900	The world population reached 1.6 billion.
	Rediscovery of Mendel's law
1905	Albert Einstein published the principles of relativity.
1909	Gene testing on *Drosophila* by Morgan
1911	Kitaro Nishida published "An Inquiry into the Good." (Nishida was the most prominent leader of and authority on specifically Japanese philosophy and ethics, which were developed based on Zen Buddhism. His philosophical system, based on "absolute nothingness," had a significant impact on Japanese culture, including the Kyoto school.)
1914	World War I (-1918)
1917	Russian Revolution (birth of the Soviet Union as a socialistic state)
1918	Spanish flu (influenza) epidemic (2% of the earth's population died.)
1935	Extraction of penicillin
1939	World War II (-1945)
1944	Oswald T. Avery, *et al.* discovered that the main body of genes consists of DNA.
1945	Atomic bombs were dropped on Hiroshima and Nagasaki.
1947	Nuremberg Code (ethical reflection of human beings on the living-body experiments conducted by German Nazis)
1948	Karl Jaspers published "*Von der Warhheit.*" He introduced the concept of "*das Umgreifende.*" He evaluated natural science, claimed, houever that it should be positioned properly within the realm of the totality.
1949	Aldo Leopold published "A Sand County Almanac." (He insisted on the importance of the conservation of nature from the viewpoint of ecosystem ethics, i.e. land ethics.)
1953	James D. Watson and Francis H.C. Crick disclosed the DNA double helix model.
1955	Reports of the ouch-ouch disease (cadmium poisoning)
1956	Reports of Minamata disease (mercury poisoning)
1961	Reports of Yokkaichi asthma (air pollution)
1962	Rachel L. Carson published "Silent Spring." (She pointed out that artificial chemical agents are accumulating in plants, animals and nature, affecting the entire ecosystem on a global scale.)
1964	Declaration of Helsinki (The World Medical Association published the Declaration of Helsinki as a statement of ethical principles to provide guidance

to physicians and other participants in medical research involving human subjects. It is revised regularly at the General Assembly of the World Medical Association once every several years.)

1966 Henry K. Beecher disclosed the actual unethical conditions of clinical trials in the U.S. in the New England Journal of Medicine.

Approvals by the Institutional Review Board (IRB) were made mandatory for medical researches involving human subjects in the U.S. (clinical trials for new drugs, etc.).

1968 Kanemi Yusho affair (PCB poisoning)

1972 The research team of Berg, *et al.* (Stanford University) succeeded in an experiment involving DNA recombination. (They made it possible to analyze and change human or animal genes on the molecular level, an impossibility until then.)

1972 Tuskegee affair (In 1930, neo-salvarsan and penicillin stopped being used experimentally on syphilis patients in African American neighborhoods. Doctors only followed up the patients. The ethical responsibility of doctors and the government was pursued.)

1978 The successful creation of a test-tube human baby (It was demonstrated that childbirth is possible without sexual intercourse.)

1979 Tom L. Beauchamp and James F. Childress published the first edition of "Principles of Biomedical Ethics." (Now in its fifth edition. An innovative book showing a specific approach to the practice of bioethics.)

1980-83 The concept of retroviral disease was established.

Discovery of adult T cell leukemia (ATL) (1980, Kiyoshi Takatsuki)

Discovery of the AIDS virus (1983, Luc Montagnier)

1981 Declaration of Lisbon on the rights of patients (Portugal)

1988 The first annual meeting of the Japan Association for Bioethics

1991 Dissolution of the Soviet Union (Bipolar conflict of ideology was disrupted. The world headed for unipolar domination.)

1996 Theo Colborn, Dianne Dumanoski and John P. Myers published "Our Stolen Future." (They showed that endocrine-disrupting chemicals, the so-called "environmental hormones," cause feminization of a male organism.)

1997 The global warming conference in Kyoto issued the Kyoto Protocol, which is an agreement made under the United Nations Framework Convention on Climate Change (UNFCCC).

Successful creation of Dolly, the cloned sheep (This opened the way for the

> application of cloning technology in the livestock industry, human cloning, and embryo stem cell manipulation in regenerative medicine.)
> 1998   A cloned cow was born.
> 2000   The world population was about 6 billion.
> 2001-2003   Decoding of the entire human genome
> Increase in the number of AIDS patients in Asia (The number of AIDS patients is increasing rapidly in Thailand, Cambodia, Myanmar and Yunnan Province in China due to poverty, narcotic drug abuse and prostitution.)
> Decoding of all rice genomes
> Premature death of Dolly, the cloned sheep

"Silent Spring" (translated into Japanese by Yanaichi Aoki, Shinchousha Co., Ltd.), which showed that artificial chemical substances accumulate in animals and plants and will affect the global ecosystem in the future, was originally published in 1962. This book made a sensation all over the world. It pressed the artificial chemical substance DDT into political consciousness for the first time. In other words, it brought about a global awareness of existent invasions through the global food chain. The Kanemi Yusho affair in 1972 was an extension of this. It was shown that PCBs (polychlorinated biphenyls), mainly used as insulating materials for electric equipment all over the world, accumulate in living organisms, causing disorders. DDT and PCBs are now known as environmental hormones (described later).

Scientists started analyzing the human genome in the latter half of the 1990s. As a result, in 2001, President Clinton published a draft of the genomic structure with Celera Genomics. Meanwhile, all genomes of the *japonica* and *indica* rice types, which are Asia's principal food, have been analyzed. Japan actively participated in the project.

In 2001 and 2002, companies in Switzerland and the U.S. published a draft of the genome of the *Nihonbare* breed, and the Beijing Genomics Institute published a draft of the genome of *indica* rice. An international team led by Japan published a draft completed in December 2002. According to these drafts, the number of genes of the rice plant is about 50,000. This genomic analysis is an example where computers and software have changed the perspective of conventional biology. The so-called "IT revolution" generated by the rapid spread and development of computers penetrated ever further, becoming more deeply ingrained in all culture bases as the new millennium drew near. In the 21st century, this new information revolution is creating new and greater tension by causing global homogenization (globalization) in economics, politics and ethics, as well as in science and information.

In the late 1990s, cloned sheep and cows were created in succession, opening up the theoretical possibility of cloning humans by the same method, if ethical all problems are cleared. This cloning technique, called "somatic-nuclear cell transfer," is epoch-making in that it utilizes various adult cells from which the nuclei, or the DNA information of the cells, are extracted. The extracted nucleus is transferred into a donated egg; this step is absolutely necessary, as it allows the transferred DNA to become the genetic blueprint of a growing embryo. The therapeutic applications of these cloning techniques look promising and diverse; new treatments are becoming possible for serious diseases in which the replacement of injured body parts is necessary.

2. Information technology revolution

The year 2000 was the turn of the century, a time when the IT revolution was progressing rapidly. It was a restless year, because no one could predict how far the IT revolution would go. The Soviet Union, the largest socialist state, disintegrated in 1991. Considering that this historic event occurred in Eastern Europe, which includes Romania, Czechoslovakia and Yugoslavia (they also discarded socialism, in that order), and a partial conversion to capitalism is now occurring in China, the bipolarization of ideologies - capitalism vs. socialism - that had continued since the Russian Revolution at the beginning of the 20th century (1917), now seems to have given way to unification. Here we see that history is a reservoir of facts that cannot be understood by means of human theories. Karl Marx and Vladimir I. Lenin did not predict this outcome, just as capitalism failed to predict the eroding of the earth by modern industry. It is impossible for us to predict the future, but history accumulates layer upon layer of consequences. The IT revolution was only made possible in the capitalistic system. IT innovations significantly promoted capitalism, which was the basis of the IT revolution. The success of capitalism has created computers. Fresh discoveries are continually being made, and the industry is fostered by means of a lot of large valuable computers that process large amounts of data in a short period of time. Information generates patents, and patents generate wealth. Thus, the wheel of capitalism, science and industry, starts to rotate illogically. The IT revolution was an unlimited and secure change justly termed a "revolution." The IT revolution is exerting its influence all over the world even in this new century, irrespective of socialism and capitalism or the differences in religions and civilizations. As long as there is a sky, information will always fall from it. The propagating power is so high that geographical borders are no longer a factor. With the IT revolution, rational knowledge penetrates everywhere irrespective of national borders, transcending nationality as the Industrial Revolution has done in the past.

Consequently, the global spread of knowledge or the wave of globalization is forcing the native cultures of regions and nations to change. It is an indisputable historic fact that the Industrial Revolution generated in Britain in the 18th century became more radical, taking the form of colonial rule and the North-South problem and changing the actual condition of world politics. The abrupt modernization which occurred in Japan after the Meiji Restoration was, in general, an acceptance of the results of the Industrial Revolution and modern science.

Thus, the IT revolution does have its positive aspects. However, the new world cultivated by the IT revolution includes new problems which belong to bioethics and environmental ethics.

For example, Celera Genomics (U.S.) blazed through the human genome analysis faster than public research teams by linking together many supercomputers with a high computing capacity from various companies. Thus, the analysis of the human genome had almost been completed as we approached the end of the 20th century. After the turn of the 21st century, people began to study its functions and applications. Applications involving genomic information include drug discovery, personalized medical care, the elucidation of the genomic structure of individuals who are likely to acquire lifestyle-related diseases (high-blood pressure, cancer and diabetes), further detection of genetic diseases, as well as farming and stockbreeding. It appears as though we can look forward to a rosy future. However, there are many bioethical problems to be considered. For example, theoretically, all genetic information about individuals can be disclosed. To whom does this information belong? Does it belong to the individual, the society or the community (nation)? Who protects this information? Should this information be kept secret? Will a new standard of privacy be formulated? We will soon be facing these problems. Science has come to know nearly all genetic information about plants and animals. The technology has passed the point of no return. When we take a look back through history, we know that objective knowledge once obtained cannot be undone. That has always been a characteristic of science. Should we inhibit or regulate this technology? Will information on individuals be kept secret by anonymity of information? Do we leave things to run their course freely, adopting the utilitarian view of benevolence, righteousness and national interest? In that case, choices are made based on the ethos of the group in question.

However, the results of genomic analyses might stimulate the advancement of eugenics in a new direction. This is the biggest concern. People are again afraid of the advent of an era where human beings are artificially selected to form superior races as industrially effective artificial breeds (like seedless watermelons or rice plants resistant to cold) through the improvement of human abilities from the standpoint of national or racial intent. This is all obtainable by genetic manipulation and breeding, as thoroughbred racehorses are obtained by breeding elite bloodlines; the German Nazi intention to form a superior race is a crucial example. History shows that human beings were born in Africa, moved to the other continents, and evolved and diversified there. As a result, racial differences appeared. This is an indisputable fact. Many are afraid that history is reversing itself in the direction of unification. In other words, we are afraid that it will become impossible to exercise our individual wills.

With regard to Internet technology, the IT revolution is strange because people do not know how far it will go. Knowledge has spread through radio waves based on Internet technology in the recent decade, inducing rapid globalization. International boundaries and geographical structures cannot constitute barriers for information as long as electronic waves can reach those locations from space satellites. No one can stop this rationalistic tendency.

Now, I will explain the state of the problem by referring to the "2000 White Paper Information and Communications in Japan." The U.S., Japan, the U.K., Germany, Canada and Australia accounted for 73.4%, 3.6%, 2.6%, 2.4%, 2.3% and 1.5% of the number of Internet hosts, respectively. The Middle East and Africa accounted for only 0.4%. At that moment, the U.S. made up the vast majority. The IT revolution started under those circumstances. This is a serious issue, because the U.S. is thereby granted sole superiority in military affairs, economics, politics, the scientific world, etc., which further aggravates the hierarchical tendency in the world, namely the North-South problem.

The fact that the IT revolution which occurred in a country conquers the world so rapidly is a surprise; this situation has not previously been experienced in history. This is also a kind of warning to human beings. It cannot be simply swept aside by utilitarian statements such as "Science is good for human beings because it offers benefits and conveniences," or "Knowledge is good for us because it eliminates stupidity." The era when people will embrace the concept of eugenics along with the technology of current life science is right around the corner. Human beings need to have a wide perspective when considering the cultural and religious risks which put human existence at risk.

3. IT revolution (globalization of knowledge) and cultural transformation

Culture is an overall system with regional peculiarities (climates, races, communities, etc.) that matures over a long period of time and that flourishes among human beings. Culture is transformed by people's interactions with different communities, the introduction and diffusion of scientific knowledge, the transformation of the ethos, etc. It is natural that culture requires a long time to change, when one considers the long period of maturation, the relationships among religions and the large amount of historic accumulation. As shown in Table 1, the world population was 1.6 billion at the beginning of the 20th century. At the end of the 20th century, it became 6 billion. We have already mentioned that the separation of isolated cultural areas was alleviated through population and physical contact between different peoples. In fact, the forced interaction of people, as well as the division and disappearance of entire countries, was observed. In this respect, the external forces driving cultural transformation must also have been affected. However, it has been pointed out that cultures have not changed significantly in spite of this. At present, the transformation of cultures may be accelerated because globalization through the IT revolution may be rapidly progressing without restraint. However, we should recognize that "knowledge" is only one among the many values possessed by cultures. In other words, it takes a long time for a culture to change when new knowledge is introduced. It is necessary for us to reconfirm that human beings are psychic existences by firmly holding on to the religious characteristics which lie at the center of our ethos, before people become viewed as simply physical existences. We only observe the effects of the IT revolution on cultures, especially the characteristic properties of cultures. That is because human beings have never before experienced the quickness and thoroughness of globalization (homogenization on a global scale) in a revolution. We cannot predict where it will settle down. Reality has always been beyond expectation and thought. That is history.

4. What is bioethics?

Bioethics is a new interdisciplinary field established in the U.S. in the 1960s and 1970s. Its emergence has several background factors. In 1947, the Nuremberg Code was issued, as a response to the unethical medical practices of human beings, such as the living-body experiments conducted by German Nazis in World War II. Taking advantage of this opportunity, several cases of unethical medical practice in the U.S. were also revealed after the war. For example, as shown in the table, the Tuskegee Syphilis Study became infamous: syphilis patients (mainly African Americans) were involved in an observation study which began in 1930 (it was not stopped until it was exposed from within in 1966). Beecher (professor of anesthesiology, Harvard University) published an exposure report titled "Ethics and clinical research" in the New England Journal of Medicine (a major medical weekly bulletin in the U.S.) introducing 22 cases of unethical clinical trials in the U.S.

All of those clinical trials were problematic because it was uncertain whether the consent of the patients had been obtained. In one trial, living cells were transplanted into 22 inpatients without informing them that they were cancer cells. In another trial, radiographic visualizations were performed on 26 babies who were 48 hours old or less in order to confirm the phenomena of urinary reflux from the bladder to the urinary duct just out of medical curiosity.

All of the cases he revealed made people mistrust the concept of doctor paternalism, which had not been an issue previously because people had trusted their doctors implicitly. Patients doubted the medical community for the first time, a community which had been a sanctuary before then. This was amplified by the human rights movement gathering momentum in the U.S. at that time. The Tuskegee scandal and the Beecher report were both exposures from within. The soundness of the American society can be seen in the respect for inside denunciations. These affairs caused America to head for autonomy, in the sense of self-control. Thus, they are good examples of how America advocates liberalism as a principle of its foundation. That is because freedom and autonomy are the bases of liberalism.

Rightly, the number of medical malpractice suits increased when the relationship of mutual trust between patient and doctor became eroded. Doctors were forced to protect themselves by law. In one sense, it could be said that the establishment of bioethics, which clarifies the import of informed consent (explanation and agreement), was a response to doctors' practical concerns. Implementing the required legal guideline is a practical method of ensuring the physician's exemption from responsibility. Therefore, bioethics in the U.S. was at first medical ethics targeting medical practices chiefly involving humans. In general, however, the concept of bioethics includes in its scope medical ethics as well as environmental ethics, targeting ecosystems and the biological environment. Especially for those of us who have been raised in Buddhist cultures, nature and the environment are extensions of human beings. Human beings and nature, or human beings and the environment, cannot be neatly distinguished. As ethics is deeply linked to culture, it is only normal that environmental ethics and bioethics should take into account differences in culture. For those whose ethical minds suffer from the invasion and destruction of the ecosystem by humans, these issues are naturally bioethics problems (in the broad sense). The word "bioethics" is formed by combining "bios," meaning "life" in Greek (the word origin of "biology", "bioscience", etc.) and "ethics," originating from "ethos," meaning "custom" or "atmosphere."

Life science, including genetic engineering, cloning technology, etc., has evolved tremendously in recent years, at an accelerated pace. The disclosure of scientific facts has been expanded to unknown fields based on the inner principle of autonomous self-expansion, an inherent characteristic of natural science. Science is liable to grow to an enormous size, far removed from the intentions of the human beings who produce it. Undoubtedly, the principle of natural science is mechanicism, and its results are based on objectivity (*logos* lies at the heart of objectivity). It demands of human beings to do more serious soul-searching than ever before regarding ethical and moral problems. Human beings contain some parts (ethics and morality) that cannot be understood by means of the "human machine" theory, which is on the same level as the "animal machine" theory.

Not only life science, but also general natural science has led to the deterioration of a large portion of the global environment and life environment, in both quantitative and qualitative ways. The results are summarily discarded as things or facts. They are making human beings face new choices in the areas of ethics, morality, law and *nomos*. This is quite rightly the business of environmental ethics and bioethics. Thus, interdisciplinary studies involving the life sciences (microbiology, medical, zoological science, botany, etc.), ethics, philosophy, religions, sociology and environmentology came to be pursued. These are new fields of human enquiry which appeared as a response to the demands of the present age.

Ethics and morality can be divided into two categories. One is ethics and morality which possess universality, or a transcendental commonality among human beings; the other is ethics and morality which are characterized regionality or diversity based on race, religion, cultures, geography, history, etc. The right understanding of ethical and moral problems that we confront must include both of these aspects. Therefore, we should consider individual matters as they are affected by culture and history, and, needless to add, we should weigh ethical standards justly.

5. What is environmental ethics?

Environmental ethics is a relatively new field which appeared in the 1960s as "bioethics." These two branches of ethics are similar because they were created when modernization after the Industrial Revolution hit a rut. Small-minded egoism and national interests, principles based on which people care only about themselves (nationalism), were dismissed from these new branches of ethics. The advent of gentler macroscopic viewpoints, which take into consideration the whole ecosystem on a global mass scale and require new paradigms, kick-started the movement of environmental ethics.

Human beings have been modifying and using nature in the process of modernization since the Industrial Revolution, believing that nature is meant to attend to them. Humanism, according to which people believe that nature exists for the sake of human beings, is spreading continuously. The idea of feeding herbivorous animals, such as cows, with meat-and-bone meals made of sheep or other cows (the cause of mad cow disease), has never occurred to those of us who live in Buddhist cultural areas. Those that engage in such feeding practices consider animals to be literally machines that produce meat. Nature has been modified by human beings in other ways, including the consumption of fossil fuels such as coal and petroleum, and the destruction of rainforests in order to harvest pulpwood, the overexploitation of animals, the recovery of land from the sea, and rock breaking for building materials. They are far too numerous to name.

Descartes thought that nature, including living organisms, is mechanical or part of a mechanism. It is due to him that the mechanicist principle or basis spread among people in the process of modernization. However, the artificial materials profusely produced by human beings in this process have upset the normal cycle of nature, as seen in the generation and extinction of natural objects resulting in environmental contamination and deterioration. Still, people at large have begun to have misgivings about the accumulation of contaminated materials that are not being removed from the earth, putting the future of the human race in danger. There are so many examples around us: industrial pollution, contamination with toxic artificial chemicals, drug poisoning, ever-lasting residual war materials which deteriorate human life, as exemplified by the potent dioxins diffused in Viet Nam, global temperature changes, and so on. Reliable data show the increase in global temperature within the past 50 years and the increase in the atmospheric concentration of carbon dioxide (CO_2) over the past 100 years, respectively. It has been noticed that the rise of the global temperature was 0.8℃ in the past century, with the past 30 years (1970-2000) accounting for 75% of that rise, or 0.6℃, and this hugely accelerated rate remains unchanged in the years around the millennium (James Hansen, *et al.*, PNAS, September 26, 2006). Carbon dioxide is a symbolic by-product of modernization emitted by automobile and airplane engines, factory chimneys and other urban industrial sources.

The idea that the accumulated layer of carbon dioxide will cause global warming appeared already in 1932 in a novel by Kenji Miyazawa, a Japanese writer (1896-1933). Pure-minded Gusco-Budori, the hero of this novel entitled "*Gusco-Budori no Denki*," or "The Legend of Gusco-Budori," hit upon the idea of creating a layer of carbon dioxide by detonating a volcano artificially to increase the temperature of a region where people were suffering the ravages of cool summers. He tried to protect the people's livelihood from the damage caused by cool summers in the novel. He visited a great doctor and asked him, "If the carbonade volcanic island were to erupt now, will it emit enough carbon dioxide to change the climate here?" The doctor replied, "I have already planned it. If it erupts now, the gas will soon be mixed with the wind in the upper layer of greater systemic circulation and encircle the entire globe. I believe the gas will prevent the diffusion of heat from the lower layer and the earth's surface and will cause the entire globe to become warmer by about 5℃ on average." This novel was written one year before the death of Kenji Miyazawa. The environmental ethics we are now discussing are the opposite of this novel. We suffer from the accumulation of carbon dioxide in the atmosphere brought about by modern industry and by the warming of the earth's atmosphere. It is possible to observe changes in the amount of carbon dioxide in the atmosphere from the viewpoint of global history by measuring the carbon dioxide trapped in the layers of ice in Antarctica. Actually, the data show that the amount of carbon dioxide in the atmosphere has been increasing since the Industrial Revolution. Finally, human beings have noticed that this crisis situation has been caused by modernization. Global warming is progressing year by year. The glaciers in Antarctica and the Alps are dwindling. Melted water is raising the sea level. Small islands around the earth are at risk of sinking below sea level. In Japan, the amount of snow in Nagano prefecture, a snowy district famous for its skiing facilities, has decreased considerably, and the lake of Suwa in the prefecture which was previously a mecca for skaters freezes over only with great difficulty. Also, in Kyoto and Osaka, we now rarely experience snow in December and January, unlike in previous years.

The Kyoto Conference, whose purpose was to prepare a protocol for the international reduction of emissions of six green house gases (GHGs) – carbon dioxide, methane, nitrous oxide, hydrofluorocarbons, perfluorocarbons and sulfur hexafluoride - was held in Kyoto in 1997. The Kyoto Protocol, under which industrialized countries will reduce their collective emissions of GHGs by 5.2% (imposed cap) compared to the year 1990 over the 2008-to-2012 period, was submitted for signing on December 11, 1997 and entered into force on February 16, 2005, following ratification by Russia on November 18, 2004. The meeting was timely, considering the critical situation of global warming and the coincident increase in GHG emissions around the planet. However, the U.S. gave priority to its national interests. Less-developed countries retained the right to maintain production levels in the future, and their interests conflicted with the aim of the treaty. As a result, the U.S. did not ratify the treaty and encountered criticism from across the world. I would say, as an ethicist, that issues at the level of national interest, regional egoism, etc., are really the work of minor politicians, given the grave state of the planet. Sadly, they lack the global perspective and a philosophy which takes into consideration the future of mankind. Ethicists and philosophers should not theorize a specific or local model if they are to act their part well by indicating an ideal future for humankind. The important fact is that the earth is now sick. Truly great, philosophical politicians who can elucidate and solve problems on a global basis are eagerly awaited at this time. The environmental deterioration carves a steady course on a global mass scale. In fact, the results of studies by the Goddard Space Flight Center and the National Aeronautics and Space Administration (NASA), published on November 27, 2002, showed that the amount of ice in the Arctic Ocean has been decreasing at an astonishing pace of 9% over the last ten years. Almost all the ice in the Arctic Ocean may disappear in the 21st century if nothing is done.

Anyway, the Kyoto Protocol is forging ahead, without the ratification of the U.S., in its global effort to reduce carbon dioxide and other GHGs. The protocol provides for a "cap and trade" system, and trading of GHG emissions is now becoming real in Japan, Canada and Europe. It covers 168 countries and at least 55% of GHGs as of November 2006. This effort, albeit bedeviled by many problems which should be solved, especially with regard to developed and developing countries, is to be highly valued for its communal activity carried out by countries all over the world dedicated to the future welfare of the earth.

Environmental ethics makes human beings reflect and try to correct the degradation or distortion of the global environment caused by modernization. In this sense, environmental ethics and bioethics belong to a more practical and social field of human enquiry. In this respect, environmental ethics innovates in a direction different from that of traditional ethics. Bioethics and environmental ethics have their own specific meanings, which reflect a new understanding that is different from that of conventional ethics, when practical workability and present effectiveness are considered. The environment is nature, the framework of the entire global ecosystem which includes plants, animals and human beings. Plants and animals have no forensic ability. It is only human beings who make an issue of ethics. They discuss animal rights, the theory of personality, etc. Human beings are responsible for making the entire ecosystem develop in a balanced and ethical manner. We, Far-Eastern Asian people, have an ethos according to which this is also good for human beings. This viewpoint seems to be necessary and essential for the wellbeing of the global ecosystem. The degradation of the environment observed on a global mass scale often causes international problems. For example, the Chernobyl nuclear reactor accident caused radiation contamination as far away as in three Scandinavian countries. The pollution spread all over the world. Radioactive rain was observed even in Japan.

For example, people eat reindeer in Finland. Reindeer received unfavorable criticism among customers at restaurants because reindeer eat moss and the venison was contaminated by radioactivity via that moss. The air is polluted by factory smoke and yellow dust emitted by heavy industries and desertification in China. It has become evident that this polluted air travels to Japan riding an air current through the stratosphere.

Meanwhile, international efforts are producing results in some fields. One of them is an effort to clarify the properties of the ozone holes over the Antarctic. It is surmised that ozone holes are generated by freon gas (used as a cooling medium) which destroys the ozone layer. If the ozone layer becomes too thin, it can no longer serve as a barrier against the ultraviolet light radiating from the sun, allowing it to reach the surface of the earth, thereby increasing the incidence of skin cancer. Many people are now part of an international movement to repair the ozone holes by stopping the production and use of freon gas, and to eliminate this artificial substance from the earth.

There are many historical examples which confirm that environmental ethics is regional. For example, there were problems such as Minamata disease (mercury poisoning), ouch-ouch disease (cadmium poisoning) and Yokkaichi asthma (air pollution) in the 1970s in Japan. Recently, the feminization of male organisms caused by the so-called "environmental hormones" (endocrine-disrupting chemicals) has become an issue. The details regarding environmental hormones will be discussed in a later chapter.

6. The AIDS problem

AIDS (acquired immunodeficiency syndrome) caused by infection with HIV (human immunodeficiency virus) is a civilization disease, because it initially spread through the homosexual community, with its sexual freedom, while in Japan AIDS was first noted as a transfusion-induced infection among patients with hemophilia who were treated with HIV-contaminated blood products. AIDS was initially a local disease in Africa (it is supposed to have originated in monkeys), but now it has spread across the globe as today's most prominent sexually transmitted disease. In 2002, the number of people who died of AIDS, newly infected people and total number of infected people was about 3.1 million, 5 million and 42 million, respectively. According to the statistics of 2006 (UNAAIDS and WHO), the number of AIDS deaths in 2006 was 2.9 million, and the recorded number of people newly infected with HIV and people living with HIV was 4.3 million and 39.5 million in 2006, respectively, showing that global treatment and prevention programs are making headway. However, the number of newly infected people in 2006 exceeds that in 2004 by about 400,000, showing that AIDS is still a severe global problem. According to the report, many of the newly HIV-infected people are young adults between the ages of 15 and 24 years; they account for 40% of new HIV infections in 2006.

"The State of the World Population 2003" (UNFPA 2003) showed that the world population is estimated to fall by 400 million by 2050 because deaths due to AIDS are supposed to increase rapidly as 2050 approaches (278 million). AIDS is the major ethical problem of the present day for the following reasons:

First, the AIDS infection is global. Second, it has spread rampantly, especially in the poor countries of Africa and Asia. Third, with regard to therapeutic agents, discrimination, as in the Tuskegee syphilis case, can occur. Fourth, the AIDS epidemic has been caused in part by the modernity of our sex culture, including homosexual sex, the buying and selling of sex, the prevalence of unsafe sex, and free sex, all based on the premise of liberalism. Fifth, the wide spread of AIDS has also been caused by poverty and backwardness, as seen especially in the sharing of narcotics syringes and needles. And sixth, in Japan, AIDS was a drug disaster that affected hemophiliac patients who were administered contaminated blood products that were poorly processed. These phenomena show that AIDS is the new ethical problem of today.

AIDS is characterized by dysfunction of immunocompetent lymphocytes (more specifically, helper T cells) infected with HIV, which is a "retrovirus" (reverse-transcriptase-containing oncogenic virus). This was revealed when Luc Montagnier (France) discovered HIV in 1983. "Retrovirus" is a generic term which refers to viruses that cause disease gradually by persisting through lymphocyte divisions in a symbiotic state. The nucleic acid of the virus, which is its main body, is converted into DNA; the lymph cells (a kind of leukocyte) have their own DNA, which carries their genetic information; when the virus infects the lymph cells, the reverse transcriptase of the virus is transformed into DNA which then becomes embedded into the original nuclear DNA of the lymph cells and the virus then replicates.

The first known case of human retroviral disease was adult T cell leukemia (ATL), discovered by Kiyoshi Takatsuki (Kyoto University) in 1980. This is worthy of special mention as an historical and honorable achievement by a Japanese. Kiyoshi Takatsuki, a clinical hematologist, proposed ATL as a new disease entity in 1980, upon observation that there was a cluster of adult leukemia cases around the southwestern region of Japan (Kagoshima, Nagasaki and Okinawa Prefectures). The specific pathological features include skin eruptions and cloverleaf-shaped nuclei in peripheral-blood lymphocytes. He came to consider this disease as a lymphoid tumor caused by a viral infection, wholly different from any of the known leukemia types. ATL is characterized by skin rashes and hypercalcemia as well. The mode of propagation of ATL is the migration of HTLV-1 (human T cell leukemia virus 1) lurking as a provirus in the infected T cell genome, and the principal propagation paths of ATL are the transfusion of blood which contains T cells, mother-to-child transmission through nursing (T cells in breast milk) and sexual transmission (T cells in semen). The onset of disease in HTLV-1 carriers is usually insidious and takes the form of ATL (4-5% of carriers develop the disease after several decades), spinal nerve disorder and uveitis, but fortunately most carriers do not develop any of these diseases. The number of Japanese carriers is approximately 1.2 million, and the mean onset age is 60 years. A global survey has shown that endemic ATL is present throughout the world, including the coast of the Caribbean Sea, Africa and South America, as well as southwestern Japan and other Asian coast regions. Takatsuki's ATL discovery gathered remarkable momentum, and clinical and virological investigations of ATL followed throughout the world; the resulting discovery was that ATL and AIDS are both diseases caused by retroviral infection. Since so far no effective remedies have been developed for ATL except bone-marrow transplantation, it is crucial for the time being to prevent infection from the standpoint of public hygiene. Such preceding advances in the investigation of ATL have greatly served the study of AIDS.

In ATL, the retrovirus (in this case, HTLV-1) causes the canceration, or neoplastic division, of T-cells. In AIDS, the clinical condition is quite different because the retrovirus (HIV) causes the disappearance (apoptosis) of T cells, which play a cardinal role in the immune system of the host individual. In other words, ATL is a neoplastic or tumorigenic transformation of leucocytes associated with an increased T cell count in the blood, while the leukocyte count in the blood is low in AIDS patients with declining immunity function exerted by T cells. Therefore, the direct cause of death in AIDS is an opportunistic infection (pneumocystis carinii pneumonia, tuberculosis, etc.). In the early stages, AIDS was an endemic disease limited to Africa. People were infected with AIDS by eating monkeys or coming into contact with the blood of monkeys. People infected with AIDS died in their area. Therefore, AIDS was regionally limited. AIDS would not have been transferred to other people if the first HIV carriers had had rigorous sexual discipline or ethos. The rampancy of AIDS all over the world is mainly caused by cultural globalization, which is the negative side of liberalism. In this sense, one can consider AIDS to be a kind of nemesis in the breakdown of morality caused by the liberalism of our times.

However, in Japan, AIDS occurred because blood components that were the media of HIV were injected into patients as a result of improper screening. The scandal of the HIV-tainted blood occurred only in Japan. It had nothing to do with punishment from heaven. It was caused by the shameful deficiencies of ministerial and corporate ethics. A reconciliation was established among drug companies, nations and patients. However, the ethical reflection of Japanese people on this matter should by never fade with time, so that similar incidents can be prevented in the future. This disaster was a good example of what should be committed to memory by the ethos (cultural convention) or ethics of the Japanese people who witnessed it first-hand.

More information about leukocytes would be helpful to the readers here, as ATL and AIDS are both diseases which affect leucocytes. There are several types of leukocytes in the blood: lymphocytes, granulocytes, etc. Lymphocytes act as eliminators of extraneous invaders (viruses, bacteria, fungi, graft cells), and are classified into T cells (about 80% of peripheral-blood lymphocytes are T cells) and B cells (up to 20%). In principle, T cells take part in cell-mediated immunity and B cells take part in humoral immunity by way of antibody production. T cells issue orders for antibody production by B cells; in addition, T cells control the overall immune system through cytokine production. While the antibodies generated by B cells directly and rapidly prevent bacteria and viruses from invading the host body from the outside, T cells eliminate cancer cells and cells which have become infected with viruses or whose antigenicity has degenerated (cell-mediated immunity). Upon the infection of an individual with a virus, T cells detect the viral antigens, order the B cells to produce antibodies and induce cytolytic T cells to kill the infected cells. The antibodies specifically combine with viruses as neutralizing antibodies to inactivate them, and cytolytic T cells annihilate the cells infected with viruses. As just described, the decrease in T-cell function leads to immunodeficiency or chronic infection, and the canceration of T cells causes malignant lymphoma with lymph node enlargement. The so-called helper T cells are referred to as CD4-positive cells (CD4 is a protein present on the helper T cell membrane). Both ATL and AIDS are diseases in which CD4-positive T cells become infected with the respective retrovirus (HTLV-1 or HIV).

A new phase in the rampancy of AIDS occurred in 2000. AIDS has been spreading rapidly in the poor regions of Asia, such as Cambodia, Yunnan (China), India, Myanmar, Thailand, and Vietnam. This is partially caused by severe poverty, a social circumstance in which AIDS is not the most feared thing. People die of poverty, famine and wars quicker than of AIDS. Therefore, people do not have an enormous fear of AIDS. The values are relative. AIDS is also caused by the enhanced use of drugs, the sharing of syringes, and prostitution. The situation cannot be easily corrected because it is related to politics and poverty. We should expand education, distribute condoms, and introduce and implement a correct ethos. We should start with these. Bioethics and environmental ethics are new branches of ethics because they are effective in practical ways.

AIDS is still a lethal disease if it is allowed to develop. The development of therapeutic agents has made progress, as shown by the introduction of reverse transcriptase inhibitors, protease inhibitors, etc. If a patient takes the drugs, he can extend the period before AIDS develops even if he is infected with the HIV virus, or at least slow down the progression of AIDS even if AIDS has developed. On the basis of international ethics, international organizations must function so that countries that can produce drugs will supply these therapeutic drugs inexpensively to poor, less-developed countries that have AIDS patients. One defect of the utilitarianism which supports capitalism is the lack of any consideration of the equal distribution of aid. This must be overcome. Morally, it is normal that rich people should help poor people in a crisis. We should avoid a "natural selection" due to poverty among human beings.

Lastly, the increasing number of AIDS cases in Japan is a problem mainly caused by the acute change of moral standards which transpired in this country after the war. The number of patients infected with the HIV virus is steadily increasing (in 1995 <200, 1996-1998 >200, 1999-2000 >300, 2001-2002 >600, 2004 >6500, and 2005 17,000); the first AIDS patient in Japan was diagnosed in 1985. The age at which people become sexually active is becoming lower in Japan as a result of vicious liberalism concerning sexual behavior. The major causes of the increased number of HIV-positive people in Japan include ignorance among young people about HIV infection, the rising trend of sexual freedom and the spread of HIV by foreigners. Poverty is not a cause of AIDS in Japan, as it is in other Asian countries. The actual reality is that the spread of AIDS is accelerated by the noninterference or irresponsibility of adults in the ethical education of young people, as a result of the corruption of the traditional Japanese moral system which had been rigidly preserved in society until WWII. And anyway, this is liberalism, and it was brought to Japan after the war by the U.S. The distance between the traditional and the newly introduced moral system was tremendous. It has been thus far impossible for Japanese people to find their way morally, in their attempt to encompass their complex history, religion and culture. However, they have begun to move at last, as shown by their election of the new Prime Minister Shinzo Abe in 2006, an active young leader who has declared his intention to revise the Fundamental Law of Education in Japan, which took effect in 1947 and remained unchanged until now. Also, under his leadership, the initial steps have been taken towards a constitutional revision whose final goal is to extricate Japan from the postwar regime. Thus, there is now hope of reestablishing a proper Japanese ethos, in which excellent traditional values and virtues will be preserved in an integrated manner along with the many Western values and virtues which have been introduced through the education of children and young people in school and in society after the war. Good customs and a sound morality are crucial for the normal development of young people in society, as anciently taught by Confucius and Aristotle. Unexpectedly, Abe suddenly resigned his post after a year, mainly because of his failing health, and was succeeded by the 71-year-old Yasuo Fukuda, elected as prime minister on September 25, 2007. Different from the prior Prime Ministers Koizumi and Abe, both of whom were reform-minded politicians grounded in market fundamentalism, Prime Minister Yasuo Fukuda seeks to establish a sense of security based on harmony, or *wa* in Japanese, as expressed in his phrase, "politics through dialogue." This *wa*, or "sense of balance," is a traditional and well-known virtue in Japan originated by Prince Shotoku (574-622), as described later. Fukuda and his cabinet are generally continuing Abe's policy, which includes the intentional cultivation of a firm moral sense after specifically Japanese standards. There is a strong expectation among the Japanese public of the reestablishment of the most appropriate and proud morality rooted in national history and culture, including religion.

AIDS has become a novel global disease, and is arguably the heaviest burden which human beings now have to bear. It is comparable to syphilis, which was transmitted worldwide in the Age of Discovery. In fact, AIDS, today's venereal disease, poses a far more serious threat to human society than ATL, another retroviral disease. In some counties in Africa, AIDS is likely to annihilate the entire population of young people. As of 2005, more than 25 million people have died of AIDS throughout the world. In 2005 and 2006, 3.1 and 2.9 million more people died of AIDS, respectively. According to the statistics of 2006, the number of adults and children living with HIV in sub-Saharan Africa is 24.7 million (two thirds of global sufferers). In India, which is the world's second-most populous country, 5.7 million people were living with HIV in 2005; in the same year, there were 650,000 in China and 17,000 in Japan.

As shown above, the background of the emergence of environmental ethics and bioethics is similar to that observed in many phases of human history. Western-inspired modernization, generally speaking, or the globalization that has occurred recently, presents us with various problems. These problems can be observed everywhere as crises of the global ecosystem. But it is human beings who know how to remedy the ecosystem from a global viewpoint. Environmental ethics and bioethics aim at the recognition and creation of new values by taking into account the diversity of cultures, histories and races on earth.

References
1) Kitaro Nishida: Zen no Kenkyu (A Study of Goodness). Iwanami Shoten, Tokyo, 1942
2) Karl Jaspers; translated by Ralph Manheim: Socrares, Buddha, Confucius, Jesus. Harcourt Brace & Company, San Diego, 1962
3) Henry K. Beecher, Ethics and Clinical Research, The New England Journal of Medicine, Vol.274, No.24, 1354-1360, 1966
4) Kenji Miyazawa: Miyazawa-Kenji Zenshu 8. Tsikuma Shobo, Tokyo, 1986
5) Peter Singer; translated by Kiyoshi Toda: In Defence of Animals. Gijyutu To Ningen, Tokyo, 1986
6) Keiji Nishitani; translated by Seisaku Yamamoto and James W. Heisig: Nishida Kitaro. University of California Press, Oxford, 1991
7) Tom L. Beauchamp and James F. Childless: Principles of Biomedical Ethics, Fourth Edition. Oxford University Press, New York, 1994

8) Gilbert C. Meilander: Body, Soul and Bioethics. University of Notre Dame Press, Notre Dame, 1995
9) Aldo Leopold; translated into Japanese by Yoshiaki Niijima: A Sand County Almanac. Kodansha, Tokyo, 1997
10) Raphael Cohen-Almagor: Medical Ethics at the Dawn of the 21st Century. The New York Academy of Sciences, New York, 2000
11) Sheldon Krimsky; translated into Japanese by Sanae Matuzaki and Yoko Saito: Hormonal Chaos. Fujiwara Shoten, Tokyo, 2001
12) Tom L. Beauchamp and James F. Childress: Principles of Biomedical Ethics, Fifth Edition. Oxford University Press, New York, 2001
13) Earth Policy Institute News, Dec. 18, 2001, Earth Policy Institute (founded by Lester R. Brown)
14) Norihiko Aoki: Hito Wo Ikiru –Experience and Insight into the New Millennium–. Tyusekisha, Tokyo, 2003
15) Timothy F. Murphy: Case Studies in Biomedical Research Ethics. The MIT Press, Cambridge, 2004

Chapter II: *DNA and Life*

The scientific understanding of life has been rapidly progressing since the middle of the 20th century. As a result, the expression "life science" is commonly used now. Life science is a field of study which investigates life using the same scientific principles and methods as those used in physics and chemistry. Life phenomena that were once a mystery are now well understood scientifically as a result of the introduction of molecular biology and molecular genetics.

It is essential that we retain the latest level of objective knowledge in life science in order to enable the rich and profound development of environmental ethics and bioethics in the future.

1. Genetic information exists in the DNA.

As is apparent from the large amount of work regarding animals and plants done by Aristotle during the Greek era, human beings have long known that life perpetuates through heredity. It was Gregor J. Mendel (1865) who first showed that heredity follows scientific laws. The correctness of his laws was reconfirmed at the beginning of the 20th century (see the chronological table in Chapter 1). If we take this into consideration, the history of the scientific understanding of life is only about 100 years old.

Individual character traits, such as height, stockiness, nose shape, skin characteristics, being beautiful, having a fine singing voice, and running fast are called "phenotypes." The phenotype of an individual is the set of all visible characteristics of that individual. Genes are invisible. At first, they were deduced scientifically and postulated as a concept. In the 20th century, genes were finally made visible as a result of the rapid progress of molecular genetics and molecular biology.

In 1944, Oswald T. Avery found that genes are mainly composed of DNA (deoxyribonucleic acid), an organic compound composed of three types of units: deoxyribose (a five-carbon sugar), phosphoric acid and nitrogenous bases (there are four types of bases: adenine, guanine, thymine and cytosine).

DNA is called a nucleic acid because it exists mainly in the cell nucleus. Although major genetic information is transmitted by DNA in the nucleus, it has become clear that a small amount of DNA exists in the subcellular organelles called "mitochondria," which reside in the cytoplasm. Basically, mitochondria are supposed to be bacteria living in symbiosis with the host cell. They produce energy through oxidative phosphorylation. The DNA of mitochondria is handed down to the offspring of the host organism directly (maternal inheritance). Research into mitochondrial DNA has allowed the investigation into human mitochondrial diseases (e.g., mitochondrial myopathies and diabetes mellitus accompanied by hearing loss) transmitted via maternal inheritance, as well as the study of the origins of human existence, through tracking of the genes carried by women.

DNA is included in a substance called "chromatin," which exists in the cell nucleus. This term was chosen because chromatin is highly stainable when cells are stained with a dye. During cell division, chromatin moves into both resulting cells by dividing into strings called chromosomes. Humans have 46 chromosomes (two homologous sets of 22 autosomal chromosomes and a set of sex chromosomes). Females have 44 autosomal chromosomes and two X-chromosomes (46,XX). Males have 44 autosomal chromosomes, one X-chromosome and one Y-chromosome (46,XY). It is easy to differentiate Y-chromosomes from X-chromosomes under the microscope because Y-chromosomes are much smaller than X-chromosomes. Compared with autosomal chromosomes and the X chromosome, the Y chromosome contains fewer genes but harbors several important genes related to male gonadal and genital development. For instance, a Y-linked gene named *TDF* (testis-determining factor) leads to testicular development of the bipotential primitive gonads of the embryo. In other words, testes are formed when there is a Y-chromosome, whereas ovaries are formed when there is no Y-chromosome. As far as the sex chromosomes go, females have XX and males have XY. It is also possible to observe the history of mankind from the male side by tracing the alteration of the DNA structure of the Y chromosome. During meiosis, germ cells (spermatocytes or oocytes) are haploid: they contain one full set of autosomal chromosomes (22) and one full set of sex chromosomes. At fertilization, one full complement of autosomal and sex chromosomes, half deriving from the mother and half from the father, is constructed to form 46, XX or 46, XY.

Turner's syndrome (gonadal dysgenesis) is a chromosomal disorder which occurs in females who have only one X-chromosome (i.e., whose karyotype is 45,X, meaning a lack of the second X chromosome; this karyotype affects about half of the patients with Turner's syndrome, while the mix of 45,X/46,XX affects one-fourth). Typical abnormalities in such patients are amenorrhea, ovarian dysgenesis and short stature. In contrast, Klinefelter's syndrome occurs in male patients who have an additional X-chromosome (47,XXY). The male functions, including the secondary sex characteristics and the production and secretion of androgens, are lower than normal. The patients are tall and thin with disproportionately long legs. They appear normal until puberty, when gynecomastia and male hypogonadism become manifest. It is possible to diagnose 45,X and 47,XXY by staining and counting the chromosomes under a microscope. These anomalies are the easiest to detect among the gene defects because one entire gene-carrying chromosome is either missing or added.

In 1953, Watson and Crick discovered that DNA has a double-helix structure. The molecular structure of DNA is like a circular staircase or a twisted ladder made of two chains of repeating nucleotides winding around one another. Each nucleotide is composed of a molecule of sugar (deoxyribose), a molecule of phosphoric acid and a base. The total length of all of the DNA in a single human cell is about 2 m. One can visualize DNA as a long and thin tube with a diameter of 5×10^{-12} cm. The outer sides are composed of units made of sugar (deoxyribose) and phosphoric acid. The inner "rungs" are composed of base pairs (the two bases in each pair are connected via a hydrogen bond). Each rung is composed of one pair of bases. The twist angle of the helical structure returns to the original position every ten base pairs. There are four types of bases which can form part of a nucleotide: adenine (A), thymine (T), cytosine (C) and guanine (G). With regard to the ratio of the four bases, they exist in an equimolecular state in any DNA. Each base pair is a combination of A and T, C and G, G and C or T and A. In other words, A is always connected to T, and C is always connected to G. To find out the structure of a DNA molecule, it is enough to know the base sequence (***ACGGACGGGGAA***) in one of the two DNA strands of that molecule. If the base sequence of one strand is determined, the base sequence of the opposing strand in the double chain is easily deduced (***TCGCTGCCCCTT*** in the above case). The opposing DNA strand is called the "complementary DNA strand." The original DNA chain is called the "sense strand" (running from the 5'-end to the 3'-end). The complementary DNA chain is also called the "antisense strand" (running from the 3'-end to the 5'-end). Typically, the base sequence of DNA is expressed by the sequence of the sense strand. DNA chains are almost always in a state where the two strands are connected with each other via their bases. They only separate into single chains (single strands) to make copies of themselves (replication) or to pass on information to RNA (ribonucleic acid) by transferring the base sequence. There are about 3.1 billion base pairs (base sequences) in human DNA. The four bases (A, T, G and C) are analogous to characters in a sentence. The important thing is their sequence; bases arranged in certain sequences form "sentences" that carry specific "meanings" (genetic information). The smallest set of genes that characterizes a biotic body is called a "genome."

2. The human genome project

The goal of the human genome study was to translate all base sequences in human DNA. The International Human Genome Project was launched at the initiative of the U.S. at the beginning of the 1990s, with the participation of European countries, Japan, China, etc. It started as a public endeavor, so to speak. In mid-course, Celera Genomics, an American venture company, joined the scientific competition and used its enormous wealth and computer technology to secure patents. The genome sequencing work proceeded faster than expected because of the competition among various public institutions and a private company. As a result, in June 2000, Celera Genomics, President Clinton and Prime Minister Blair announced in a joint announcement that the rough mapping work (draft) of the human genome structure was almost complete. Reports on the results of the human genome study by two groups were separately published in "Scientific American" (weekly scientific magazine in the U.S.) and "Nature" (scientific weekly magazine in the U.K.) in February 2001. In April 2003, the deficiencies in the mapping of the human genome were remedied and they announced that the human genome sequencing work was complete. Mankind had mapped all of the base sequences of human DNA. We are now in the post-genome era. We have made the transition to the application of the genome, in other words, to the scientific interpretation of the meaning of the sentences written in characters (codes) called "bases." For example, we can determine from the bases of the genome many characteristics of proteins, their interactions, the relationship among the genes which serve as their templates and the meaning of base sequences that were previously assumed to be meaningless. Immediate applications include therapies, disease prevention, and the prognostic development of new drugs. There are many advantages to this technology. However, it is certain that this knowledge also has adverse effects. There are major ethical problems. The human genome project started in 1991 and its completion was declared in 2003. During this period, many facts became clear from the research findings of the U.S. government agencies coordinated by the NIH, the competitive research findings of U.S. venture companies, and the partial contributions of other nations. The key points are as follows. ① All 3.1 billion base sequences of human DNA have been clarified. The number of human genes revealed in the structure is about 31,000, the same as the number of genes coding a mouse and smaller than that coding a rice plant. It was smaller than expected; the number of genes coding a fruit fly is 13,000. In general, not all bases of a DNA molecule are part of a gene. Some become genes (exons) while others do not (introns), according to the base sequence. The portion of the base sequence which comprises genes accounts for 5-10% of all DNA. ② 1/400 to 1/1,000 of the bases show individual variations. These variations are called "single-nucleotide polymorphisms" (SNPs). The number of SNPs in humans is about 1.4 million. SNPs can be used to determine the risk of developing lifestyle-related diseases (high-blood pressure, diabetes, etc.) and the likelihood of subtle individual variations such as mathematical acumen, poetic talent, musical talent, and physical capabilities. It is expected that customized drug administration tailored to the individual constitution will be realized in the future. Persons who are likely to experience side effects, who are insensitive to drugs because the body eliminates them too rapidly or who are hypersensitive to some drugs can be identified based on the presence of SNPs. ③ Chimpanzees and humans share 98% of their gene sequences. The homology between a mouse (house mouse) and a human is about 80%. In the gene sequence, there are some genes commonly conserved among different species (having a common ancestor), while others are responsible for species diversity. This diversity attests to the long process of evolution, which started after life appeared on Earth and living organisms adapted to changes in their environment, forming species. Diversity has a serious significance in the life of each organism. ④ The base sequence of human DNA contains a portion that is similar to the base sequence of bacteria. It is unknown whether this is caused by horizontal propagation or by evolution. Future research will answer this question. ⑤ The main stuff of life, or living organisms, is the DNA. The genetic information in the DNA survives through the self-duplication of the DNA and its translation into proteins, which are reflected in the functions of cells. This system works not only in animals but also in plants. Major plants for which genomic analysis has been completed include Arabidopsis (gene number: 25,000 or more) and the rice plant (gene number: about 32,000), which is the principal food of Asian people. The four bases constituting the DNA are, so to speak, characters in a sentence. There are "sentences" specific to plants, flies, animals and humans, all formed using these common characters. In principle, a part of the character array specific to one species can be brought into the character arrays specific to others (plants, animals, humans). If the base sequences are changed, the phenotypes can be changed. This idea has been implemented in gene therapies in the medical field and in the genetic modification of foods in the agricultural field.

3. DNA replication and transcription

Living organisms, from humans to bacteria and viruses, propagate by making copies of themselves. This is called "replication." The main stuff of living organisms is DNA. The default shape of DNA is a double helix. When replicating, the two DNA strands separate into single chains, and each single chain functions as a template for the production of a complementary DNA strand. If the original DNA chain is "***CAAGG***", the complementary base chain is "***GTTCC***".

The two single-stranded DNA chains reunite into a double-stranded DNA molecule after producing the complementary DNA and completing the replication.

This pathway for the transmission of genetic information to descendants is found not only in cell division, but also in the replication of DNA viruses, etc. There are DNA viruses and RNA viruses. The difference is whether the genetic information of the virus is stored in DNA or RNA. A virus has a nucleic acid at its core. Typically, there is a protein sheath around the viral nucleic acid. A virus only carries nucleic-acid information and cannot generate by itself the energy required to replicate, so it self-propagates by borrowing the replication mechanism of a host cell. The process of replication of a DNA virus is as follows: infection of a cell by the virus → elevation of the DNA polymerase concentration in the host cell → replication of the viral DNA. For example, in the blood of a patient in which the hepatitis B virus (a DNA virus) is active, the concentration of DNA polymerase is raised by the virus. Quantitative measurement of DNA polymerase is clinically used as an indicator of the pathologic stage of the hepatitis B disease in the patient.

"Transcription" is the conversion of the genetic information in DNA into RNA according to the "central blueprint" in which the DNA directs the synthesis of the RNA (messenger RNA) on the DNA template; after being transported from the nucleus to the cytoplasm, the thus synthesized RNA in turn directs the synthesis of amino acids and proteins, a process known as "translation." RNA has the same nucleic acid structure as DNA, except that the sugar in RNA is a ribose instead of a deoxyribose and uracil (U) replaces thymine (T) as one of the two pyrimidines of RNA. In addition, RNA is not a double-stranded helix like DNA in most organisms. Therefore, RNA is not three-dimensional, and is folded inside the cell.

As shown in Table 2, another difference between DNA and RNA is that T (thymine) in DNA is replaced by U (uracil) in RNA. RNA has no T bases. However, the other three bases (A, G and C) are common to both nucleic acids. Therefore, if the base sequence in DNA is "***ATGCAAT**," the transcription to RNA is "***UACGUUA**" under the paired conversion rule of A to U, T to A, G to C, and C to G. Thus, the base sequence of the RNA in transcription corresponds to the base sequence of the antisense strand of the DNA. The only difference is that the T in DNA is replaced by U in RNA. The DNA information transcribed into RNA is miscellaneous and vast. Therefore, the parts containing unnecessary information are cut off (splicing), and the remaining parts are rebuilt into compact mRNA (messenger RNA). mRNA exits the nucleus and synthesizes protein from amino acids in the ribosomes of the cytoplasm. The enzyme which performs the transcription from DNA to RNA is "transcriptase." There is also an enzyme that performs transcription from RNA to DNA, i.e. in the reverse order. It is called "reverse transcriptase." DNA can be obtained by allowing reverse transcriptase to act on the mRNA after it is separated. The resulting DNA is called "cDNA" (complementary DNA). As this cDNA is derived from mRNA, cDNA shows the location of an activated gene on the base sequence. If the cDNA is separated (cloning) from the cell, proteins (hormones, hormone receptors, etc.) can again be synthesized in a test tube using the RNA.

Table 2 Comparison of two nucleic acids DNA and RNA.

Nucleic acids	Formal name	Sugar	Base	Form	Location	Function	Viruses (representative examples)
DNA	Deoxyribonucleic acid	Deoxyribose	T: Thymine A: Adenine G: Guanine C: Cytosine	Double-stranded helical structure	Nucleus, Mitochondria	Carrier of hereditary information	Hepatitis B virus, Adenovirus, EB virus
RNA	Ribonucleic acid	Ribose	U: Uracil A: Adenine G: Guanine C: Cytosine	Single-stranded	Cytoplasm, Nucleus	Transmission of hereditary information (in the case of RNA viruses)	Hepatitis C virus, ATL virus, AIDS virus

Some viruses have RNA instead of DNA as their nucleic acid. In this case, the hereditary information exists in the RNA. RNA viruses include retroviruses. A retrovirus synthesizes DNA through the reverse transcription of the viral RNA with the help of the reverse transcriptase existing in the host cell. This DNA is wedged into the DNA of the host cell and maintains its parasitic status by accompanying all subsequent cell divisions. ATL (adult T-cell leukemia, discovered by Kiyoshi Takatsuki) and AIDS (acquired immunodeficiency virus, discovered by Luc Montagnier) are famous examples of retroviruses. Reverse transcriptase inhibitors are being developed as a type of therapeutic agent against AIDS.

Hereditary information is read into the DNA base sequence (the sequence of A, T, G and C forms the DNA chain). RNA undertakes the role of conveying hereditary information in the nucleus and mitochondria to a protein synthesizer in the cytoplasm. The DNA base sequence is transmitted to the RNA (transcription, the effect of RNA polymerase). This RNA conveys the DNA's messages to the cytoplasm for the synthesis of proteins in the ribosomes.

The mechanism of protein synthesis common to all living organisms is as follows: DNA (hereditary information) → RNA (message propagation) → protein synthesis (function or reaction of cells). This is the so-called "central blueprint." Enzymes, hormones and their receptors, which are crucial for the functioning of cells, are proteins which are coded in the corresponding genes stored in the DNA. For instance, if specific genes for human insulin or human growth hormone mutate, these hormones may not be produced or may be insufficiently active, causing diabetes mellitus or pituitary dwarfism, respectively.

The information determining the order of the amino acids in the protein is in the DNA base sequence; when proteins are needed, the DNA information is translated and proteins are synthesized. Each amino acid is specified by a sequence of three bases (which form a codon).

ATTCA	isoleucine		TTTC	phenylalanine
ATG	methionine (initiator codon)		TTAG	leucine
ACTCAG	threonine		TCTCAG	serine
AATC	asparagine		TATC	tyrosine
AAAG	lysine		TAAG	(stop codon)
AGTC	serine		TGTC	cystine
AGAG	arginine		TGA	(stop codon)
			TGG	tryptophan

GT**TCAG**	valine	CT**TCAG**	leucine
GC**TCAG**	alanine	CC**TCAG**	proline
GA**TC**	asparagine acid	CA**TC**	histidine
GA**AG**	glutamic acid	CA**AG**	glutamine
GG**TCAG**	glycine	CG**TCAG**	arginine

The bases in the squares can be variable.

Fig. 1 Correspondence between the DNA base sequences (codons) and the amino acids.

For example, the first and second bases are the same for the following four DNA codons: CGT, CGC, CGA and CGG. Only the third base in each codon is different. All four of these codons code the amino acid arginine. This means that it is the first two bases of a codon that define the amino acid. As shown in Figure 1, the two codons AGA and AGG also code arginine. Thus, several types of codons order the same amino acid to be produced. To take another amino acid as an example, GGT, GGC, GGA and GGG are four of the codons that specify glycine. In this case as well, the first two bases are constant. Figure 6 shows the changes in the production of amino acids when a base in a codon mutates. The mutation causes no problem even if, say, AGA changes into AGG, as shown in ① to ③, because the same arginine is coded at the amino-acid level. However, as shown in ① to ⑤, the amino acid changes from glycine to arginine if GGG changes to AGG. In some cases, this single amino-acid mutation may affect the conformation and function of the entire protein.

Some examples of diseases caused by such mutations will help to illustrate this phenomenon. The 6th codon of the β-globin gene on the 10th chromosome is normally GAG. If this mutates to GTG, the amino acid changes from glutamic acid (normal) to valine (Glu6Val). As β-globin is a constituent protein of the hemoglobin in red blood cells, the mutation of β-globin can cause a malfunctioning of the red blood cells, resulting in hemolysis, hematuria and ischemia. Homozygosity for the mutation causes "sickle cell anemia," which is a severe genetic disease characterized by hemolytic anemia and the appearance of elongated and crescent-shaped red cells (Fig. 3) in the peripheral blood. This disease is not seen in Japan, but is frequently observed in equatorial Africa (about 30% of the population is affected).

Multiple endocrine neoplasia type 2 (MEN2) is an autosomal dominant hereditary disease. It is characterized by a high incidence of medullary thyroid cancer (MTC), which is a tumor of the calcitonin-producing parafollicular cells of the thyroid. MTC usually develops in childhood, and other neoplastic tumors, including pheochromocytoma in the adrenal gland and hyperparathyroidism in the parathyroid gland, can associate to form MEN2. Mutations are present in the *RET* gene on the 10th chromosome in about 90% of the population. The most frequent mutation is at codon 634. The normal TGC (cystine) is changed into TAC (tyrosine), CGC (arginine), or TGG (tryptophan). Abnormality in this *RET* gene is linked to the generation of multiple cancers, because the *RET* gene is one of the proto-oncogenes that we inherently possess.

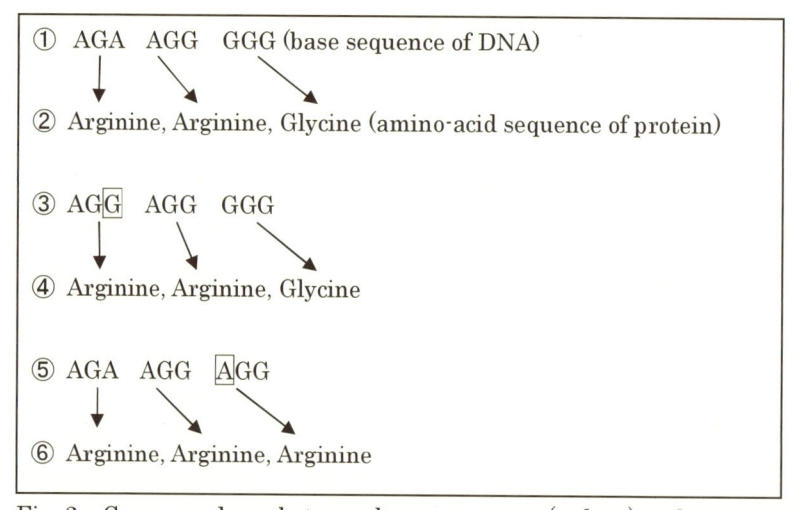

① AGA AGG GGG (base sequence of DNA)

② Arginine, Arginine, Glycine (amino-acid sequence of protein)

③ AG[G] AGG GGG

④ Arginine, Arginine, Glycine

⑤ AGA AGG [A]GG

⑥ Arginine, Arginine, Arginine

Fig. 2 Correspondence between base sequences (codons) and amino acids.

Normal red blood cells   Sickle cells

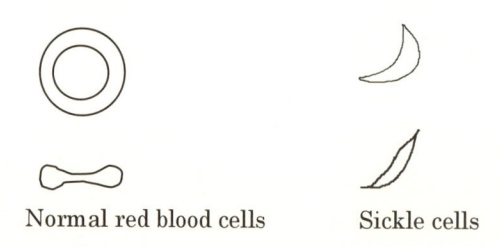

Fig. 3 Shape of red blood cells.

---

① Medullary thyroid cancer (mutation observed in 90% or more of the population)
- Thyroid nodule→Radical surgery is required at the early stage because it is often malignant.
- Elevation of calcitonin (in blood)

② Adrenomedullary tumor
- Pheochromocytoma
- High-blood pressure→Often malignant
- Elevation of catecholamine (in blood and urine)

③ Parathyroid tumor
- Hyperparathyroidism
- Hypercalcemia→Kidney and ureteral stones

④ Tumors of the mucosa (mouth, lips and gastrointestinal region)

Either ③ or ④ is associated.

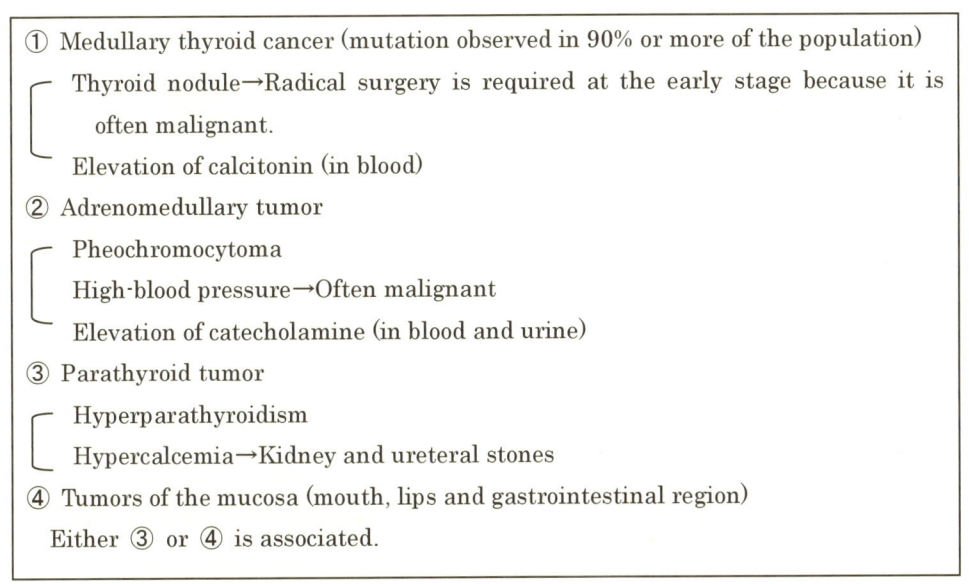

Fig. 4 Configuration and characteristics of MEN2.

The protein specified by the *RET* gene is a receptor on the surface of the cell. It is a ligand, which is a kind of growth factor. The receptor has tyrosine-kinase activity. This is the structure of oncogenes. When this receptor protein is changed due to a mutation in the *RET* gene, cell growth occurs spontaneously by bypassing the binding of the ligand to the receptor. This is canceration, and it occurs in multiple endocrine organs. The most frequently affected region is the C-cells, or parafollicular cells, of the thyroid (medullary carcinoma), the second is the adrenomedullary cells (pheochromocytoma) and the third is the parathyroid cells (hyperplastic parathyroid, which causes elevated blood calcium).

Abnormalities in the *RET* gene are most frequently observed at codon 634. Other frequently affected codons include 609, 611, 618, 620, 630 and 634 (the extracellular proteins of the receptor are coded by these codons), and 768, 790, 791, 804, 883, 891 and 918 (the intracellular proteins of the receptor are coded by these codons).

If an abnormal *RET* gene is diagnosed, the thyroid cancer must be thoroughly removed in the early stage. Any remaining cancer can cause death. Testing for *RET* gene mutations is indispensable in the diagnosis of MEN (multiple endocrine neoplasia) in the U.S. Investigation of family histories is also useful for early detection and treatment. Informed consent should always be obtained for such genetic testing. A counseling system should also be established for mutation-positive cases. Japan is rather behind in this ethics aspect. The *RET* gene tests are associated with preventative operations and techniques that will save lives if ethical standards are met.

There is additional information given by base sequences; for example, the codon ATG in the DNA codes the amino acid methionine, which also orders the start of translation and is known as the "start codon." The three codons TAA, TAG and TGA do not code amino acids and give the order to stop translation; they are called "stop codons." The term "codon" is used not only for DNA base sequences, but also for RNA base sequences. The RNA stop codons are UAA, UAG and UGA.

I mention here an interesting scientific fact discovered recently regarding the relationship between diseases and base sequences. Three bases form a codon. A codon is also called a triplet. If there is a mutation where the number of a specific triplet increases abnormally in a gene, the amino acid coded by the triplet may be over-synthesized in the cytoplasm. For example, the triplet CAG encodes the amino acid glutamine, as shown in Figure 5. The disease caused by the over-repetition of CAG in a gene is called "polyglutamine disease," as coded protein product possesses additional polyglutamine tracts. Such abnormal proteins are assumed to be toxic to neural cells, causing neurodegenerative diseases. There are at least nine known types of disease in which the pathological expansion of CAG repetition occurs in different genes. The most famous is Huntington's disease. In this progressive and ultimately fatal disease, the Huntington gene has as many as 67 exons encoding a protein comprised of 3114 amino acids; it is located on the short arm of the 4th chromosome (4p16.3), and there is a mutation in the first exon which yields an over-repetition of the CAG motif. The number of repeats (...CAGCAGCAGCAG...) of the CAG triplet in the gene is normally 35 or less. Individuals with 40 or more repeats will almost invariably develop Huntington's disease (full penetrance), while individuals with 36 to 39 repeats may remain asymptomatic or develop the disease late in life (variable penetrance). The mutant protein resulting from the over-repetition of CAG causes cell death through its accumulation in the nuclei of neural cells. Clinically, Huntington's disease presents with movement abnormalities such as balance difficulties and clumsiness, and cognitive abnormalities such as personality change, dementia and psychiatric disorders. Usually, the onset of the disease is between the ages of 35 and 50, with death occurring 15-20 years after disease onset. The greater the number of CAG repetitions, the earlier the age of onset. This disease is inherited by half of the children of affected parents in an autosomal dominant fashion. Thus, Huntington's disease is one of the most prominent clinical diseases in the context of "DNA and life," and its definite diagnosis is now feasible though genetic testing, in which the CAG repetitions in the first exon of the Huntington gene are counted. However, as this is an adult-onset disease, is fatal, or essentially incurable with the present medicine, and has 100% penetrance, molecular testing for confirmative diagnosis of Huntington's disease should be employed very carefully, especially for presymptomatic children and younger individuals; the transplantation of embryonic stem cells may be used to treat this disease in the future. The availability of a multidisciplinary support system, including pre-test and post-test counseling, is mandatory for the performance of DNA testing. This is another important ethical issue related to this disease.

Other polyglutamine diseases include spinocerebellar ataxia (in which the affected gene is located on the 6th chromosome) and spinobulbar muscular atrophy (in which the affected gene is located on the X chromosome). Recently, diseases caused by abnormal increases in the number of other base triplets have been found. They include fragile X syndrome, caused by an abnormal increase (more than 200; normal value: 54 or less) in the number of CGG triplets, myotonic dystrophy, caused by an abnormal increase (more than 80; normal value: 30 or less) in the number of CTG triplets, and Friedreich's ataxia, caused by an abnormal increase (more than 200; normal value: 34 or less) in the number of GAA triplets. These, together with the polyglutamine diseases, are generically called "triplet repeat diseases."

Thus, some fundamental rules of the living world have been revealed: the information governing the life of cells is located in the genes on the DNA strand, qualitative and quantitative abnormalities in the bases constituting the DNA of the genes cause diseases, and genetic information is transmitted to the descendants.

4. Animals can be cloned from the somatic cells of mature animals.

In the natural world, there are naturally occurring scientific experiments, so to speak. For example, we know that human clones called "twins" (monozygotic twins) are often born. A fertilized egg divides into two eggs and both of these differentiate into adult individuals without genetic change. Therefore, the genomes of monozygotic twins are identical. This natural model clearly shows that an adult can be copied if the genome is kept the same. Experiments, where an animal copy of the original adult DNA donor with the same phenotype as the donor is produced by artificially removing the genome from a differentiated adult cell of the donor and transferring it into the enucleated oocyte of a female adult, followed by the implantation of the artificial zygote into the uterus of another female for embryo development, have been conducted with higher mammals such as sheep and cows. Many such experiments have been successful recently. The fertilized egg differentiates into the adult cells which make up the adult individual, such as liver cells, skin cells, eye cells, or mammary gland cells. Even at this mature stage, the genomes in all cells are the same, regardless of the cell type. However, although they have copies of the same genome, different genes are silenced in different types of differentiated adult cells (e.g., liver cells or breast cells). People had long supposed that it was impossible to make copies of adult organisms from the genomes of differentiated cells. In 1996, Wilmut (Roslin Institute, UK) removed the nucleus from a breast cell of a six-year-old female sheep and placed it in an egg collected from a female sheep of another ancestry through nucleus interchange. Then, he implanted the synthesized egg in the uterus of a third sheep. This sheep, whose womb was borrowed, became pregnant and gave birth to Dolly, the famous cloned sheep. Dolly had the same genome and phenotype as the six-year-old sheep from which the nucleus was taken. Figure 5 outlines this process.

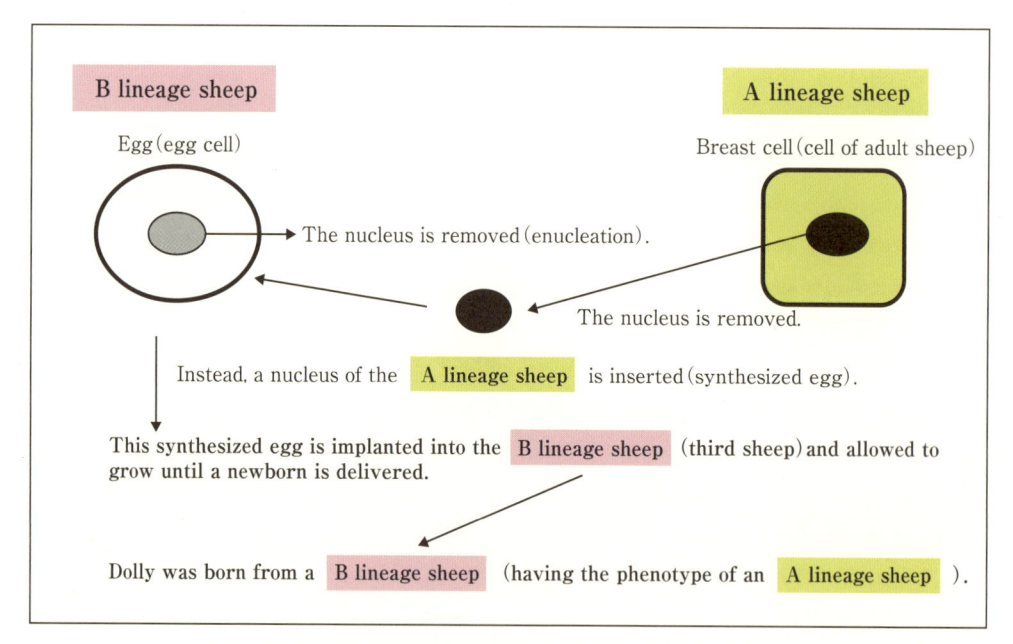

Fig. 5   Scheme of the cloning of the sheep Dolly.

This accomplishment was publicized in "Nature" in 1997. It was innovative because it used the nucleus of a somatic cell (breast cell) of a mature sheep instead of the nucleus of a fertilized egg or embryonic cell at an early stage of development. In 1998, a group from Kinki University in Japan succeeded in creating cloned cows (Noto-go and Kaga-go) using the same method. After that, cloned cattle were being delivered all over

Japan. The total number exceeded 3,000 at the beginning of 2003. Such nuclear transplantation methods utilizing adult somatic cells as DNA sources have been successful in mice, cats and dogs thereafter, although the rate of successful births of thus constructed clones has been generally low. However, this cloning technology is expected to be applied in the future in various ways for the benefit of humankind, for instance in the production of high-quality cattle meat in the dairy field or in harvesting a sizeable volume of pharmaceutical bio-factors from the milk of cloned cattle. In a more familiar vein, patients will be able to replace their malfunctioning organs, such as muscles (muscular atrophy), nerves (spinal injury), and pancreas (diabetes mellitus) with cloned cells, tissues or organs derived from their own DNA, where theoretically no graft-versus-host reaction occurs since the transplant and the host are immunologically the same. Regrettably, Dolly, the cloned sheep, died in March 2003. It was unknown that cloned animals have a short life span and that they inherit the age of their donors. Still, the breakthrough of animal cloning showed that an animal can be copied (cloned) even by using DNA from the somatic cells of mature animals. The technology has reached the stage where humans can be cloned from adult human cells. The origin of the word "clone" is the Greek word " κ λ ω ν ," meaning "twig" or "to burgeon."

5. Human ES cells

Fertilization is a syncretization of the DNA from a male sperm (genetic information in a sperm cell) and the DNA from a female egg (oocyte) (genetic information in an egg cell). When an egg is fertilized, cell division commences as a result of stimulation by yet-to-be-clarified factors existing in the egg. The genetic information guiding embryo development and cell differentiation thereafter is contained in the newly syncretized DNA. Early embryogenesis goes through the two-celled, four-celled, eight-celled, morula and blastocyst stages, as shown in Figure 6. An embryo is a fertilized egg in the initial stage of development, after it starts to divide. The individual cells of the embryo during the early cell-division stage are called blastomeres. In *in vitro* fertilization (IVF), one of these blastomeres is utilized for pre-implantation genetic diagnosis (PGD); the rest of the cells are allowed to continue to grow into a fetus after being implanted into the uterus. Generally, a human fertilized egg becomes a blastodermic cluster in five to seven days after fertilization, and nidates (attaches itself to the womb) six days after fertilization. After implantation, the embryo differentiates into a fetus and develops as birth approaches. In general, the human embryo is called a "fetus" after two months of pregnancy, in order to distinguish the two stages of growth. An ES cell (embryonic stem cell) is a stem cell originating from an embryo. When ES cells having the same DNA are split repeatedly in a test tube and are separated into homogenous cell lines, ES cell "strains" or "lines" are said to be established. Studies of ES cells have advanced far, especially in mice. As an extension of this, the establishment of new human ES cell strains is constantly being reported since 1998, and studies on human ES cells have turned into an international industrial competition for the futile world of extensive application to general biology and medicine. In fact, the peak of the human genome project has passed, and it is no exaggeration to say that international scientific competition has shifted its attention to human ES cells. The application of human ES cell technology is expected to open the door to huge business opportunities in multiple fields such as medical transplantation, regenerative medicine and more effective studies on drug metabolism using human cells. We, as individuals, originated from fertilized eggs that have divided and differentiated. An individual grows as the number of cells increases via cell division. A cell acquires special functions as a result of cell differentiation. For example, early embryogenic cells differentiate into nerve cells, hormone-secreting cells, blood cells, liver cells, etc. The source of this division and differentiation is the ES cells. Stem cells are so named because they are like the stem of a tree. Each branch is a type of differentiated cell.

The embryo used for establishing ES cells is a clump of cells (blastocyst) at the initial stage of division of a fertilized egg (Fig. 6). As differentiation has not yet started, the cells at this stage (5-7 days after fertilization) are pluripotential, or able to differentiate into any type of cell. The cells composing the inner cell mass of a blastocyst are teased away and then transferred to petri dishes for *in vitro* culturing. When homogenous cells, which can proliferate endlessly and be kept alive *in vitro* by constantly supplying nutrients, are separated, they are called ES cell strains. Concerning human ES cells, one of the major ethical problems is that they can only be obtained upon the destruction of an embryo, which can develop into a normal baby if allowed to do so.

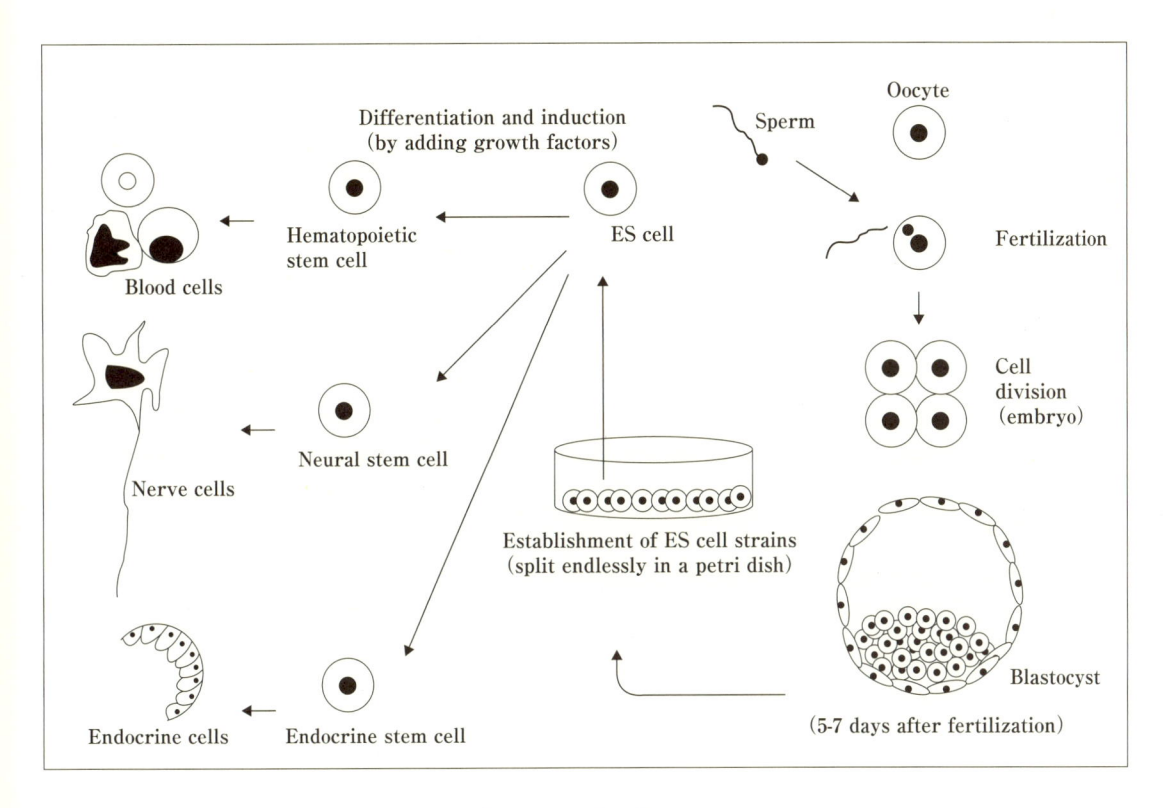

Fig. 6 Separation and differentiation of human ES cells.

　　Once ES cells are separated, their further differentiation can be induced *in vitro*. ES cells can be made to differentiate into nerve cells, liver cells, cardiac muscle cells, endocrine cells, blood cells, etc., by adding special hormones and growth factors to the culture. To make this easy to understand, this process can be explained in a very simplified, if abrupt, manner, as follows. In the future, doctors will perform heart and liver transplants with organs, tissues or cells differentiated from ES cells. Likewise, Parkinson's disease, a common neurodegenerative disorder characterized by the reduction of dopaminergic neurotransmission within the brain, will be treated by implanting ES cell-derived brain cells which can secrete dopamine. Diabetes mellitus, characterized by a lack of insulin, will be treated by implanting ES cell-derived pancreatic β-cells which can secrete insulin. Also, instead of performing bone-marrow transplantations as they are currently performed for hematopoietic diseases, doctors will implant hematopoietic stem cells originating from ES cells. Thus, ES cells can make our dreams come true in many fields of regenerative medicine.

However, human ES cells are obtained through the destruction of embryos, i.e. human fertilized eggs which have begun to split. More precisely, an embryo which has already developed into a hollow ball called a "blastocyst" (Fig. 6) is necessary to establish human ES cell lines because the co-culturing of the inner cell mass (ICM) derived from the blastocyst eventually makes it possible to generate human ES cells. Currently, some supporting humoral factors derived from ICM cells are speculated to function. Therefore, there are serious ethical problems to be solved in that we have to kill embryos, albeit at an early stage of life. As fertilized embryos represent the germination of life, it is needless to say that human self-regulation based on respect for life on both religious and ethical grounds is primarily required in the manipulation of fertilized embryos for research purposes. In every country where research into human ES cells is officially accepted, the source of human embryos is the extra fertilized eggs resulting from test-tube fertilization, or *in vitro* fertilization (IVF), and grown into blastocysts after the donor's consent has been obtained. IVF and IVF-linked pre-implantation genetic diagnosis (in which a single blastomere from an embryo is extracted and the rest of the embryo is left intact), as an option of IVF, are now well-established technologies. They are employed for producing babies and detecting their possible genetic disorders. In pre-implantation genetic diagnosis, the biopsy of a single blastomere is usually performed earlier than in the blastocyst stage, and it is generally accepted that the biopsy does not interfere with the normal growth of the embryo from which a blastomere is separated. These technologies surrounding IVF are now so advanced as to be applied to the establishment of human ES cell lines, based on successful results obtained in mice. As this method is analogous to the one used in IVF-associated pre-implantation genetic diagnosis, which has been widely accepted since it does not destroy embryos as previous methods have done, the ethical problems are less severe. Now, a single blastomere obtained from an early embryo at the 8 to 10 cell-stage can be used. In any case, it is true that the utilization of human ES cells promises to open up a whole new world to explore from the scientific viewpoint. Hopefully, valid procedures for harvesting human ES cells will be established after the inherent ethical problems have been solved and the world has successfully passed through the narrow gorge guarded by science and ethics.

In November 2007, astonishing and cutting-edge data were presented by Shinya Yamanaka and his colleagues at Kyoto University (*Cell*, 131:861-72). According to those data, human pluripotential cells behaving like human ES cells can be generated merely by reprogramming human adult skin cells through the viral transduction of defined transcription factors into those cells. The technique was elegantly applied to human cells based upon the same team's successful experiments conducted with mice. The methods are cutting-edge because they utilize adult, or differentiated, somatic cells, which makes it theoretically possible to obtain patient-specific and disease-specific stem cells best suited for the treatment of human genetic diseases including Huntington's disease, Alzheimer's disease, muscular dystrophy, and so on; further, and most importantly, this technique allows us to dispense with human oocytes in the whole procedures. Although we still have many barriers to overcome, we are undoubtedly one step closer to the ideal goal of treating intractable human genetic diseases using stem cells obtained from the patient, which means we will be able to resolve both the ethical and the tissue-rejection problems associated with tissue/organ transplantation.

References

1) Donald Voet, Judith G. Voet; translated into Japanese by Nobuo Tamiya, Masami Muramatsu, Tatsuhiko Yagi, and Hiroshi Yoshida: Biochemistry Vol 1. Kagakudojin Co., Tokyo, 1994

2) Keiko Nakamura: Seimeikagaku. Kodansha, Tokyo, 1996

3) Robert K. Murray; translated by Nobuto Jyodai: Harper's Biochemistry 25th Edition. Maruzen, Tokyo, 2001

4) Carina Dennis, Richard Gallgher; translated by Asao Fujiyama: Human Genome. Tokumashoten, Tokyo, 2002

5) Richard Fortey; translated by Masataka watanabe: Life, A Natural History of the First Four Billion years of Life on Earth. Soshisha, Tokyo, 2003

6) John Sulston, Gergia Ferry; translated by Keiko Nakamura: The Common Thread A Story of Science, Politics, Ethics, and the Human Genome. Shuwa System, Tokyo, 2003

7) Nature, Vol 409, No 6822, 2001

8) Science, Vol 291, No 5507, 2001

9) Arlene Y. Chiu and Mahendra S. Rao: Human Embryonic Stem Cells. Humana Press, Totowa, 2003

10) Lenny Moss: What Genes Can't Do. The MIT Press, Cambridge, 2003

11) Nature, Vol 444, No 7115, 2006

Chapter III: *Greek Culture and Its Significance for the Later Development of Science and Ethics*

Ancient Greece was a large cultural area that included domains, or ranges, of cultural exchange, such as Asia Minor (then called Ionia, with the ancient city Miletus as one of its major settlements), southern Italy, Sicily, Africa, etc. In voyages and commerce, human beings had to deal with the vast atmospheric phenomena of the sea, as well as astronomical phenomena, and they became increasingly displeased with the hitherto dominant mysticism surrounding the universe and nature. Consequently, they started to think rationally. At first, simple doubts about the world (the natural or phenomenal world) generated natural philosophy. The aim of this philosophy was to find an invariable and unifying principle lying at the root of all miscellaneous phenomena, such as the generation and change of things. At that time, science and philosophy (metaphysics) were the same. Ancient people chiefly observed nature. Therefore, medicine, geography, geometry, mathematics and astronomy appeared, and they all employed the basic methods of natural science. Observations then brought forth the inductive method. In addition, excellent science, art and literature were established in ancient Greece. Although there was no prose literature in ancient Greece, sophisticated works were created in the fields of poetry, drama, sculpture and architecture. Thus, in the ancient Greek era, people were free to develop in a wide range of fields. This had a significant impact on the progress of culture and civilization from the Renaissance to the present age. Therefore, it is very important to understand the human activities of the ancient Greek era, especially the ethos of natural philosophy that formed the foundation of Western science at the time; this Western science has led to the westernization and modernization prevalent today.

1. Greek natural philosophy

The early Greeks started to inquire into the nature of primary matter (*archè*), which is the unifying principle of all things and of their movement in the natural world. They wanted to find a stable unifying principle at the root of miscellaneous natural phenomena. This tendency of thought was fundamental to the Greek world. Their style of rational thought was a kind of materialism. Human thought became independent of conventional mythology. This meant that human beings tried to construct rational thought, which was the beginning of philosophy (questions regarding existence, or metaphysics) and natural science (rational questions regarding the natural world, or physics). In the Greek era, especially the era of early natural philosophy, philosophy and natural science were intertwined. In other words, a philosopher was a thinker who sought knowledge and at the same time a scientist who performed cause-and-effect analyses of natural phenomena. Since philosophy and natural science both started from simple human questions about the environment and the outer world (including the physiology of their own bodies), they were alike. A philosopher was basically a mathematician or scientist ascribing to the Greek ethos prevalent at that time, represented by the question, "What is the primary matter?". The philosophers of those days who were interested in varied environments were persons of superlative wit who were universally recognized as great thinkers. They were often religiously charismatic (e.g., Pythagoras, Empedocles). The people who belonged to the intellectual group of this age were as follows:

Thales (625-545 B.C.)

Thales believed water to be *arché* (primary matter). In other words, he believed that all things are generated and changed according to the transformations of water (unitarian materialism). It was his belief that all things are generated by water and return to water when they perish. *Arché* is an example of a reduction to a unifying principle. Therefore, explanations of natural things and phenomena were always accompanied by thoughts of genesis and annihilation. Thales also excelled in geometry. He discovered many geometric facts, such as the fact that the base angles of an isosceles triangle are equal, that the angle of a diameter at the circumference is 90°, and that the sum of the internal angles of a triangle is 180°. Thales was a natural philosopher who was active mainly around the Nile and the Mediterranean Sea. He performed scientific observations based on causality in various fields of practical science, such as geography, meteorology and astronomy, through which he concluded that "water is the primary matter."

Anaximander (610-545 B.C.)

Anaximander was a pupil of Thales, and at first he naturally perpetuated the belief that *arché* is water. However, he later defined a common eternal substance from which water and fire were generated. This was the unlimited basic matter (*apeiron*), which is ageless primary matter (*arché*) and is transformed into everything existing in the world.

Anaximenes (?-about 500 B.C.)

Anaximenes believed *aer* (air) to be the primary matter (*arché*). He believed that *arché* can change in quality (can become thicker or thinner). He concluded that air changed into water and fire when it got thicker and thinner, respectively.

These three philosophers were from Ionia. Ionia was also called "eastern Greece," because it occupied the Mediterranean region of what is now Turkish territory (Asia Minor). There were Mesopotamia and Babylonia to the east of Ionia. They were also affected by the advanced culture of Ionia. Ionians were maritime merchants. Therefore, they excelled at practical sciences such as astronomy and mathematics. These three philosophers were said to be of the "Ionian school," as they were active in Ionia. Meanwhile, Pythagoras was active in western Greece (the currently Italian territories of Sicily and southern Italy). Sicily was then called Sikelia (Sicilia). It was a territory of Greece, which then included southern Italy. To this day, Sicily has many Greek stone temple ruins.

Pythagoras (was active around 582 B.C.)

Pythagoras was born on the island of Samos near the western coast of Asia Minor. The city of Miletus was nearby on the opposite shore, and was the base of the Ionian school. To the south lay Cos, where Hippocrates was born. Pythagoras was taught by Anaximander (Miletus) when he was young. Soon, he broke away from the materialistic thought of the Ionian school and moved to Croton (Greek territory at the time) in southern Italy. His inclinations were mystical rather than materialistic in regard to *arché*. He believed that mathematical principles underlie the movements of celestial bodies, music, beauty and the order of nature. Numbers were, so to speak, *arché* in his view.

Pythagoras was a religious charismatic (he founded the Pythagorean community) and taught people the catharsis of the psyche. He believed that music is required to effect catharsis. He thought that human beings in the world should devote themselves to the pursuit of psychic catharsis, and that the psyche returns to God at the moment of catharsis. He organized a religious community (the Pythagorean community), which was designed as a full-fledged society. This community followed the tenets of Orphism. Its members adhered strictly to strange laws: eating beans was forbidden, and so was touching white hens, eating hearts, picking up anything that had fallen from a table, etc. The members of this closed occult community conducted research into mathematics, natural science and theoretical medicine, as well as holding secret ceremonies.

Pythagoras was active in southern Italy (it was called Magna Graecia, and included Sicily at the time) and was a child of his time in that the nature of *arché* (primary matter) preoccupied him. However, Pythagoras was different from the exponents of the

Ionian school, in that he used mathematical and geometrical principles to understand *arché*. He found beautiful principles hidden in nature, such as those governing the movements of celestial bodies and music. He gleaned a deity beyond human understanding. It was almost the focus of a religion. He considered the earth to be a globe; he did not think that the earth is the center of the universe, but a celestial body revolving around the sun. The Pythagorean community was both materialistic and idealistic, but more idealistic than materialistic. It influenced Plato (theory of Ideas) and Aristotle (theory of *eidos*), because Pythagoras looked at what was behind physical objects and phenomena. The Pythagorean community believed that the psyche (soul) can exist without the body. In this respect, the Pythagorean theories had a profound effect on Plato.

Alcmaion (500-428 B.C.)

Alcmaion was a pupil of Pythagoras in Croton in southern Italy. He conducted numerous autopsies and knew about the nerves emanating from the brain, including the optic nerve; he also knew that perceptions are sent to the brain and that intelligence is generated by the brain. In fact, Alcmaion was a mathematician belonging to the Pythagorean community, as well as an excellent empirical physiologist.

Heraclitus (540-475 B.C.)

Heraclitus was deeply committed to the Ionian school. He considered fire to be the primary matter (*arché*). He thought that generation and extinction followed the following course: air → water → earth → fire (→ air →); he also believed that all of these elements can be ultimately interchanged, as the primary substance is fire. He considered that all things are exchanged for fire, just as all products are exchanged for gold.

Another innovation of Heraclitus was that he emphasized the fact that all things change. He said, "We can never step into the same river twice," and in the same way, time passes inexorably, day and night. He believed yesterday was already part of the past, morning is flowing towards us afresh and only change is real. The aphorism **"Panta rhei"** ("Everything flows") was passed down to posterity by Heraclitus. In the beginning, *arché* existed. Substances come into existence and disappear based on *arché*. That was the basic thought common to all members of the Ionian school, including Thales, Anaximandros and Anaximenes. If *arché* is represented by a single substance, the phenomenal world cannot be explained unless we suppose the generation and extinction of everything from *arché*.

However, Heraclitus felt that fire is more mysterious and deserves more religious reverence than conventional *arché*. It is an interesting that the teachings of the Buddha presented the same basic concept of the impermanence of all things, as in metempsychosis, and that the Buddha was active far away in the Orient.

Anaxagoras (500-428 B.C.)

Anaxagoras conceived infinite *spermata* (seeds) to be *arché*. He imagined that all things exist from the beginning and denied the concept of generation and change.

His thoughts affected atomism. He believed intelligence (*nous*, or mind) to cause the movement of the *spermata*. Thus, he brought mind to the conventional concept of *arché* (primary matter) for the first time. It was Anaxagoras who realized that the moon shines because it reflects the sun's light and that the sun is not a god, but a burning rock. Anaxagoras was from Ionia. However, he had a great impact on Athenian philosophy (the idealism of Socrates and Plato).

Empedocles (493-433 B.C.)

Empedocles was a member of an aristocratic political family of Siracusa (Akragas) in Sicily (Sikelia). He is known as the founder of rhetoric (debating skill). Empedocles was a poet endowed with varied talents. His thoughts have been preserved until now in fragmentary remains of his poems.

He was the first to abandon monism, the assumption that a single substance is the primary matter (*arché*). Instead, based on the thoughts of his predecessors he distinguished four root elements: earth, water, fire and air. He believed that they are not interchangeable. To him, the four roots really exist as substances that are neither generated nor eliminated. This was the source of the so-called four-element theory. Notice that the word "element" does not refer to the elements of modern chemistry such as "hydrogen" or "oxygen." It refers to elementary substance (*elementa*). They are types of *arché* that were a popular part of the mental landscape at that time.

One innovation of Empedocles was to apply the principles of movement to the four elements. The power which combines the four elements is "love." The ideal state where love exerts its effect unimpeded is the "sphere." If love functions ideally, the four elements are well blended and stable. Meanwhile, the force that functions in the direction of the separation of the four elements is "strife." The four elements become unstable when affected by strife, and form individual substances in the phenomenal world. Empedocles abandoned the idea of generation and change, and thought that all things are brought forth by the unification and separation (love and strife) of the four "roots." This four-element theory explained the phenomenal world more easily than the conventional single-substance theory, and became popular at the time.

Plato referred to the thoughts of Empedocles in his work *Timaeus*. Hippocrates, a physical and contemporary of Plato, cited the thoughts of Empedocles as the basis of his theory of the four bodily humors. Aristotle also mentioned this theory in his own works.

Thus, the four-element theory was very attractive and survived the Middle Ages until the actual elements began to be discovered in the 18th century (H and O; water: H_2O). Empedocles excelled in poetry, philosophy, politics and medicine, and was charismatic. A relationship with Orphism (the Pythagorean school) is also indicated. As he was an all-round scholar, there are many legends about him. Among these, there is an anecdote in the *Ars poetica* by Horatius (65-8 B.C.) that he killed himself by diving into Mt. Etna, the infamous volcano in Sicily (Sikelia), in order to become an immortal god. The great eruption of Mt. Etna made worldwide news in October 2002. The volcano has remained active in Sicily since the age of Empedocles. There is a legend that Empedocles stopped an epidemic that occurred in a colony in Sicily by digging new channels to open up the ditches and curtaining valleys to prevent winds from blowing.

Democritus (470-400 B.C.)

Democritus was from Abdera, a small town in northern Greece. He thought that atoms (indivisible matter, *atomos*) are the primary matter (*arché*).

He lived at the same time as Socrates (470-399 B.C.). The ethos of the speculative quest for the primary matter was started by Thales (an empiricist and mechanicist) and continued down to Democritus (a theoretical thinker). An atom is a thing that cannot be divided and is homogeneous. It has always existed without generation or destruction. The shapes, sizes and other characteristics of atoms determine the characteristics of substances. In philosophical terms, atomism is connected to materialism. Atomism was a response to the demands of the times; it was deemed necessary to increase the number of ultimately indivisible substances (*arché*) from the four of Empedocles (water, air, earth and fire). Leucippus from Miletus was the first to invented atomism, but it was Democritus who systematized it.

The quest of natural philosophy for *arché* from Thales to Empedocles was unable to weather the criticism formulated by the Eleatic school, which focused on a certain type of ontology. In this Eleatic ontology, everything exists or nothing exists, what does not exist does not exist at first, and nothing is created from nothing. Parmenides (544-501 B.C.) from Elea in southern Italy was the leading figure of the Eleatic school. At that time, Leucippus conceived the idea of vacancy (the existence of nothingness) or space. In other words, "nothing" is a kind of existence. Nothing also exists; vacancy also exists. Looking at it in this way allows physical objects to be divided without contradiction. Afterwards, this developed into the atomism of Democritus. This thinking process shows that the Greeks were very intellectual, logical, self-corrective and constructive. They formed a thinking pattern directly linked to that of modern people, those who modernized the world.

2. Philosophy of the psyche

Under the influence of Anaxagoras, Athens became the new center of philosophy in about 450 B.C., after Ionia. Philosophy started to diverge from natural philosophy. The interest of philosophy shifted to speculative contents (idealism), mainly concerning the psyche.

Socrates (470-399 B.C.)

The simple materialism originated by Thales was introduced into society as utilitarian illuminism. If we assume that utilitarian illuminism was the core of the Greek ethos, a significant shift from materialism to idealism can be observed in Socrates. In other words, he adopted a method of idealism in which the truth is obtained by making an induction from concrete phenomena to a universal concept with the help of *logoi* (words). In the beginning, Socrates studied natural science and mathematics. However, his chief interests were ethics, morality and the virtues. There are no true remnants of his own work. His thoughts were made known to the world through the works of Aristophanes and his own pupil, Plato.

Socrates was a logician who excelled in the methods of dialogue (dialectic). Like a mediator, he helped people to gain insight into their errors and to practice correct thinking through questions and answers. In his life, he pursued the highest goal, philosophy (to love (*philo*) wisdom (*sophia*)).

Plato (427-347 B.C.)

Plato was a pupil of Socrates and left numerous works. He accepted the knowledge that was popular at the time (e.g., the four-element theory of Empedocles). He was absorbed by idealistic philosophy, which he considered to be more valuable than physics. For example, he believed that the physician's task is to care for bodies, while the philosopher's is to care for the psyche. He thought that the principles of mathematics are important and that the psyche (mind, soul, spirit) is something over and above the human body. Those were the views in which he was affected by Pythagoras. The school of Pythagoras at Croton in the southern Italy, called Magna Graecia at the time, preceded Plato by a century. One of the Pythagorean was Empedocles, the author of poems expressing the assumption of four eternal "roots" are moved by the two driving forces of Love and Strife; another was Alcmaion, who dissected animals.

Theory of Ideas

Plato conceived of "Ideas" (forms, original forms), which are existences belonging to the invisible extrasensory world, while matter and phenomena belong to the visible sensory world. For Plato, the cognitive faculty corresponding to the visible and invisible world were perception and intelligence, respectively.

What we perceive in the phenomenal world is just a simulacrum of the Ideas. For example, a perfect circle belongs to the world of Ideas. The circles we draw and see are imperfect simulacra. Philosophical, ethical and religious temptations occur when human souls recall the world of Ideas. The Ideas are the purpose of phenomena. Ideas are ordered in a hierarchy. The highest Idea is that of the Good. Thus, Plato established a dualistic cognitive theory based on perception and thought. This duality also consists of the visible (the world that is the target of perception) and the conceptual (world of Ideas) worlds, on the basis of objectivity as the aim of perception and thought. The mind (psyche) belongs to the world of Ideas. It was Plato who emphasized and pioneered the conceptual world. Forerunners of the theory of Ideas included Pythagoras and Anaxagoras. However, it was Plato who started the systematization (idealism) of the mind (psyche).

Uranology and cosmology

Plato was recognized as being a leader of idealism at a later age. He developed a cosmology in his *Timaeus*. Plato was also interested in mathematics. As it is well known from the fact that he visited Sicily several times, he was significantly affected by the Pythagorean school. In *Timaeus*, Plato described his idealistic cosmology, which he had developed under the influence of Pythagoras. Plato's astronomy was a system of the universe where spheres and circular motion are Ideas.

Simple questions about existence were focused on the outer world and natural phenomena in the Greek era. As a result, the physics and philosophy of the *arché* were developed (the lineage from Thales to Democritus). That was the characteristic of the Greek ethos. Soon, fundamental doubts began to appear in connection with the inner aspect or mind of humans, and this generated a philosophy of the psyche (Anaxagoras,

Socrates and Plato). Both lines of philosophy have developed until now, each pursuing its own separate goal.

The two philosophies coexisted with each other in the field of inquiry dedicated to the elucidation of human beings, and were thus inseparably connected. They are both important for the contemporary investigation of the body and the mind. Body and mind are discussed in the fields of religion, philosophy, psychic medicine, psychology, and in connection with specifically contemporary issues such as organ transplants, brain death, bioethics and environmental ethics.

God placed water and air in the mean between fire and earth, and made them to have the same proportion so far as was possible (as fire is to air so is air to water, and as air is to water so is water to earth); and thus he bound and put together a visible and tangible heaven. And for these reasons, and out of such elements which are in number four, the body of the world was created, and it was harmonized by proportion, and therefore has the spirit of friendship; and having been reconciled to itself, it was indissoluble by the hand of any other than the framer. (*Timaeus, The Complete Works of Plato*, vol.1, Iwanami Shoten Publishers)

These they took and welded together, not with the indissoluble chains by which they were themselves bound, but with little pegs too small to be visible, making up out of all the four elements each separate body, and fastening the courses of the immortal soul in a body which was in a state of perpetual influx and efflux. (*Timaeus*)

The truth rather is that the soul which is pure at departing draws after her no bodily taint, having never voluntarily had connection with the body, which she is ever avoiding, herself gathered into herself. And what does this mean but that she has been a true disciple of philosophy and has practiced how to die easily?" (*Phaedo, The Complete Works of Plato*, vol. 1, Iwanami Shoten Publishers)

Meletus and Anytus will not injure me: they cannot; for it is not in the nature of things that a bad man should injure a better than himself. I do not deny that Anytus may, perhaps, kill him, or drive him into exile, or deprive him of civil rights; and he may imagine, and others may imagine, that he is doing him a great injury: but in that I do not agree. (*Apology, The Complete Works of Plato*, vol. 1, Michitaro Tanaka, trans., Iwanami Shoten Publishers)

Aristotle (384-322 B.C.)

Aristotle was the son of Nichomachus, who was the physician of the King of

Macedonia and belonged to the guild of the Asclepiads. Aristotle was a pupil of Plato, just as Plato had been a pupil of Socrates. He remained a member of Plato's Academy until he was 37. Although Aristotle was initially educated at Plato's Academy, he later covered a range of nature far wider than Plato had done, and he attained numerous achievements in physics (natural science), in particular biology, zoology and comparative anatomy, as well as metaphysics. The close relationship between these two great men lasted for 20 years. At the age of 42, Aristotle was appointed tutor to Alexander the Great.

He theorized about the pyramidal hierarchy of life with humans at the apex. He adopted a philosophy of teleology, which in essence maintains that god is above humans.

Aristotle actively studied physiology, embryology and anatomy, and left an evolutionary theory with humans at the apex. He was seen as a naturalist, and he did indeed display a wide-ranging curiosity about the world. However, he thought that intelligence originates in the heart, so he also bequeathed errors to posterity.

Aristotle conceived of "eidos" (form), in contrast with the "Ideas" of Plato, which are an idealistic substance. They are similar as far as their metaphysical definition is concerned; i.e. both *eidos* and Idea can only be understood through the psyche with extrasensory principles of substances. However, the Ideas exist apart from substances, while *eidos* was thought by Aristotle to exist within substances. This is an ontology characteristic of Aristotle, who introduced the empirical method to biology (anatomic investigation and observation).

According to Aristotle, a substance is an integration of *eidos* and matter. Pure *eidos* is God. Pure matter is *arché*. Substances are in between them. They are controlled by *eidos* and vary both in quality and in quantity. The world is understood in terms of teleology. Substances (inorganic substances, plants and animals) are always aiming for a higher *eidos*. In other words, every *eidos* is part of a single hierarchy with god at its apex. This was the structure of the universe for Aristotle. He took over the theory of four-fold *arché* (primary matter), which was the mainstream of Greek thought. He thought of four new causes to explain the generation and extinction of substances. They were *hylé* (material cause), *eidos* (formal cause), *arché* (efficient cause) and *telos* (final cause). His system was a criticism and modification of his teacher Plato's theory of Ideas. Aristotle thought that the Ideas of Plato stood apart from substances, and could not explain the movements occurring in the natural world. It was a criticism generated by his understanding of the actual world as a biologist.

God, which is the "the unmoving mover," exists at the end of the chain of final causes. According to Aristotle, nature, including humans, living organisms and

Chapter III : *Greek Culture and Its Significance for the Later Development of Science and Ethics* 57

inorganic matter, is ordered in a hierarchy suited to the accomplishing of an end. God makes this possible. Aristotle concentrated on biology, because he wanted to prove that there is a divinity (order and beauty) hidden behind nature; he also wanted to investigate the beautiful structure of the world. Its beauty indicated that all of nature is disposed of and created in a manner suitable to the accomplishing of an end.

Aristotle gave greater importance to empirical biology than Plato. Aristotle had a strong motivation to prove the actual workings of teleology. At that time, astronomy depended largely on mathematical speculation because people had no telescopes. Therefore, Plato, who thought the earth revolves around other celestial bodies, was ahead of Aristotle in this regard.

The huge system of biology that Aristotle created as a result of his experimental studies is still astounding today. Everybody feels that he was a person of multiple attainments unequalled in history, including our current age.

For example, the anatomical knowledge of human internal organs (such as the heart, blood vessels, lungs, liver, kidneys and bladder) is presented in *Historia Animalium*. The observed that animals belong to various species, such as seals, elephants, pumas, camels, horses, cattle, deer, goats, dogs, cats, boars and pigs. In his observations he distinguished between soliped and cloven-hoofed animals, as well as types of teeth.

His accomplishments include developmental and embryological studies on cuttlefish, urchins, actinians, crevettes and fish, as well as studies on birds, insects, the sexual behavior of dolphins, fish parasites, swine and bovine diseases, and human and animal birth. He was a physiologist as well as a biologist, covering a wide range of fields. The metaphysics of Aristotle was established on this empirical biology. He was significantly ahead of his teacher, Plato, in this respect. Specifically, he maintained an astounding consistency between his theories and the actual world. Aristotle developed a system of logic and ethics as a philosopher who enjoyed speculation and showed an obsessive interest in all phenomena of the actual world.

Aristotle was also different from Plato in his evaluations of poems and poets.

For Aristotle, poems are associated with creation (*poiesis*) which reverberates into the future. A poet is different from a historian, because a poet is not only a person who describes facts, but also a person who exhibits an insight into the future while he describes these facts. That is, a poet can become engaged in the world of Ideas. Conversely, Plato thought that a human (soul) can recall the world of Ideas, but he can never reach it, and that adoration of the world of Ideas is the urge to philosophize.

Aristotle's thoughts on ethics are expressed in his *Nicomachean Ethics*. The central issue in this work is the nature of virtue, or what the good is, something that had also preoccupied Plato. According to Aristotle, there are two kinds of virtues, intellectual and moral. The former group consists of *techné* (art, technical expertise), *epistemé* (systematic knowledge), *phronesis* (practical wisdom), which is required for practical reasoning and experience, *sophia* (wisdom), and *nous* (intelligence), which has the greatest affinity to the divine; the latter group of virtues includes many familiar attitudes of the mind, such as courage, courtesy, truthfulness, friendship and justice. The five intellectual virtues are transmitted through teaching and training, while the moral virtues are acquired through habit or in an *ethos*. Performing just acts habitually renders a person just, and so forth for other moral virtues. *Phronesis*, for which Aristotle is famous, plays a central role as the decisive factor in moral behavior or action, as shown in his wider discussion on moral virtues. Aristotle was epoch-making and is still influential now, in showing that virtue is a state of the soul and the means to the good and truth. The principle underlying each moral virtue is moderation, i.e. neither excess nor deficiency, and is called the Golden Mean. However, the happiness obtained as a result of the practice of moral or practical virtues alone is limited, and only with the aid of intellectual virtues, including intelligence, can we attain the highest kind of happiness.

Thus, teleological physics originates from Aristotle, who was a great intellectual and biologist, and excelled in all fields of inquiry existing at that time, such as metaphysics, ethics, logic, politics and physics. He has dominated physics for the past 2000 years with his strong powers of persuasion.

3. The Medicine of Hippocrates
Hippocrates (460-370 B.C.)

The *Corpus Hippocraticum* was edited by the pupils of Hippocrates, "the great doctor." In it we can access the huge record of his scientific observations.

Hippocrates lived during the same age as Democritus (atomist) and Socrates (idealist). He himself was never a speculative philosopher; he seems to have disliked philosophical speculation.

His work suggests that he rejected the philosophical speculations and technical terms that were popular at the time. Hippocrates was a natural and medical scientist because he observed phenomena comprehensively and formed his deductions based on his records. His objective descriptions of diseases are correct, and some are valid enough even today (epidemic parotitis, convulsions, tuberculosis).

However, this was the Greek era, and no experimental validations were performed. Hippocrates borrowed the essential parts of other theories about diseases as they were. It is therefore unavoidable that his own theories were limited.

He explained diseases by means of a theory of the four bodily humors (blood, phlegm, yellow bile and black bile); this theory is a reflection of Empedocles' theory of the four elements.

He believed that disease occurs when the four bodily humors are unbalanced. Hippocrates also used the phrase "natural healing power."

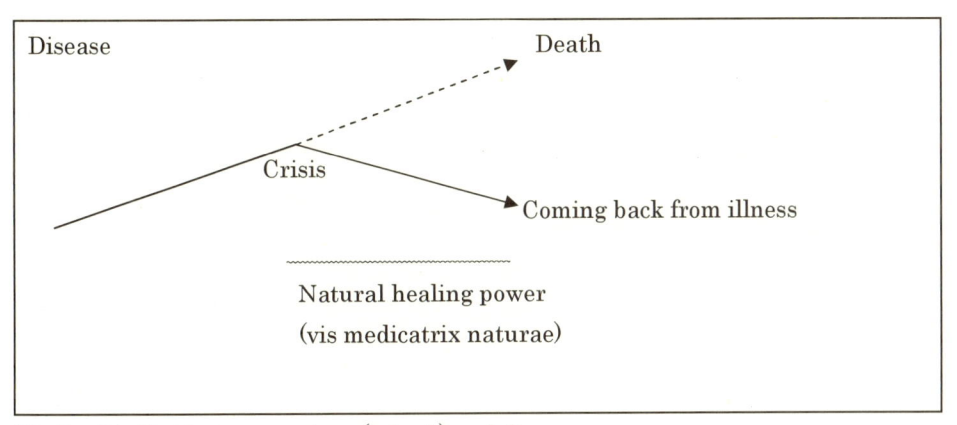

Fig.7   Conflict between nature (*physis*) and disease

A disease emerges from the natural state as a result of a derangement. However, we have the power to return to the natural state, as shown in the figure.

The task of the physician is to help the natural healing power to eliminate the disease by prescribing an appropriate diet and lifestyle to the patient. Fever, general malaise and other symptoms are simply responses of the sick organism fighting off invading stimuli. If these symptoms are overcome before crisis erupts, the disease is self-limiting. In this case, nature (*physis*) means "what exists originally," as used in the English idiom "by nature." The original (natural) state is health. The figure shows how a patient recovers from a disease with the help of natural healing power. The diverging point of outcome in the course of a disease is called a "crisis" (critical period).

In accordance with the theory of the four bodily humors, physicians gave laxatives and diuretics, and performed phlebotomies to control the bodily humors.

Of course, Hippocrates' theory of medicine was rather scanty. However, he excelled at the scientific observation of symptoms and pathology, and at constructing an empirical medicine based on it. In other words, he excelled at making prognoses and prescribing therapies by making rational inductions from his rich experience of disease.

Hippocrates was a prominent scientist. For example, he made it clear that epilepsy (called the "Sacred Disease" at the time) is caused by a brain disorder and that the intellect is generated by the brain and not by the heart or any other organs that were thought to be the source of the intellect.

It is thus with regard to the disease called Sacred: It appears to me to be neither more divine nor more sacred than other diseases, but **has a natural cause** from the same origins as other affections. Men regard its nature and cause as divine out of ignorance and wonder, because it is not at all like to other diseases.
(*On the Sacred Disease*, Section 1, in *Hippocrates: On Ancient Medicine*, translated into Japanese by Masanori Ogawa, Iwanami Bunko)

But **this disease seems to me to be no more divine than others**; but it has its nature such as other diseases have, and a cause whence it originates...
(ibid., *On the Sacred Disease*, Section 5)

But **the brain is the cause of this affection**, as it is of other very great diseases, and in what manner and from what cause it is formed, I will now plainly declare. The brain of man, as in all other animals, is double, and a thin membrane divides it through the middle, and therefore the pain is not always in the same part of the head; for sometimes it is situated on either side, and sometimes the whole is affected; and veins run toward it from all parts of the body, many of which are small, but two are thick, one from the liver, and the other from the spleen. And it is thus with regard to the one from the liver: a portion of it runs downward through the body on the side, near the kidneys and the psoas muscles, to the inner part of the thigh, and extends to the foot. It is called the vena cava. The other runs upward by the right veins and the lungs, and divides into branches for the heart and the right arm. The remaining part rises upward across the clavicle to the right side of the neck, and is superficial so as to be seen.
(ibid., *On the Sacred Disease*, Section 6)

Whoever having undertaken to speak or write on Medicine, have first laid down for themselves some hypothesis to their argument, such as hot, or cold, or moist, or dry, or whatever else they choose (thus reducing their subject within a narrow compass, and supposing only one or two original causes of diseases or of death among mankind), are all clearly mistaken in much that they say; and this is the more reprehensible as relating to an art which all men avail themselves of on the most important occasions, and the good operators and practitioners which they hold in especial honor. For there are practitioners, some bad and some far otherwise, which, if there had been no such thing as Medicine, and if nothing had been investigated or found out in it, would not have been the case, but all would have been equally unskilled and ignorant of it, and everything concerning the sick would have been directed by chance. (ibid., *On Ancient Medicine*, Section 1)

This story is not appropriate for people who are accustomed to hearing of naturalness of human bodies exceeding the extent of medicine. That is because **I never say humans are air. I never say humans consist of fire, water, earth or other substances that apparently do not exist in human bodies.** Let them say, however, I think the people saying that are wrong because they have different stories though they use the same concept. They have a single preposition in the concept (they say a substance consists of a single element. The part and the whole are made of air). However the names are different. People say the part and the whole are made of air, fire, water or earth. Each person shows useless evidences. **They use the same concept. However, their assertions are different. It shows their knowledge is wrong.**
(ibid., *On the Nature of Man*, Section 1)

The whole constitution of the season being thus inclined to the southerly, and with droughts early in the spring, from the preceding opposite and northerly state, ardent fevers occurred in a few instances, and these very mild, being rarely attended with hemorrhage, and never proving fatal. **Swellings appeared about the ears, in many on either side, and in the greatest number on both sides, being unaccompanied by fever so as not to confine the patient to bed; in all cases they disappeared without giving trouble, neither did any of them come to suppuration, as is common in swellings from other causes. They were of a lax, large, diffused character, without inflammation or pain, and they went away without any critical sign.**

They seized children, adults, and mostly those who were engaged in the exercises of the palaestra and gymnasium, but seldom attacked women. Many had dry coughs without expectoration, and accompanied with hoarseness of voice. **In some instances earlier, and in others later, inflammations with pain seized sometimes one of the testicles, and sometimes both; some of these cases were accompanied with fever and some not; the greater part of these were attended with much suffering. In other respects they were free of disease, so as not to require medical assistance.**
(ibid., *Of the Epidemics*, Section 1)

Hippocrates was born on Cos, a small island in Ionia located to the south of Samos, where Pythagoras was born. Among the ancient Greeks, the worship of Asclepius, the god of medicine, for healing was prevalent. In those days, the healing procedures at the temple of Asclepius consisted of fasting, a ritual bath, prayer, seeing a play, and dreaming in the *adyton*. The temple usually extended over a large area, housing a theater, a stadium and a gymnasium, and was supplied with abundant running water for baths and treatments as well as religious activities. The principal temples of Asclepius were widely distributed in Epidaurus, Cos, Cnidus, North Africa, and later Pergamum in Asia Minor and on the acropolis in Athens. The Asclepiads, who were said to be the descendants of Asclepius, were originally priests at the temple of Asclepius and naturally had a great opportunity to learn from the sick. Hippocrates was also a priest of the Asclepius temple on Cos, but, instead of concentrating on magic and philosophy, he directed all of his attention to the observation of patients and described the course of diseases in scientific ways. There was a medical school on Cos, and Hippocrates and his disciples were so prominent as physicians throughout the Greek world, including Athens, that Plato and Aristotle quoted him in their writings. The Oath of Hippocrates given below has been used as the ethical standard of doctors in many medical academies until the middle of the 20th century. In the latter half of the 20th century, a concept of medical ethics which gave the patients a great deal of autonomy came to the forefront. As a result, Hippocratic paternalism does not have a large influence today. However, some Hippocratic concepts are still relevant, including, for example, the duty of confidentiality, not administering lethal chemicals, prioritizing the patients' welfare, and fairness. On Cos even today, at the vacant lot of the temple of Asclepius, priestesses in ancient Greek garb hold Oath ceremonies for tourists.

I swear by Apollo, the physician, by Aesculapius, Hygeia, Panacea, and all the gods and goddesses, that, according to my ability and judgment, I will keep this Oath and this stipulation — to reckon him who taught me this Art equally dear to me as my parents, to share my substance with him, and relieve his necessities if required; to look upon his offspring in the same footing as my own brothers, and to teach them this art, if they shall wish to learn it, without fee or stipulation; and that by precept, lecture, and every other mode of instruction, I will impart a knowledge of the art to my own sons, and those of my teachers, and to disciples bound by a stipulation and Oath according to the law of medicine, but to none others.

I will follow that system of regimen which, according to my ability and judgment, I consider for the benefit of my patients, and abstain from whatever is deleterious and mischievous.

I will give no deadly medicine to any one if asked, nor suggest any such counsel; and in like manner I will not give to a woman a pessary to produce abortion. With purity and with holiness I will pass my life and practice my art.

I will not cut persons labouring under the stone, but will leave this to be done by men who are practitioners of this work. Into whatever houses I enter, I will go into them for the benefit of the sick, and will abstain from every voluntary act of mischief and corruption; and, further, from the seduction of females or males, of freemen and slaves. Whatever, in connection with my professional service, or not in connection with it, I see or hear, in the life of men, which ought not to be spoken of abroad,

I will not divulge, as reckoning that all such should be kept secret. While I continue to keep this Oath unviolated, may it be granted to me to enjoy life and the practice of the art, respected by all men, in all times. But should I trespass and violate this Oath, may the reverse be my lot.

(ibid., *Oath of Hippocrates*)

4. Comparisons between Plato, Hippocrates and Aristotle

The figure shows the relationship between Plato, Hippocrates and Aristotle, whose lives partially overlapped in terms of chronology.

Plato was one of the figures most strongly affected by the Pythagorean school. He excelled at mathematical reasoning. He considered the world to be a beautiful ordered structure with the Ideas as the basic principle or deity. He used the method of deductive speculation. Plato had much to say on uranography (descriptive theory of the heavens). Uranography at the time was more mathematical speculation than physics. Plato, who was skilled at uranography, proposed that the circle and the globe are perfect shapes and therefore divine. As such, he already thought the earth is a globe which orbits other celestial bodies. Pythagoras was an excellent mathematician and religious charismatic, while Plato was ultimately a teleologist who put god above everything else. Aristotle was Plato's successor in this respect. Plato believed that the method of observing and recording observations, as the scientist Hippocrates had done, is merely useful in clarifying the sensory world or phenomena. Plato emphasized mathematical logic and applied deductive thinking, and so he felt that Hippocrates' description of the world, with its sketchy details, is, so to speak, ridiculous. It was markedly different from description of the psyche (idealistic world) that Plato was developing as his life's work. In fact, Plato described his view of physics chiefly in *Timaeus*, a late dialogue from his huge body of work. He mentioned Hippocrates very little in *Timaeus*; in fact, Hippocrates' name only appears as the name of a physician.

Meanwhile, Hippocrates rejected speculative philosophy. Hippocrates said that, in treatments for existing patients, he could use nothing from the theories of Pythagoras, Empedocles, and other forerunners, or Socrates and Plato, who developed theories of speculative philosophy with no roots in reality.

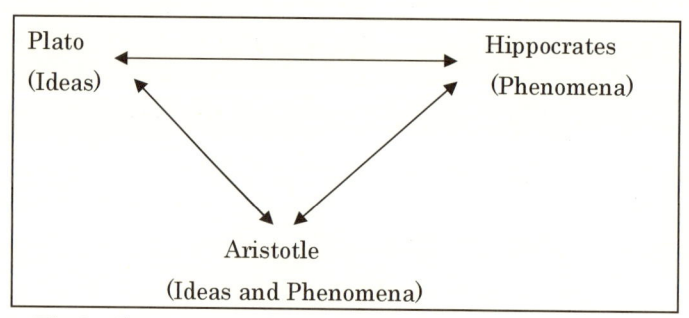

```
Plato                          Hippocrates
(Ideas)                        (Phenomena)

            Aristotle
       (Ideas and Phenomena)
```
Fig.8   Comparison of Plato, Hippocrates and Aristotle

Hippocrates emphasized the observation of individual patients. While this strategy did not necessarily improve the treatments, the patients were treated in a scientific manner because this was the most effective way to determine the prognosis of diseases. Aristotle adopted theories from both Plato and Hippocrates. He was a philosopher and the first systematic empirical biologist in the world. His biology covered a wide range of phenomena, including the embryology of eggs, comparative embryology and the anatomy of animals. We can see his theory in his *On the Generation of Animals*, *On the Parts of Animals* and *The History of Animals*. Plato wrote most of his works between the ages of 60 and 80, when he died. Aristotle died when he was 62. Despite that, Aristotle left a body of work comparable to or greater than that of Plato, chiefly because he was brought up in a favorable economical and educational environment, and plenty of books and materials were later supplied by his pupil, Alexander the Great.

Aristotle was born in 384 B.C. into a family of physicians in Stageira, a small city in the north of Greece. His father was the court physician of the King of Macedonia. His family had many documents and books, and employed many teachers. He spent his adolescence studying at Plato's Academy, the Academeia (Athenai), from the age of 17 to the age of 37. He left Athenai when Plato died in 347 B.C. He transferred his activities to Asia Minor and Macedonia in the north of Greece. In 342 B.C., he became the tutor of a 14-year old student who would later become "Alexander the Great." He stayed in Macedonia until 335 B.C. In 336 B.C., Alexander the Great ascended to the throne and began to govern Greece. At that time, Aristotle returned to Athenai again and ushered in the golden age of Greek enlightenment, which included philosophy and physics (the age of the Lykeion). "Lykeion" was the name of a place, but it also denoted the school where Aristotle educated his disciples in rivalry with the Academeia of Plato. Disciples who gathered at the Lykeion were called "Peripatetics," because they applied their minds to speculation while walking around the cloister of the school. Aristotle's most fruitful years were spent mainly at his school, the Lykeion; this period lasted for 12 years, until the fall of Alexander the Great (reign: 335-323 B.C.). All human endeavors, such as biology, physics, ethics, philosophy, logic, politics, theology, and poetics, were investigated and integrated into one system by this one person named Aristotle. This was the first such unification. Plato and Hippocrates left massive bodies of work that could be said to be revolutionary in Greek history, yet Aristotle was greater because he completed a great and improved system of physics and metaphysics.

5. Hellenistic Rome

The Hellenistic era lasted from 336 B.C. (the coronation of Alexander the Great) to 30 B.C. Culturally, it was a fusion of Greek and Eastern culture. It was an era when the Greek culture centered in Alexandria expanded into other regions of the world.

Herophilus (335-280 B.C.)
Herophilus was a great believer in Hippocrates; he lived in Alexandria and was a grandson of Aristotle. He founded the Alexandrian school with Erasistratus (mentioned below) and developed the world's most advanced physiology at that time.

He dissected many human bodies and made many anatomical discoveries. For example, he was able to differentiate between the veins and the arteries, and attributed the pulsation of arteries to the beating of the heart. He also differentiated nerves from blood vessels and showed that a cut nerve causes paralysis. He was the first to distinguish the cerebrum from the cerebellum, and believed the brain to be the center of the nervous system and the source of the intellect. He agreed with Hippocrates in this, and disagreed with Aristotle, who considered the heart to be the source of intellect. In addition, he showed the locations of the stomach and the intestines in the abdomen and named the "duodenum." The duodenum is the part of the intestinal tract immediately following the stomach. It was so named because its length is equal to the width of twelve fingers placed side by side.

He was also an empirical clinician, a second Hippocrates. He made objective observations of patients and diseases, as Hippocrates had done. He treated patients based on his experiences, not speculation. Herophilus adopted the attitude of Hippocrates, but he was even greater than Hippocrates because of his anatomical achievements. He is known to the contemporary world as the person who founded pathological anatomy.

Erasistratus (310-250 B.C.)

Erasistratus was also active in Alexandria. He established a system of physiology, which includes the differentiation between the cerebrum and cerebellum, the anatomy of the brain, the differentiation between sensory nerves and motor nerves, and the recognition of sensation by the brain. He showed correctly that the arteries emanate from the heart. However, he thought that *pneuma* (vital spirit) circulates around the body. His concept was that the *pneuma* in the body originates from the *pneuma* pervading the universe. His anatomy of the heart was so correct that even the tricuspid valve is mentioned.

Galen (131-201 A.D.)

Galen (Galenus in Latin) was an enthusiastic admirer of Hippocrates and greatly influenced medieval medicine. He was born in Pergamum in Asia Minor. Galen was a physician who lived about 600 years after Hippocrates.

Pergamum is a famous city where the magnificent temple of Aesculapius was built; the temple still stands today.

Historically, Galen took over the philosophical thoughts of Plato and Aristotle. Medically, he was a successor of Hippocrates. He modified the systems of his Greek predecessors very little, and tended to adopt their systems as he found them. We can say that Galen himself had no extraordinary achievements of his own; he adopted Greek knowledge. Yet, he infused teleology into those Greek theories. Because of this, he was thought to be an authority on medicine in medieval times, despite the many errors of his medical theories.

He is credited as having written commentaries on the complete works of Hippocrates, thus popularizing the medicine of Hippocrates and handing it down to the present generations. However, Galen also passed down the errors of his predecessors uncritically. For example, he perpetuated the four-humor theory, and so he did not advance beyond Plato or Hippocrates. His interpretation of nature was teleonomic because he was also considerably influenced by Aristotle. Like Aristotle, Galen committed the error of believing that the heart is the source of intellect. He thought that the basic principle of life is *pneuma*, as Erasistratus had done. He also confronted and criticized Erasistratus in his interpretation of *pneuma*. This shows that pneumatism was a widely accepted theory after the time of Erasistratus, deeply penetrating the world of thought. Thus, Galen was a great intellectual and literary person who borrowed and spread the achievements of his predecessors.

The number of existing works by Galen is larger than that by any other scholar of his age. Therefore, his profound effect throughout the Middle Ages is understandable. Some of Galen' works were passed down to posterity, as shown below.

1) Experimental physiology based on anatomy

Human dissections were prohibited at the time. Galen built his experimental physiology using mainly monkeys. As a result, he found that the pulse is generated by the contractions of the heart, and that the arteries are filled with blood, not with *pneuma* as Erasistratos had claimed. He demonstrated these facts empirically.

2) Experiments on cutting nerves

He showed that aphonia (gruff voice) can be induced by cutting the recurrent laryngeal nerve. He also revealed the relationship between the location of a cut and the resulting paralysis in experiments involving the cutting of the spinal marrow.

His theory of teleological biology was in agreement with the theology that governed the Middle Ages. It spread not only to Christian countries, but also to Islamic countries (Arabic countries). When we closely examine his theory, we find many errors. However, he had an enormous effect on the Middle Ages as the successor to the great Hippocrates. Therefore, we can say that his contribution to human knowledge had both drawbacks and advantages.

Metaphysics and theology based on teleology prospered in the Middle Ages. If the Greek era and the Middle Ages are understood in succession, we see that, while physics (materialism, causation and mechanistic theory) and metaphysics (idealism, the science of religion, philosophy and ethics) appeared at the same time in ancient Greece, physics declined while metaphysics prospered, due to the strong impact of theology; in the Middle Ages, even "unscientific science" did well, such as astrology and alchemy.

6. The lessons of Greek culture

Greek culture is characterized by the simple and generous confidence in human wisdom. This wisdom surpassed the mythical religions and animism that tended to be recognized by other civilizations.

There was as yet no monotheistic god in the Greek era. The Greeks worshipped specifically Greek pagan gods. Therefore, there were none of the rigid commandments typical of monotheistic religions. There was a religious community, such as the Orphic one. However, it was at best a kind of society.

The ancient Greeks were lively seekers of *arché*, the unifying principle of physics. Their interest in this principle was more ardent than their concern for religion. They spontaneously asked questions such as "What is *arché*?" or "Why is *arché*?" and looked to nature for the answers. This is why natural sciences based on mechanicism, causality and mathematics were developed.

A characteristic of Western wisdom is that such a free "flight of wisdom" was possible. This is the radical difference between the Western and Eastern wisdom.

East Asian people are in the grip of religions such as Shinto, Buddhism, Confucianism, Taoism, Brahmanism and Hinduism. On an individual basis, the scientific mentality and its results have flourished; however, they have never stepped beyond religion and the circle of the collective or contemporary ethos.

In other words, East Asian people do not like analysis and are likely to maintain ambiguous totalities (called "conformity" from the moral standpoint). Western people are likely to analyze, simplify and reduce data to their essence. That is the greatest difference between Eastern and Western wisdom. The difference can be broadly called a bipolar confrontation, although this might be too simple a comparison.

We cannot say which kind of wisdom is better. Instead, we recognize that the two are indispensable to each other, when reflecting on the present and the past of mankind. Our objective is that East Asian and Western people should help each other and use their collective wisdom to benefit all human beings on this planet in the 21st century.

References

1) James S. Elliott: Outlines of Greek and Roman Medicine. John Bale, Sons & Danielson, Ltd., London, 1914
2) Henry O. Taylor: Greek Biology and Medicine. Marshall Jones Company, Boston, 1922
3) W. Windelband; translated into Japanese by Takashi Ide and Michitaro Tanaka: Plato. Omura Shoten, Tokyo, 1924
4) Arthur J. Brock: Greek Medicne. J.M. Dent & Sons, London, 1929
5) A. Cornelius Benjamin: An Introduction to the Philosophy of Science. The Macmillan Company, New York, 1937
6) Francis Adams: The Genuine Works of Hippocrates. Baillierere, Tindall & Cox, London, 1939

7) William Arthur Heidel: Hippocratic Medicine. Columbia University Press, New York, 1941
8) Seiichi Hatano: Seiyo Shukyo Shisoshi, Greece 1. Iwanami Shoten, Tokyo, 1942
9) Benjamin L. Gordon: Medicine throughout Antiquity. F. A. Davis Company, Philadelphia, 1949
10) J. Burnett; translated into Japanese by Takashi Ide and K. Miyazaki: The Philosophy of Plato. Iwanami Shoten, Tokyo, 1952
11) George Sarton: A History of Science Vol.1. The Norton Library, New York, 1952
12) Michitaro Tanaka: Socrates. Iwanami Shoten, Tokyo, 1957
13) G. S. Kirk, J. E. Raven, M. Scofield: The Presocratic Philosophers 2nd Edition, Cambridge University Press, New York, 1957
14) W. K. C. Guthrie: A History of Greek Philosophy Vol. 3. Cambridge University Press, New York, 1957
15) Hippocrates; translated into Japanese by M. Ogawa: On Ancient Medicine. Iwanami Shoten, Tokyo, 1963
16) S. W. Dampier: A History of Science. Cambridge University Press, New York, 1969
17) D. O'Brien: Empedcles' Cosmic Cycle. Cambridge University Press, New York, 1969
18) G. Sarton: A History of Science Vols 1& 2. The Norton Library, 1970
19) W. K. C. Guthrie: Socrates. Cambridge University Press, New York, 1971
20) Owsei Temkin: Galenism - Rise and Decline of a Medical Philosophy -. Cornell University Press, London, 1973
21) A. J. Bronto: Greek Medicine. J.M. Dent & Sons, New York, 1977
22) C. E. Millerd: On the Interpretation of Empedcles. Garland, 1980
23) M. R. Wright: Empedcles The Extant Fragments. Yale University Press, New Haven, 1981
24) Michitaro Tanaka: Platon II, Tetsugaku (1). Iwanami Shoten, Tokyo, 1981
25) Frederick Sargent II: Hippocratic Heritage - A History of Ideas about Weather and Human Health -. Pergamon Press, New York, 1982
26) Michitaro Tanaka: Kodaitetsugakushi (History of Ancient Philosophy), Tsikuma Shobo, Tokyo, 1985
27) Michael Frede: Essays in Ancient Philosophy. University of Minnesota Press, Mineapolis, 1987
28) Galenus; translated by Kyoko Taneyama: The Function of Nature. Kyoto University Press, Kyoto, 1988
29) H. Diels, W. Kranz: Die Fragmente der Vorsokuratiker II. Weidmann, Zurich, 1989
30) Mirko D. Grmek; translated by Mireille Muellner and Leonard Muellner: Diseases

in the Ancient Greek World. The Johns Hopkins University Press, Baltimore, 1989
31) Friedo Ricken: Philosophy of the Ancients. University of Notre Dame Press, London, 1991
32) R. S. Bluck; translated into Japanese by Katsutoshi Utsiyama: Plato's Life and Thought. Iwanami Shoten, Tokyo, 1992
33) Julius Moravcsik: Plato and Platonism − Plato's Conception of Appearance and Reality in Ontology, Epistemology, and Ethics, and its Modern Echoes −. Blackwell, Oxford, 1992
34) Aristoteles; translated by Jinsuke Matsumoto and Michio Oka: Poetics. Iwanami Shoten, Tokyo, 1997
35) Aristoteles; translated into Japanese by Saburo Shimazaki: The History of Animals (1). Iwanami Shoten, Tokyo, 1998
36) Aristoteles; translated into Japanese by Saburo Shimazaki: The History of Animals (2). Iwanami Shoten, Tokyo, 1999
37) Aristoteles; translated into Japanese by K. Boku: Nichomachean Ethics. Kyoto University Press, Kyoto, 2002

Chapter IV: *Japanese Religion*

All cultures in the world have some religion at their core.

Religion, as it is mentioned here, is taken in a broad sense and ranges from historically well-developed religions possessing systematized dogmas or holy scriptures that still continue to have a profound effect on modern times (i.e. China-centered religions, Buddhism, Christianity and Islam) to primitive forms of religion which express themselves simply in prayer to a wide range of physical objects and phenomena. A commonly observed feature of these religions could be said to be the inherent "religious feelings" or the devotion of human beings as actual existences directed toward supernatural or transcendental existences in the phenomenal world. Indeed, human beings have not been able to live without such religious feelings since the beginning of time, and this is true of modern people as well.

Aristotle in ancient Greece defined human beings as "reasoning animals." After that, the definition changed to "social animals," "tool-using animals," etc., depending on the viewpoint taken, although some of these definitions do not conform to current findings. Metaphysically speaking, human beings are the most clearly different from other animal species in that only humans have "religious feelings," which reveal themselves in daily human attitudes and actions. Although animals other than humans can also use tools and organize societies, no animal other than humans can experience "religious feelings." In fact, the feeling of religious awe is exclusively seen in humans.

For what do humans experience religious feelings, then?

For instance, in Mahayana Buddhism, which was founded in India by the Buddha, or Shakyamuni (566-486 B.C.), and transmitted to China and Japan as well as through Christianity, the object of faith is quite apparent. On the other hand, the target of Chinese classical thought or religions (the doctrine of Yin-Yang and the Five Elements, Taoism, Confucianism) has generally been Heaven (天). Heaven in ancient China was thought of as a humanized divinity, as seen in the Yin (殷) dynasty (16th-11th century B.C.) and its successor, the Chou (周) dynasty (1066-256 B.C.). Later, in the era of two great minds, Confucius (孔子, 552-479 B.C.) and Lao Tzu (老子, 604-517 B.C.), Heaven became an impersonal deity, i.e. a more fundamental, almighty and absolute entity.

Viewed broadly, Chinese society has been mentally and thus politically controlled by the Confucianism established by Confucius and Mencius (孟子, 372-289 B.C.). Confucianism could be described as a system of morality or thought which stresses the importance of the form of things and the law. The antithesis of Confucianism is Taoism, as developed by Lao Tzu and Chuang-tzu. It is a philosophical stance which emphasizes noninterference, simplicity, naturalness and the lack of intension as means to the attainment of the virtual happiness connected to Tao or the Way. Both of these great thought systems were generated very early in Chinese history, and they affected each other dynamically. Subsequently, Buddhism was imported from India into China during the 1st century B.C. and prospered there even as Confucianism and Taoism continued to flourish. Buddhism rose to the top during the Tang period in China, while Confucianism was reactivated during the Sung dynasty by Chu Hsi (1130-1200) in the form of Neo-Confucianism, a current which supplemented the weak points of the original Confucianism by borrowing metaphysical ideas from Taoism and Buddhism. It could be said that the belief system in China evolved soundly through mild and deep syncretism among these three religions. Historically speaking, Japan, ever since its foundation, has been affected significantly by Chinese culture and civilization. It is therefore natural that Japan was profoundly influenced by Buddhism, which was transmitted by way of China, and by original Chinese worldviews such as Confucianism and Taoism as well as the doctrine of Yin-Yang and the Five Elements.

For example, the Tokugawa government in the Edo period (1600-1867) exclusively adopted as the state religion the Chu Hsi school of Confucianism which was remodeled as Neo-Confucianism, thereby building the foundation of the Japanese feudal system. Actually, the Japanese government established after the Meiji Restoration enforced the basic virtues of Confucianism, such as politeness, devotion, loyalty and benevolence toward people, in association with Shinto (the classical Japanese religion), up to the end of World War II. Other virtues of Confucianism include justice, wisdom and faith. There are still many Japanese people whose given names include *kanji* (Chinese characters) which signify the virtues emphasized by Confucius; this is ample proof that Confucianism has had a substantial effect on the foundations of Japanese society.

Japanese people today ordinarily use idioms constituted from the word "heaven" (天 in Chinese and pronounced *ten* in Japanese). These include *ten-mei*, meaning "mandate from heaven," *ten-batsu*, meaning "punishment from heaven," *ten-pu*, meaning "gift from heaven," *ten-sai*, meaning "heaven-given talent," another *ten-sai* with a different Chinese character for *sai*, meaning "catastrophe sent from heaven," and so on. These expressions have become ordinary phrases in everyday life in Japan and have thus been deeply woven into the culture of the present Japanese people. In Confucianism, Heaven is the generator and principle of all things. Lao Tzu and Chuang-tzu, the main developers of Taoism, insisted on abandoning artifice in order to be oneself and rejected legislation because, if human beings abide by laws, they cannot perform what Heaven intends for them naturally in the form of *ten-i* (the will or mind of Heaven). This emphasis on naturalness and freedom has profoundly aroused the sympathy of modern people, and, accordingly, Taoism has currently gained a high popularity worldwide.

We could point out that Heaven, or 天 in ancient China, was personified and was thought to possess a powerful will to generate every event or phenomenon in the universe. The only thing humans could do was to contemplate and appreciate the will of Heaven in a refined state of mind. This philosophical concept appeared very early in the history of China, earlier than the rise of Taoism and Confucianism, and can be dated back to the Yin period (16th-11th century B.C.).

Religion is the most important factor characterizing a society, race or nation in terms of its ethnicity.

For example, the two major religions that have governed the religious feelings of the Chinese are Taoism and Confucianism, as described above, both of which characteristically affirm this world as it is, or the actual life of people. Neither of them preaches belief in the afterlife. It is true that Taoists believe in the power of mountain hermits; however, this is not at all equivalent to the salvation of the mind freed from the physical body, as typically seen in the Buddhism so deeply ingrained in Japanese culture. The good of Confucianism includes ancestor worship, family prosperity, giving birth to boys, keeping the family intact, building a reputation in order to reward one's parents, and so on.

When we look at the popularity of various religions among the Chinese people, it seems Taoism has gained more acceptance than Confucianism, presumably because the secularized form of Taoism is easier to understand and its tasks are easier to perform. The enjoyment of the actual life in its natural form, for instance, long life, sexual intercourse, etc., was looked upon with approval in Taoism. This led people to try to unveil the secrets of perennial youth and long life; by becoming mountain hermits themselves, they would cultivate longevity and also try to salvage their fathers, mothers and ancestors. Lao Tzu, who formulated the doctrine of Taoism, rejected Confucian ethics and artificiality. Basically, Taoists leave everything to nature without straining themselves. Concerning this, there is a similarity between Taoism and Zen Buddhism, which is self-reliant in its practice of attaining Buddhahood. In general, Taoism engendered the natural or continental generosity characteristic of the Chinese people.

However, in Japan, which is situated near China but is separated from the Chinese continent by a sea, it was Buddhism and not Chinese thought that has flourished. As a matter of fact, esoteric Buddhism disappeared in China and prospered in Japan in the form of Shingon Buddhism, founded by Kukai (774-835), who brought Chinese esoteric Buddhism to Japan in 806. Several creative forms of Japanese Buddhism evolved in the Kamakura era. Two sects of Zen Buddhism, Rinzai and Soto, were among them. Zen (Ch'an) was first transmitted to Japan in the latter part of the 12th century from the Southern Sung. Zen, as a rather new sect of Buddhism, was eagerly accepted by the *samurai (bushi)*, or warrior class, which was newly rising in Kamakura during the latter part of the Heian era in Japan and politically replacing the aristocratic government of Kyoto. Zen appealed to the new class because of the strictness and self-dependency of thought and practice. Since then, Zen has continuously grown in the mind of the Japanese throughout its long history until now, to occupy the core of contemporary Japanese culture in the form of the tea ceremony, traditional flower arrangement, short verses like *waka* and *haiku*, the concepts of *wabi* and *sabi*, *teien* (Japanese garden), *bushido*, meditative philosophy, and so on.

The Japanese national character (thoughts, behaviors, conception about the afterlife, and other cultural elements as a whole) observed now is the result of the integration of a specific climate (island country, temperate monsoon climate, remote region in the Far East, etc.), a specific history (spanning about 3,000 years, beginning with the Jomon and Yayoi periods and reaching down to the present age) and a specific religious ethos, all of which have interacted and gradually yielded what we recognize to be the Japanese identity.

In the international homogenization process called "globalization," the national character of the Japanese is now being called into question. The Japanese identity cultivated for so long has been on trial at the contact points with foreign or incompatible cultures. Today, Japanese people are being forced to change their ways and attitudes more than ever. After World War II, the entire nation experienced a feeling of deep despondency and a terrible sense of emptiness when they lost their spiritual support and the prevalent "communal common sense," which was derived from a blend of Shinto, Confucianism, Taoism and Buddhism. People still feel apprehensive and uneasy, as if a baby has been sent out into the world unprotected. It is a matter of deep concern and anxiety whether to let the transformation proceed freely and naturally, as in the liberal individualism which has been introduced after the World War II, or to reconstruct our specific configuration in which all history, religion, culture, and of course present status within the global reality are reflected, and, most importantly, of which we are conscious and proud in everyday life.

At this time, it is very important for us Japanese to look back into the past at

Japanese religion and develop a proper understanding of the historical facts related to that religion in order to grasp rightly the characteristics of the Japanese as historical beings, which would enable us to make a correct personal decision regarding the future. The religious ethos which evolved in Japan, an island country, is outlined below against the background of its history. New religions, such as Christianity, that were imported in the modern age will not be mentioned here.

1. The syncretization of religions

The main characteristic of Japanese religion is that it is a comparatively peaceful mixture ("syncretization") of transmitted religions and Shinto, which is the indigenous belief system originating from the Jomon period (10th-4th century B.C.).

Buddhism was the largest foreign religion to enter into the mix. Buddhism had a sophisticated philosophical logic, a robust religious system and vastness, and generated a large number of cultural elements in Japan. Buddhism was developed in India. It was brought to China around the time of the birth of Jesus, and gradually became syncretized with Chinese thoughts (Confucianism and Taoism), after which it was imported to Japan in the 6th century. In other words, Buddhism already included Chinese elements when it was brought to Japan.

In Japan, a synthesis of Shinto and Buddhism took place. In many cases, Buddhism, an advanced religion at that time, induced in native Shinto a gradual transformation. In China, Confucianism and Taoism accepted Buddhism, a foreign religion, with a similar mildness. This may be a characteristic common to all Asian religions, or it may be the result of the mellowness of Buddhism itself, which advocates mercy. Buddhism itself underwent the same experience in the 6th century B.C. Buddhism had its roots in the Vedas, Brahmanism and the belief in ancient Hindu gods, which were incorporated into Buddhism. For example, Cetaka (明王) became a guardian god of Buddhism; Brahman, a god of Brahmanism, became Brahma (梵天) in Buddhism. Similarly, Indra of Brahmanism became Sakra devanam Indra (帝釈天) in Buddhism. Sarasvati or Benzaiten (弁才天) was the wife of Brahma. It is also true that Shitenno (四天王), who are the guardian gods of Buddhism, can be traced back to Hindu gods. As such, Buddhism has always been tolerant and flexible within itself and with other religions. The indigenous religions that originally existed in Japan were generally primitive, as typically seen in earlier Shinto, or took the form of pantheistic animism. Under Shinto, people believed that spiritual beings manifesting themselves as gods, spirits and souls which cannot be reached through normal cognition, exist at the basis of nature (rocks, trees, waterfalls, grass, mountains, seas, etc.) and natural phenomena (the wind, clouds, rain, thunder and volcanic eruptions). The simple sense of awe and belief in the power of nature evolved into this primitive Shinto when agricultural communes and settlements were established in Japan (the Yayoi period, 300 B.C.-300 A.D.). People prayed during Shinto rites for good harvests and the safety and prosperity of their colonies. They also built sanctuaries. However, there was no doctrine in Shinto comparable to Buddhist or Chinese thought.

In the Kofun (tumulus) period (3rd-7th century A.D.) or the Asuka period (end of the 6th century-7th century) following the Yayoi period, the indigenous religion of Japan, or early Shinto, remained in this primitive state. The main feature of this primitive form of religion was to place a high value upon partnership between humans and nature. People found nature spiritually meaningful. Under these animistic circumstances, Taoism, Confucianism and Buddhism as well as their highly advanced cultural elements were imported from mainland China to Japan in the 5th, 6th and 7th centuries. The politics, economics and religion of Japan all developed under the strong influence of foreign cultures. People largely spent their time importing mainland cultural elements, and thus many Japanese official diplomatic delegations were sent to China during the Sui (隋) and Tang (唐) dynasties in the 6th and 7th centuries. The gap between Japanese culture and mainland culture at the time is estimated to be as large as, or more significant than, in the Meiji period when the Japanese government accepted the tide of Western-style modernization on a clean slate state after the Meiji Restoration. When we look back at this historic process, we see that the religious syncretism which occurred in Japan is significantly different from the hostile processes caused by the invasion of monotheistic religions such as Christianity and Islam. In other words, no religion suppresses or annihilates the others in Japan and the other countries of East Asia.

In this process, it deserves to be mentioned that Japan's indigenous Shinto peacefully accepted Buddhism in a manner specific to natural religions, and also that Buddhism as a newcomer has had the salient trait of benevolence ever since it was developed in India. In fact, until now Buddhism has always been tolerant of other cultures and religions. Of course, it is only natural that there were collisions and conflicts at the forefront where the heterogeneous cultures first encountered each other. However, I am saying that the conflicts as well as the reconciliations surrounding Buddhism have been relatively peaceful.

Such religious tolerance has sometimes appeared to be a distinctive ethnic trait of Japanese people thereafter, and thus seems to intrinsically control modern-day Japanese life. It is an ethnic trait that has been cultivated historically. It seems that this tolerance has allowed Japanese people to survive on small islands during their long history. Viewed in this light, such tolerance could be said to be a major characteristic of the Japanese people.

2. Shinto: the indigenous religion of Japan

In ancient, rice-growing Japan, people began to establish permanent colonies. The first indigenous religions went through various stages of animism and gradually evolved into Shinto. Generally, the deities of Shinto are called *kami*, or *kamigami* in the plural. Actually, Shinto (神道) means "the way (道) of *kami* (神)".

The profound appreciation of the harvest, the feeling of awe for nature (the water, the sun, the climate, the earth etc.), and the hope of safety and continuation of the colonies generated religious feelings. The indigenous religions of Japan characterized by nature worship and ancestor worship developed based on these religious feelings.

Many things in nature were worshipped, including mountains, rivers, lakes, water, waterfalls, seas, forests, rain, winds, thunder, the stars, the moon and the sun. People believed that there are supernatural beings or gods (souls or spirits called "*kami*" in Japanese) in them. Japanese indigenous religions had the following features: ① the harmonious coexistence of nature and humans, ② feelings of awe for nature, and ③ the concept of animism ("*anima*" means "psyche") expressed as a belief in many gods.

The original form of Shinto is referred to as primitive Shinto. In the Yayoi period, people started to plant rice and agricultural colonies were formed in many regions across Japan. People buried the dead close to their homes and the veneration of forefathers entered folklore. Primitive Shinto spontaneously developed in this way. At the beginning, people chiefly worshipped elemental gods, ancestral spirits and the village god (the god of a clan as a social unit), and led Shinto religious ceremonies at the *himorogi* (sanctuaries). There is always a sanctuary for this purpose in every colony discovered by archeologists. The concept of souls of the dead became fused with that of ancestral spirits and changed into the concept of *kami* over the years. People referred to the place where the spirits live as "another world." This place was in the mountains, in the sea or below the ground.

To lead a religious ceremony at a sanctuary meant to have a relationship with the gods, and living people were inspired by this communion. Living people cultivated a tight relationship with the gods through the ancestral spirits.

In Shinto, people believe that dead people change eventually into gods after passing through several unstable stages of the soul. Therefore, Gods (spirits) exist close to the living and watch over them. When a foreign religion, Buddhism, was imported to Japan, it fused with native Shinto in a process called "syncretization." In current Buddhism in

Japan, there is a habitual conception or faith that dead people become *hotoke* (*butsu*), or Buddha, as the ultimate state. This concept was not found in original Buddhism and may be due to the influence of Shinto, as some modification of Buddhism was naturally required when it came to Japan where Shinto prevailed. Also, the Shinto concept of "another world" was transformed easily into the Buddhist belief that a "Pure Land" exists in the West where Amitabha, or Amida, resides and can be reached through Buddhist memorial prayers for the deceased.

The Yamato dynasty (4th-7th century) was the first to rule a unified Japan, having authority over the local ruling families. Each local ruling family worshipped its own guardian god in a dedicated shrine. The major local ruling families included the Mononobe, Soga, Nakatomi, Ohtomo, etc. The Mononobe family governed all shrines, while the Ohtomo clan controlled the military system and the Soga clan supported Buddhism.

Buddhism was imported to Wa (the older name of Japan) in 538 during the reign of Emperor Kinmei, from Paekche(百済), a kingdom located in the southern part of the Korean Peninsula and ruled by King Seimeioh. On the Korean Peninsula at the time, Koguryo(高句麗)and Silla (新羅)were located to the north and east of Paekche, respectively. Buddhism was transmitted to Koguryo in 372 and to Paekche in 384. The three nations on the peninsula had a tense relationship with one another at that time. King Seimeioh died in battle in 554. Many people immigrated to Japan from the Korean Peninsula after Paekche became a ruin, bringing with them many advanced cultural elements, including Buddhism.

The great Soga family introduced and popularized Buddhism in Japan in a positive manner. However, there was serious antagonism at that time between the Soga family, which admired Buddhism, and the Mononobe family, which was conservative and had opposed the importation of Buddhism during its first 50 years in Japan. It was an inevitable conflict generated in a situation where a foreign advanced culture, Buddhism, was introduced into a less developed country (Japan, or Wa) which already had a native religion (Shinto).

The first full-scale Buddhist construction in Japan is believed to have been the Hoko-ji temple in Asuka (the Asuka-dera temple, erected in 596). Soga-no-Umako (Umako of the Soga family) constructed this temple in the Paekche style with the help of priests and carpenters brought from the mainland. It was originally a private temple (*uji-dera*) of the Soga clan, but it was transferred to Heijo-kyo (an old name of the capital Nara) to become the Gango-ji, an authorized temple, in 718. Taking this opportunity, individuals or clans from the continent scrambled, in a veritable boom, to build their own private temples as the Soga had done. Thus, people came to believe in Buddhism, which gradually expanded and became a constant part of their lives during the Nara period (710-794).

During the Yamato dynasty, the nation and the royal families of Japan were protected mainly by the official system of Shinto, which benefited from the powerful political support of the Mononobe clan (a protector of Shinto). However, after Buddhism was gradually brought to the center of politics, the Mononobe declined and the Soga began to prosper, as they were admirers of Buddhism. They began handling the diplomacy of the Imperial court by succession. As a result, Buddhism and its concepts of the Buddha, the *dharma* and the priesthood were transmitted from the clan to the Imperial court, and the belief in the Japanese gods (pagan gods), which had prevailed until then, began to decline.

Shinto is greatly indebted to Buddhism for the introduction of ideograms (Chinese characters, or *kanji*), as well as for the new construction technologies brought to Japan. Buddhist texts originally written in Pali or Sanskrit were translated into Chinese first, which caused Mahayana Buddhism to develop extensively because Chinese characters were highly evolved ideograms capable of transmitting the complex philosophy implied by the Mahayana *sutras*. Thus, Chinese characters were effective in putting the doctrines and holy scriptures of Buddhism into broad circulation among the peoples of Asia. Indeed, as a means of communication, Chinese characters at that time are comparable to today's IT.

Empress Suiko (592-628), who inaugurated the Asuka period (592-645), was the daughter of Emperor Kinmei. She empowered Prince Shotoku (574-622), her nephew, to handle the affairs of state as the prince regent. Both of them were descendants of the Soga clan.

"*Wa*" (和、倭、わ)

Prince Shotoku attached a great deal of importance to the emerging Buddhism as well as to the indigenous Shinto for the guardianship of the nation. His sense of proportion, i.e. employing both religions without leaning to either side, was rightly seen as the harmony or "*wa*" stated in his declared code. This "*wa*" later became a characteristic virtue of the Japanese attitude. Besides being a capable statesman, he was an excellent scholar as well, and published a guidebook for the Buddhist scriptures. He built the Shitenno-ji temple in 593 (in Osaka) and became actively involved in further introducing Buddhism. Temples all over Japan were managed by his government and now functioned as a means of announcing ministerial decrees and programs. In 603, he established the first system for ranking officials, according to which each official was categorized into one of 12 ranks. Furthermore, he established the "Seventeenth Article of the Constitution" in 604. The first article states: "Harmony is to be valued." The second article stipulates: "Respect the Three Treasures, which are the Buddha (仏), the *dharma* (法) embodied in *sutras*, and the priests (僧), or the monastic organization." He erected the Horyu-ji temple and sent Japanese official diplomatic delegations (Imoko and others) to Sui (隋) China in 607, with the aim of importing continental cultural elements.

In this way, he was actively engaged in protecting and enhancing Buddhism in his politics, and also brought into it useful aspects of Confucianism and Taoism. As a politician, Prince Shotoku is today thought of as an unbiased pragmatist.

For example, in developing his 12-level ranking system, he employed a nomenclature inspired by six virtues of Confucianism, i.e. integrity, benevolence, politeness, faith, justice and wisdom, and divided each of these into two (high integrity, low integrity, high benevolence, low benevolence, etc.).

The theological word "*ten-noh*" (天皇, emperor) of Taoism had already been introduced into Japan at the time (according to Koji Fukunaga). It is also said that the belief in mirrors and swords as symbols to be used in religious ceremonies appeared under the influence of Taoism. The belief in the powers of mountain hermits, originating in Taoism, was imported and syncretized with Buddhism. A trace of the earliest syncretism between the two religions can be seen today in the *ko-shin-do* (Taoist shrine) built on the temple grounds of the Shitenno-ji (Buddhist temple) in Osaka.

In this way, Prince Shotoku, who was the regent, first decreed that conformity or harmony be treasured. Then, he put this conformity into practice himself. In retrospect, conformity, or "wa" (和), has been in the mind of every Japanese person and at the heart of Japanese culture since his days, and is still very much a part of modern Japanese life.

"*Wa*" (和, harmony, conformity) leads to "*wa*" (倭), a word which has been used to refer to Japan since long ago. "*Wa*," "*wa-jin*," "*wa-shu*," and "*wa-koku*" are the words used in the *Gisho, Gokannjo, Shinsho, Sosho* and *Zuisho* (Chinese history books); all refer to Japan and its related meanings. In the old days, people in China, a large country with an advanced culture, used this term in a disparaging way to describe Japan and the Japanese. The article "*wa*" (和) is defined in the *Daijiten* (*The Encyclopedic Dictionary*, Mannen Ueda, *et al.*, 1965, Kodansha) as "the other name of Japan." " "*Wa*" (倭) was used in ancient China and was later changed to "*wa*"(和)," according to the *Daijiten*, and "*wa-shu*" means "Japanese people." "*Wa*" means "dwarf," the *Daijiten* continues. "*Wa*" also means "to tone down," "to obey," "harmonious," "no conflict," "warm," "gentle" and "peaceful." The article "*wa*" has connotations such as "submissive" and "respectful." The Chinese characters "和," "倭," "山迹" and "大和" have all been pronounced "Yamato" in Japanese until now. The Japanese syllabary character "わ," pronounced "*wa*," is derived from the flowing style of writing the Chinese character "和" (*wa*).

Looking back over history, one can say that *wa* has actually been the name and substance of Japan. Indeed, *wa* was employed dually as the name of Japan and the virtue which Prince Shotoku held in the highest esteem.

The word "*wa*" in "*wa-shiki*" ("Japanese-style"), "*wa-shoku*" ("Japanese food"), "*wa-fuku*" ("Japanese clothes"), "*wa-shitsu*" ("Japanese-style room"), etc., all reveal the characteristic Japanese dislike of taking a definitive and unilateral ethical stance; Japanese people would rather try to ensure consensus in advance or pull strings behind the scenes in an attempt to bring the matter at hand to a successful conclusion for everyone involved. It is highly important to note that Prince Shotoku practiced "*wa*" or harmony himself in his politics of combining Japan's indigenous Shinto with foreign religions (Taoism, Confucianism and Buddhism). In other words, *wa* is a virtue of the Japanese people adopted at the birth of Japan and constantly cultivated throughout its lengthy history.

From the period of Prince Shotoku to the Nara period (710-794), many Buddhist temples (Tachibana-dera, Daian-ji, Kofuku-ji, etc.) were built and foreign cultures were actively imported. Meanwhile, people tried to change Shinto to enable it to survive the rapid social and political transformations taking place; the influences of Buddhism, Confucianism and Taoism were grafted onto Shinto in a positive manner. The conflict between the Soga clan and the Mononobe clan ended at this time, as the government clearly manifested its preference for Buddhism. Under such circumstances, Shinto started to incorporate Buddhist ideas without hesitation, and ultimately succeeded in modifying itself substantially in order to survive. So, many Japanese people today have both Buddhist and Shinto altars in their homes; they give offerings on both altars at the same time and pray to the gods and the Buddha alternately at home. Western people, who are monotheistic, seem unable to understand this type of activity. However, this custom of harmony has been firmly ingrained in modern Japanese life. This syncretization of Shinto with Buddhism was initiated by the government during the reign of Prince Shotoku.

In the same period, many temples (Jingu-ji) were attached to shrines as a result of the syncretization of Shinto and Buddhism. Kihi-jingu-ji in the Echizen district, Usa-jingu-ji in Kyushu, Kashima-jingu-ji in the Hitachi district and Tada-jingu-ji in Ise are all examples of this religious fusion, where Shinto gods became the *bodhisattvas* (菩薩) of Buddhism. Then, these gods were elevated to the same level as that of the Buddha in accordance with the theory of *honji-suijaku*. "*Honji*" means the Buddha, and "*suijaku*" means a god derived from the Buddha. In other words, the Buddha came to Japan to become a Shinto god, according to this theory. "Gongen" was considered an avatar of the Buddha in the theory of *honji-suijaku*. In this way, many shrines were fused with temples in the form of *Jingu-ji*, and hereby the large information network through which the government's policies were communicated across the country was completed.

Shrine Shinto

People began performing religious ceremonies in shrines in the 3rd and 4th centuries A.D. Therefore, Shinto is sometimes called "shrine Shinto." Shrine Shinto includes Imperial Family Shinto and general Shinto. Ise Shinto at the Grand Shrine of Ise is the most important, serving as the center of Imperial Family Shinto.

The supreme god of Imperial Family Shinto is the Goddess of the Sun or Amaterasu. General Shinto, by contrast, has many objects of faith. They include the sea, mountains, water, wind, fire, and so on (the Kumano, Suwa and Sengen shrines, etc.). The Kamo, Munakata, Usahachiman, Kashima, Kasuga and Ohtori shrines hold ceremonies for the repose of ancestors. The Ohishi, Nogi and Meiji shrines hold ceremonies for the repose of particular individuals. At the Sumiyoshi-taisha, Inari-taisha and many other shrines, people pray for business prosperity and good progress in schoolwork. Here, *taisha* means a grand shrine. Izumo shrine, or Izumo-taisha, located in the Izumo district which is an out-of-the-way place of Japan is one of the oldest and most well known. It is disproportionately big for the place and it is located in a deep forest. It was dedicated to Okuninushi-no-Mikoto, a relation of Amaterasu who are both mythological gods described in *Kojiki*, the oldest piece of literature about Japan written by Yasumaro Ohno in 712.

There are Shinto sects other than those mentioned above, and they were founded mainly by charismatic individuals inspired by Shinto. Historically, they sometimes came into conflict with the political establishment and were clamped down on (e.g., *Ohmoto-kyo*). The shrines of general Shinto are varied and branched as shown above, with almost no regard for principles. Shrines of enormous diversity were built under the influence of this polytheistic animism.

Shrine Shinto evolved from popular natural religion. In the Nara and the Heian periods, Shinto was systematized and became a well-integrated component of society and culture by borrowing the structure of Buddhism. The most typical example is *honji-suijaku*. In the Edo period, the Chu Hsi school, or Neo-Confucianism, was adopted as the national religion. At that time, Shinto was actively syncretized with Confucianism to form a nationalistic symbol. As a result, Shinto functioned well, just like Confucianism, during the feudalistic period dominated by the *samurai or bushi*. In the latter half of the Edo period, Mabuchi Kamo (1697-1769), Norinaga Motoori (1730-1801) and Atsutane Hirata (1776-1843) began the restoration of Shinto and the intensification of the study of old Japanese thought. The result was nationalistic Shinto. They envisioned a return to original Japanese Shinto and tried to eliminate the influences of foreign religions such as Buddhism, Confucianism and Taoism. They looked to *Kojiki*, or "Record of Ancient Matters," and *Nihonshoki*, or "Chronicles of Japan," for guidance.

However, this was tantamount to a regression, a return to the period before Prince Shotoku in defiance of the historical reality, and therefore a concealment of the facts. It was naturally an unreasonable theory for the Japanese people, who had already profoundly integrated foreign religions into their lives; they could not go back to the pre-Shotoku state. However, this revival of Shinto in the Edo period was kept alive thereafter as a specific stance, namely the general trend of nationalism and imperialism. It was supported by the militaristic Japanese government following the Meiji Restoration.

State Shinto

Taking over the favorable treatment of Japanese classics in the later Edo era, the Meiji government adopted and dealt well with Shinto as an official religion because it was appropriate for its militaristic policies. The anti-Buddhism movement officially proceeded to destroy Buddhist temples and statues and separate Buddhism from Shintoism. Governance in the Meiji era was, basically, the application of religion or state Shinto to politics. The creativity typical of original forms of spirituality could not be expected to flourish in such a controlled religion. Freedom and creation, which are indispensable components of original religions, disappeared from state Shinto. After World War II, the separation of state and Shinto was stipulated (Decree regarding Shinto, 1945). Since then, Japanese Shinto has again started to develop freely among people, as it had once done.

Japanese people have never abandoned Shinto ceremonies, even after the government stopped supporting Shinto in 1945. A wide range of Shinto ceremonies still color the lives of Japanese people. Each region has a shrine for its village god, and people continue their ancestor worship and attend Shinto ceremonies, including New Year's visits to shrines, cerebrations for 3-year-old boys and girls, 5-year-old boys and 7-year-old girls, a variety of annual festivals (*matsuri*) as well as purification ceremonies for new building sites to calm the local guardian spirits (*jichin-sai*). These religious manifestations are still a vigorous part of Japanese culture. This is the current state of Shinto in Japan.

According to the Internet website of the Association of Shinto Shrines, the number of shrines in Japan in 2002 was 70,074. The shrines include Hachiman, Inari, Suwa, Izumo, Kumano, etc. They have in common *torii* gates, *tamagaki* fences and front shrines (*haiden*) as well as main shrines (*honden*).

Shinto is characterized by the simple worship of ancestors and nature, without any doctrines or scriptures. Shinto has no founder (charismatic individual) such as the Buddha (Buddhism) or Confucius (Confucianism). The gods of Shinto have survived a long and tumultuous history until now, because Japanese people are under no religious control (i.e. there are no dogmas or scriptures). Shinto is thoroughly assimilated in the lives of present-day Japanese people, constituting a part of their potential religious feelings. The religious ceremonies of Shinto include ceremonies for purifying building sites, weddings, funeral rites, New Year's visits to shrines, a gala day for children of 3, 5 and 7 years of age, and portable shrine (*mikoshi*) processions, spring festivals (rice-planting season), autumn festivals (harvest season), summer festivals, god precincts in modern buildings, etc.

When asked what religion they espouse, modern Japanese people say they have no religious affiliation. Actually, the religious ceremonies mentioned above are inextricably integrated in their everyday lives.

3. Buddhism

In the Asuka period (593-710), Prince Shotoku, appointed regent by Empress Suiko, promoted an open-door policy in matters of religion. As a result, he accepted foreign religions such as Confucianism, Taoism, and Buddhism; and these religions brought with them a wide range of cultural elements. The imported religions were actively syncretized with native Japanese Shinto. Especially Buddhism had highly advanced doctrines, scriptures and cultural elements (Buddhist architecture and construction technology, civil engineering, arts and crafts). Japanese people were surprised at the spirituality, visual grandeur and practical benefits of Buddhism, things which were lacking in Shinto. Therefore, Shinto needed to change by accepting the strong influence of Buddhism. Shinto imitated the systemic doctrines and building styles of Buddhism because Shinto had no doctrine or scripture of its own.

Buddhism appeared around 500 B.C. on the Ganga River in northeastern India. The founder of Buddhism was the Buddha (566-486 B.C.). He is also called "Shakuson" or "Shakyamuni." "Buddha" was originally his name, but it is used to mean the state of enlightenment or Buddhahood, which is reached after religious austerities; it is also used to denote Buddha-like figures. He preached and practiced compassion and eventually attained enlightenment (*nirvana*). Buddhism split into two schools after his death. One was the conservative school, which strictly adhered to the Buddha's laws and focused on performing ascetic practices according to his instructions (Hinayana Buddhism). The other was the school which tried to create written interpretations of the Buddha's life and words; it is called Mahayana Buddhism, and it extended to peripheral nations such as China, Korea, Japan and Central Asia via those scriptures. Tibetan Buddhism is a branch of Mahayana Buddhism, or may be called the third school of Buddhism, because it was transmitted directly to Tibet across the Himalaya Mountains.

Sutras (Scriptures, 経, *kyo* in Japanese)

Buddhism was first imported to China in the 1st century B.C., and its scriptures were actively translated into Chinese in the 2nd century, about 600 years after the Buddha's death. Many Buddhist scriptures we see now are records of the Buddha's actions and preachings, created by his students after his death. The first scripture of Mahayana Buddhism was the *Prajna-sutra (Hannya-kyo,* or Wisdom Sutra*)*, estimated to have been completed in approximately year 0 of the Christian Era, while the *Kegon Sutra* was written in the 1st or 2nd century A.D. These are called the initial scriptures of Mahayana Buddhism. The *Prajna-sutra* is noted for its theory of *sunya* (emptiness, voidness, 空, *kuh* in Japanese) and the phrase "All matter is void, voidness is form" (色即是空 空即是色, "*Shiki soku ze kuh, kuh soku ze shiki*" in Japanese). The concept of "voidness" had a significant impact on Chinese people when the *Prajna-sutra* was first imported into China, because the Taoist concept of "non-being"(無, "*mu*" in Japanese) already prevailed in China. Naturally, the similarities and the differences between Voidness and Non-being were a source of deep concern for Chinese religious figures.

The *Nehan-kyo (Mahaparinirvana-sutra)*, which is famed for its phrase "all the living things, even trees and plants, have the capacity to attain Buddhahood" ("*Issai-shujo-shitu-u-bussyo,*" or "一切衆生悉有仏性," in *kanji*), was created a short time after the initial scriptures of Mahayana Buddhism were written.

The *Lotus Sutra (Hokke-kyo)* is one of the major scriptures of Mahayana Buddhism in which the Buddha promises the salvation of all sentient beings; it was translated into Chinese by Kumaarajiiva (344-409 A.D.) and then transmitted to China, Korea and Japan. In Japan, Prince Shotoku created commentaries for three scriptures, including the Lotus Sutra, with the aim of popularizing them. The Tendai sect of Buddhism, founded by Saicho in the early Heian period, and the Nichiren sect of Buddhism, founded by Nichiren in the Kamakura period, put much faith in the Lotus Sutra as their basic scripture. In China, the Lotus Sutra was the basis of the *Hannya-kyo (Prajna-sutra), Yuima-kyo (Vimalakirti-sutra)* and *Kegon-kyo (Kegon Sutra)*.

The *Dainichi-kyo*, or the Great Sun Sutra (*Mahavairocana Sutra*), and the *Kongocho-kyo* (*Vajrasekhara-sutra*) are basic scriptures of esoteric Buddhism, and were created in India in the 7th century A.D. (the latter phase of Mahayana Buddhism). They were translated into Chinese during the Tang dynasty. Esoteric or Tantric Buddhism, which is different from exoteric Buddhism, seeks to understand the principle (secret core) of the universe by focusing on concrete objects. It makes much of the rituals and arts, besides the doctrines. *Vairocana* (*Vairochana*), or Birusyana-butsu, is the principal image of the *Kegon-kyo,* while *Mahavairocana* (great *Vairocana*), or the *Dainichi-nyorai,* is the main image of esoteric Buddhism.

Zen Buddhism was transplanted to China by Bodhidharma in the 6th century, where it became syncretized with specifically Chinese religions such as Taoism and Confucianism. As Zen was dependent neither on religious images nor on any specialized *sutra* to enable enlightenment, it was near to Taoism, which was individualistic and rejected all legislation. Furthermore, both religions have in common the attachment to this world more than to any other world. In Sung China, all Buddhist sects except Zen fell into decline because of the rise of Confucianism and the Mongolian pressure from the north. It was in this era that Zen was brought to Japan by Eisai (1191) and Dogen (1227). Zen depends basically on the *Lotus Sutra.*

"*Nyorai*" ("*tathaagata*") in Mahayana Buddhism has the same meaning as "Buddha," a being who is completely within the truth. *Dainichi-nyorai (Mahavairocana)* is the highest Buddha and is assimilated with the sun under the influence of Hindu culture. Elements such as burning holy sticks for invocation (fire worship under the influence of Zoroastrianism) and *tantra* (holy scriptures and magic words) in esoteric Buddhism are traces of India. The *mandala* (a geometrical figure with a center and a periphery; many *buddhas* are arranged around the Dainichi-nyorai) stands for diversity and forgiveness.

The diversification of Buddhism was generated mainly by students who developed and added to Buddhist theories after the Buddha's death over the course of time. The

Buddha's ashes were distributed among *stupas*. *Stupas* are somewhat like modern-day tombs, but the Buddha's original teachings do not include the concept of *stupas* and the reverencing of bones.

Mahayana Buddhism

Mahayana Buddhism is also called "Mahaasaaghika Buddhism." Mahayana practitioners seek to salvage common people, not to benefit themselves exclusively, and rely heavily on faith. Mahayana Buddhism left many Buddhist statues and Buddhist scriptures, which allowed Buddhism to survive throughout its long history by innovating constantly. Hinayana and Mahayana Buddhism are only different in their methods of ascetic training and in the attitudes of priests toward common people. They have in common the religious purpose of achieving enlightenment and entering the truth (*dharma*). Hinayana Buddhism, which is the other main branch of Buddhism, is also called "Theravada Buddhism." It is conservative because it places great emphasis on ascetic practice. Hinayana Buddhism has not been popular in Japan, although several of its schools were imported during the Nara period. Hinayana adepts strictly adhere to Buddhist precepts (e.g., remaining celibate) and ascetic practices to attain Buddhahood. Their behavior seems to come closest to the original *dharma* teachings of the Buddha.

Mahayana Buddhism had the largest influence on Japanese culture. It also spread to the west from India, and became mixed with the cultures of Persia, Turkey and Greece, leaving many Buddhist temple ruins which still exist, such as those in Gandhara. Broadly speaking, the Buddhism of Central Asia was the same as the Mahayana Buddhism imported to Japan via China. The images of the Buddha preserved in the caves of Central Asia resemble the Great Buddha of the Todai-ji temple, which was constructed at the order of Emperor Shomu (reign: 724-749) in cooperation with the priest Gyoki in 735. People were impressed at the gentle eyes of the Great Buddha and immediately understood the nature of Buddhism with its tremendous culture. The position of Buddhism as a new religion was immediately established among the populace.

Prosperity of Mahayana Buddhism in Japan

Mahayana Buddhism originated in India at around the time of the birth of Jesus. It is characterized by a well-thought-out philosophical doctrine. Naagaarjuna (150-250) developed the doctrine of Mahayana Buddhism, especially the theory of *sunyata* (空, *kuh*), while Asanga (4th century) and his younger brother, Vasubandhu, contributed to the establishment of *vijnana* (識, *shiki*). Indian Buddhism was transferred to China in the 1st century B.C. and Chinese Buddhism was formed there under the influence of Taoism and Confucianism. For instance, enlightenment (*satori* in Japanese) was accepted at first as Tao (the Way) or a virtue. In the Sui (581-619) and Tang (618-907) periods, Chinese Buddhism flourished and reached its peak, while in the later eras of the Sung (960-1279) and the Ming (1368-1644) it declined due to the predominance of Confucianism and Taoism. After the doctrines of Chinese Buddhism became more profound, it split into several sects such as Jodo, Zen, Tendai, Kegon and Shingon (*mantra*).

Buddhism was imported to Japan via the Korean Peninsula. Seimeioh (Baekje) donated a Buddha statue and some Buddhist scriptures to the Imperial court in 538 during the reign of emperor Kinmei. Indian Buddhism continued to develop in India for several centuries and was exported to China in the 1st century B.C. It changed under the influence of Confucianism and Taoism, which already existed there. Then, it was imported to Japan. In other words, Buddhism was imported to Japan about 1,000 years after it was originally developed in India.

Originally, Buddhism aimed at supreme enlightenment, *nirvana*, and at reaching the "Other Shore," on which humans are the delivered from the four earthly sufferings: birth, old age, illness, and death. *Gyo* was the ascetic exercise required for this liberation to take place.

The original Buddhism generated in India spoke of *vimukti* (emancipation) or *samsara* (transmigration of the soul, metempsychosis), and did not adopt a serious view of the body. Buddhism was syncretized with Confucianism, Taoism and Shinto in the historical and geographical processes through which Buddhism was transferred to China, Korea and ultimately Japan during the great time span of two and a half millennia. During these processes, the notion of body also changed. For example, there was no concept of tombs (a place where the soul dwells, an extension of the body) in the age of the Buddha. In modern-day Japan, funeral services and tombs are closely related to Buddhism, and a series of Buddhist ceremonies and customs are closely interwoven to form the Buddhist way of life.

Buddhism, when imported to Japan, entered into the heart of politics, as described earlier in relation to Prince Shotoku. In the Nara period (710-794) after the Asuka period, six schools came to constitute national Buddhism: Hosso, Sanron, Kegon, Ritsu, Kusha and Jojitsu. They were collectively called the "Nanto Rokushu." They were imported by pundits who traveled to Tang China. These pundits did nothing to save the people or make their lives better; they learned Buddhism only for the aristocrats. Nara

Buddhism was protected by the Imperial court. Priests had the privilege of being given temple estates from the court and grew in power so much that they frequently intervened in politics. So, both politics and religion were corrupt in the latter part of the Nara period.

Emperor Kanmu (reign: 781-806) constructed the city of Heian-kyo (Kyoto) and transferred the capital from Nara to Kyoto. He eliminated the influence of the priests in politics and created conditions in which the new Heian Buddhism prospered. This new Buddhism was not of the urban type like the Buddhist sects of Nara; its headquarters were in the mountains. Tendai-shu based on Mt. Hiei and Shingon-shu based on Mt. Koya were representative schools of Heian Buddhism. Saicho and Kukai, who studied in Tang China, brought back Tendai-shu and esoteric Buddhism (which afterward became Shingon-shu in Japan), respectively, along with Buddhist scriptures.

Saicho (767-822) had the support of Emperor Kanmu. He was sent to Tang China by the Imperial court to study the Tendai doctrine. He went with an embassy to Tang China in 804 and studied the Tendai doctrine on Mt. Tendai. He returned to Japan in 805. At this time, he brought the Buddhist scriptures (*Lotus Sutra*) of Tendai-shu (exoteric Buddhism) and other related matters in response to the expectations of Emperor Kanmu. Some documents of esoteric Buddhism were also brought back. Saicho started the Japanese branch of Tendai-shu at the Enryaku-ji temple on Mt. Hiei north of Kyoto after he returned to Japan. It was based mainly on the *Lotus Sutra*.

Meanwhile, Kukai (774-835), who was seven years younger than Saicho, went to Tang China with the same embassy as Saicho (but on another ship). His rank was lower than that of Saicho. Kukai's specific purpose was to learn the arcane knowledge of esoteric Buddhism and the related Buddhist scriptures, such as *Dainichi-kyo (Mahavairocana Sutra, or* the *Great Sun Sutra)* and *Kongocho-kyo (Vajrasekhara-sutra)*. Esoteric Buddhism in China was in the midst of frenetic development. Before his departure, Kukai had already learned some of the scriptures that had been partially imported to Japan and noticed this new trend in China. In 805, a year after Kukai entered Tang China, he was initiated into esoteric Buddhism by Keika, who was an orthodox practitioner of esoteric Buddhism in China. Keika was on the verge of death and died shortly after initiating Kukai (December 805). Kukai was very lucky indeed to have received his initiation from Keika before the master's death. On his deathbed, Keika eagerly recommended Kukai to return to Japan early and start propagating esoteric Buddhism in Japan. In obedience to Keika's advice, Kukai returned to Japan in 806, earlier than expected, bringing with him many scriptures and tools of esoteric Buddhism. He brought back much more knowledge of orthodox esoteric Buddhism than

Saicho, who had already returned to Japan in 805.

Esoteric Buddhism declined in China after the death of Keika, but blossomed remarkably in Japan. When Emperor Saga (reign: 809-823), the second prince of Emperor Kanmu, ascended the throne in 809, the Imperial court expressed strong support for Kukai and made Mt. Koya the sacred ground of Shingon esoteric Buddhism. The Japanese branch of Tendai-shu (basically a form of exoteric Buddhism using the *Lotus Sutra* as its holy scripture), founded by Saicho was later converted to esoteric Buddhism in retard to Shingon-shu. This was called "*Tai-Mitsu*" (台蜜), while Shingon esoteric Buddhism was called "*To-Mitsu*" (東蜜).

Shingon esoteric Buddhism, which prospered in Japan, was almost an original creation of Kukai, who was a successor of the orthodox practitioners of esoteric Buddhism in Tang China. Esoteric Buddhism is the opposite of exoteric Buddhism, including Nara Buddhism. In exoteric Buddhism, priests study Buddhist scriptures, which are the words of the Buddha, and perform ascetic practices in order to achieve enlightenment or become "Buddha." In contrast, esoteric Buddhism involves the mysticism and the belief in gods or elements of magic that had long existed in India before Buddhism arose. India had an original and ancient form of mysticism or tantrism, which was gradually adopted by Brahmanism, Hinduism and Buddhism.

Esoteric Buddhism (Mahayana esoteric Buddhism) flourished in the latter stages of Mahayana Buddhism in India during the 6th-8th centuries, and the *Mahavairocana Sutra* (the *Great Sun Sutra*, or *Dainichi-kyo*) and the *Vajrasekhara-sutra* (*Kongocho-kyo*) were created in the early 6th century. Esoteric Buddhism, which was brought to Japan in 806 by Kukai, was different from the preceding Nara Buddhism because it aimed at the attainment of Buddhahood in this world. In esoteric Buddhism, or the Shingon Buddhism of Kukai, everyone is assumed to have the capacity for *satori* (enlightenment) or becoming a Buddha. This concept was completely novel and produced its own term: "*sokushinjyobutsu*," meaning that an ordinary person could become a Buddha in his own body by reaching enlightenment. Esoteric Buddhism has Dainichi-nyorai (Mahavairocana) as the most important among many Buddha-like figures (*butsu* and *nyorai*). Esoteric Buddhism, or Shingon, was also specific in stressing rituals and arts as well as doctrines. *Tantra*, or the secret spells of Shingon, were derived from ancient India.

In the Heian period (794-1192), the aristocratic Fujiwara clan, related to the Imperial court by marriage, prospered. The Heian period is also called "the period of the royal dynasty." The Fujiwara clan was founded by Fujiwara (Nakatomi)-no-Kamatari and his son, Fujiwara-no-Fuhito. It reached the height of its prosperity during the lifetime of Fujiwara-no-Michinaga (966-1027) in the middle of the Heian Period. Kofuku-ji in Nara was the guardian temple of the Fujiwara clan, and the Kasuga-taisha shrine housed its guardian god. The two religious facilities are adjacent to each other. They speak to us of the dominance of the Fujiwara clan, which ultimately abused its authority. During this stable period of the Heian dynasty, the syllabograms called "*hiragana*" or "*onnade*" were formed; at first, their purpose was to serve as women's handwriting. This epoch-making invention brought forth the creation of literary works of high quality by the women at the court, which covered a wide range of genres, including diaries, essays, *waka* (short poems) and even novels. A series of *waka* anthologies were created by Imperial command. They include *Kokinshu*, which was the first such anthology with a famous foreword written in *hiragana*, and *Shin-kokinshu*, the last of the series.

In the middle of the Heian period, the Tendai priest Genshin (Eshin Sodzu, 942-1017) wrote *Ohjo-yoshu* (*Essentials of Going to the Pure Land*) to teach the masses Pure Land Buddhism, expressing his thought in a set of famous short phrases such as "*gongu-jodo*" and "*onri-edo*," which mean the aspiration to be reborn in the Pure Land and the abhorrence of this corrupt world, respectively. He considered this world to be incorrigibly corrupt and preached to the masses that they should seek life in the Pure Land by simply repeating the *nembutsu*, or the name "Amida." His thoughts were a prelude to the Jodo-shu and Jodo-shin-shu founded by Honen (1133-1212) and Shinran (1173-1262), respectively, during the period from the end of the Heian dynasty to the Kamakura, when religion focusing on the salvation of the aristocracy declined. Kamakura Buddhism, which sought to save the common people who had not been saved by aristocratic Buddhism and to win the devotion of the *samurai*, began to prosper.

Kamakura Buddhism

Jodo-shu (the Pure Land sect of Buddhism) and Jodo-shin-shu (the True Pure Land sect of Buddhism) are both Buddhist sects uniquely established in Japan by Honen (1133-1212) and Shinran (1173-1262), respectively. These sects had characteristics specific to Japan in that they delineate proper conduct in view of salvation through faith in Amida, the Buddha of the Pure Land; the aim is to reach the Pure Land in the West through prayer. The concept of faith in the Pure Land had already been articulated by the Tendai monk Genshin (942-1017) in the Heian period. He wrote *Ohjo-yoshu*, or "Essentials of Going to the Pure Land," in which he presented the philosophical basis for the subsequent rise of Jodo-shu. However, Honen and Nichiren espoused an innovative form of Buddhism which was significantly different from the Buddhism of the Heian period. In Jodo-shu (founded by Honen) and Jodo-shin-shu (founded by Shinran), even women and evil men were thought to be capable for salvation simply by reciting the *nembutsu* phrase "*namu Amida Butsu.*" There was no need for people to understand the difficult Buddhist scriptures as required by previous Buddhist sects. That is, their approach was novel, in that it was popular and allowed the easy participation of ordinary people. A series of great philosophical works stressing the practice of *nembutsu* was published: *Ohjo-yoshu* (985, by Genshin), *Senchaku-hongan-nembutsu-shu* (1198, by Honen), *Kyogoshinsho* (1224, by Shinran), etc. In the period between the end of the Heian era and the Kamakura era, people believed that the end of the world was at hand (the *mappo* concept). Amid such public unrest, the *samurai*, or *bushi*, class was reaching new heights of prosperity, taking the place of the court nobles. People waited for a new Buddhism which would save those who were beyond all help due to the constant wars and wide-spread famine.

Other types of Kamakura Buddhism included the Japanese Rinzai-shu, founded by Eisai (1141-1215), the Japanese Soto-shu, founded by Dogen (1200-1253), and Nichiren-shu (reaching the Pure Land by chanting "*namu myo-ho-renge-kyo*"), founded by Nichiren (1222-1282). Rinzai and Soto are both Zen sects of Buddhism imported from the Sung and became popular in *bushi* circles, while the Nichiren sect of Buddhism was the most radical and nationalistic in Japanese history. All these three sects had the same characteristics as Jodo-shu and Jodo-shin-shu, in the sense that they were innovative and appeared as a result of necessity, stemming from people's desire. Young people with religious inclinations saw the conservative Heian Buddhism grow corrupt and power-hungry, and they wanted to reform it. For example, Eisai was originally a priest of the Tendai-shu and belonged to Enryaku-ji at Mt. Hiei near Kyoto; he went to Sung China when he was 28 years old (in 1168) to perform ascetic practices on Mt. Tendai where the head temple of the sect was located, aiming to reform Tendai-shu in Japan. However, there was no Tendai-shu in China anymore. Instead, the Zen sect (southern Zen) as a novel trend of Buddhism had begun to gain influence in China under general social conditions in which a new Confucian sect, the doctrine of Chu Hsi, was becoming popular. About 20 years later, in 1187, Eisai revisited Sung China to study Zen this time, and stayed there for five years. He came back to Japan in 1192 with Rinzai Zen (southern Zen). This new form of Buddhism, Zen, and his idea of importing it, were looked down upon at first by the Imperial Court in Kyoto, the court nobles and the established Tendai priests on Mt. Hiei; the Zen sect had to take root outside Kyoto and thus won adepts mainly among the *samurai*, or *bushi*, in Kamakura.

He erected the Shofuku-ji (1195), the first Zen temple in Kyushu, then the Jufuku-ji

(1200) in Kamakura and the Kennin-ji (1202) in Kyoto with the support of the Shogun of Kamakura, Minamoto-no-Yoriie. All sects of Kamakura Buddhism provided easy methods of salvation that could be implemented by everyone. Religion was no longer only for the privileged classes as in the Heian period. Even common people could turn to religion for help in the Kamakura period (1192-1333). In fact, religion was largely only for the common people in this era, becoming the core of a public movement. This was the birth of a type of Mahayana Buddhism specific to Japan, absent in China and India.

The history of Buddhism and its influences on Japan will now be outlined.

Buddhism was originally a primitive religion developed in India. This primitive Buddhism was modified as it incorporated the original Hindu gods, the Vedas, the Upanishads, Brahmanism and local occultism. After Christ was born, Buddhism spread outside India and changed depending on the route it took. Hinayana Buddhism (performing ascetic practices mainly to benefit oneself in terms of approaching Buddhahood) was exported to Thailand, South Vietnam, Myanmar, Sri Lanka, etc. Mahayana Buddhism (discussing Buddhist scriptures and performing ascetic practices mainly to benefit others) was brought to China, Tibet, Korea, Vietnam and Japan. Mahayana Buddhism was also exported to Central Asia, where different Buddhist cultures were developed through blending with the indigenous cultures in each region. For example, esoteric Buddhism, which arose in India at the end of Mahayana Buddhism, was transferred to China in the 8th century and brought over to Japan in 806 by Kukai. It prospered so outstandingly in Japan while it waned in India and China that Japanese esoteric Buddhism has its own name, "Shingon Buddhism" (or "Shingon"). A new religious center was erected at Mt. Koya, located in a mountain range in the Kii district. Emperor Saga (reign: 809-823) became a strong patron of Kukai and permitted him to use this huge mountain for his esoteric Buddhist religious activity. Kukai and his followers erected here a magnificent series of buildings in the Shingon style housing religious institutions, which included the Kongobu-ji temple and a great pagoda. This place developed then into the center of Japan's specific form of esoteric Buddhism, so that we can say that Shingon is synonymous with Mt. Koya. Recent comparative studies of religions show that the Shingon esoteric Buddhism founded by Kukai is very different from Tibet's esoteric Buddhism.

A variety of forms of Japanese Buddhism in the later Heian, Kamakura and Muromachi periods were subsequently generated from the necessity to fulfill the strong desires of the common people at critical junctures in history. They caught people's religious imagination and competed with each other in terms of philosophical innovation; thus, each of them grew prominent at one time or another. They also set fire to other temples using their political leverage, while armed priests fought each other. Here, these Buddhist sects seem to be different religions at first glance, but, originally, they were branches of the Buddhism originating in India.

In the Heian period, the Buddhism imported from the continent, including Tendai and esoteric Buddhism, prospered with the support of the Imperial court and the nobility. This Heian Buddhism was basically designed for consumption by the upper classes, and priests offered the aristocracy psychological support by performing incantations to protect them from disasters. From the end of the Heian period to the Kamakura period, inferiors overthrew their superiors and the end-of-world syndrome was acute among the people (*mappo*: the world had been predicted to deteriorate 1,500 years after the Buddha's death). Under these dire circumstances, various sects of Japanese Buddhism were developed with the aim of salvaging the common people. These sects included the Jodo-shu founded by Honen, the Jodo-shin-shu founded by Shinran, the Ji-shu founded by Ippen, the Nichiren-shu founded by Nichiren, the Rinzai-shu founded by Eisai, the Soto-shu founded by Dogen, and so on.

They were Japanese revisions or original developments of Buddhism. Zen sects (Rinzai-zen and Soto-zen) played a large role in developing the Japanese thought on nature, as seen in the concepts of *wabi* (poverty, simplicity, tranquility), *sabi* (aged and quiet beauty as a part of nature) and *mujo* (impermanence). Zen lives on in many ways in the current Japanese culture, especially in the field of art, calligraphy and the tea ceremony. Typical Japanese philosophers such as Kitaro Nishida, Daisetsu Suzuki and Keiji Nishitani developed their own philosophical standpoints through Zen meditation. It deserves special mention that their legacy is still a source of emotional comfort in modern-day Japan.

The cultural elements imported from Western countries during the modernization of Japan include philosophical and religious ideas. When considering the Japanese identity, the accomplishments of the three people mentioned above are precious because they were truly original and specifically Japanese in their work. It is notable that all of them were affected by Buddhist thought, in particular Zen.

Buddhism as a whole declined during the Edo and Meiji eras. Instead, New Confucianism, imported from Sung and Ming China, flourished. The Tokugawa government adopted the Chu Hsi school (a branch of Confucianism philosophically reconstructed through the incorporation of classical Taoism) as the national religion. Teachers used the *Analects* of Confucius and texts related to Confucianism at temple schools to educate the children of the *samurai*. The Meiji government issued the

"Buddhism-Shintoism separation decree" (1868) to prohibit Buddhism. The government abolished Buddhism and gave preferential treatment to Shinto as a national religion. It also suppressed the part of Shinto that did not worship emperors. National Shinto was a formalistic and compulsory religion generated from the syncretization of Shinto with Confucianism. However, the government could not really eliminate Buddhism, despite concerted attempts. By this time, Buddhism had pervaded every aspect of people's lives.

Since the end of World War II, politics based on national Shinto is prohibited. The political suppression of Buddhism has also been eliminated. At the end of World War II, Japan adopted a liberal policy and the principle of separation of politics and religion.

In real life, we can see many Buddhist temples, artifacts and customs around us in Japan, even though Buddhism was suppressed for about 70 years, from the beginning of the Meiji period to the end of the World War II, under a system of state support for Shinto. Japanese people cannot live without Buddhism because Buddhist culture is an integral part of their lives. This is no surprise, considering the long historical evolution of Buddhism in Japan, as described above. There are many words in the Japanese language related to Buddhism, such as "*hotoke*," or "*butsu*," "*nyorai*" and "*bosatsu*" (*bodhisattva*). *Hotoke* is an incarnation of the Buddha. There are many *hotokes or butsus*, and they form a big "pantheon." "*Nyorai*" is used in the same way as "Buddha." There are different types of *nyorai*, such as Amida-nyorai, Yakushi-nyorai, Dainichi-nyorai and Shaka-nyorai. Further, there are many Buddhist images watching over Japanese people, such as Kanon-bosatsu, Monju-bosatsu, Fugen-bosatsu, and Jizo-bosatsu, and these are worshipped by the populace even today.

4. Confucianism

Confucianism is a religion which focuses on human morality, order in particular. Individuals are part of communities (families, relatives, villages, societies and nations) governed by moral rules. Confucius (551-479 B.C.) established Confucianism in northern China, which is a cold region with crops such as oat, millet and Italian millet. Broadly speaking, people in northern China emphasize the ethics of community life, in contrast to people in southern China, where individualism is emphasized. People in northern China are topical and dogmatic, and they readily embraced the Confucian ethics of decency, piety and loyalty.

In Confucianism, there are five basic virtues: benevolence, justice, politeness, wisdom and faith. Among these, benevolence (仁) is assumed to be the highest virtue. Benevolence refers to the perfect character, or the constant tenderness of the wise man or the ruler. Justice is the virtue through which public order is maintained. Politeness is the autonomous rule to respect one's elders. Wisdom is cognitive ability. And faith is genuineness or candor.

Confucianism values order, and is characterized by strong paternal governance, as manifested in the commemoration of one's ancestors, for instance. Persons in authority have often adopted Confucianism as the national religion. In the old days, Butei in the Han dynasty in China, the Rhee dynasty in Korea, the imperial system after the Taika Restoration in Japan, other Asian countries affected by Chinese dynasties such as Vietnam and Ryukyu (now called Okinawa) and the Shogunate government of the Edo era in Japan all adopted Confucianism for its political benefits. Confucianism was imported to Japan early in its history, during the reign of Emperor Ojin (27-310), more than 300 years before the importation of Buddhism.

In Japan in 603, Prince Shotoku established the first system for ranking officials, and officials were given one of 12 ranks. In defining the 12 ranks, he used six virtues of Confucianism (integrity, benevolence, politeness, faith, justice and wisdom), and divided each of them into two grades (high integrity, low integrity, high benevolence, low benevolence, etc.). Prince Shotoku took an active part in building the Shitenno-ji and Horyu-ji temples to introduce Buddhism. Meanwhile, he prized highly the business-like advantages of Confucian bureaucracy. Clearly, Confucianism and Buddhism were already so profoundly syncretized during the reign of Prince Shotoku that they could not be separated thereafter.

5. Taoism

Taoism began as an ontology or a cosmology of the universe, and as time passed it aggregated with folk beliefs native to the Han people in China. The doctrine was based on the beliefs of the Tao school headed by Lao Tzu (reported to have been born in 604 B.C., 50 years earlier than Confucius) and Zhūang Zi, both of whom were philosophers in ancient China during the Chou dynasty (1066-256 B.C.). The founder of the sect is thought to be Lao Tzu, who left a philosophical theory of Taoism. The original thought of the Tao school was based on the concept of *tao*, a concept which emphasizes life in the natural state. Tao is Non-being or the original state, where everything, including Being, is generated and where everything ultimately returns. Non-being is the mother of Being, and Being gives birth to all things. These original metaphysical beliefs of the Tao school were quite profound in the 6th century B.C., but they did not evolve so much as to stir up a religious movement among the common people, and it was only afterwards in the Later Han dynasty (25-220 A.D.), when Chodohryo appeared, that the religious aspect of Taoism extended its influence over the lives of common people as a popular religion affirming this world. Taoism in its popularized form was also called "*Gotobeidō*" or "*Tenshidō*." Currently, Taoism in the broad sense involves the two aspects of the philosophical and the religious, as well as faith in a variety of deities beneficial to the earthy pursuits of people. "Taoism" in English refers to the philosophical views of Lao Tzu. Here, "*tao*" means "Way," i.e. the natural state before things became differentiated; it is Mother Nature or the original state of potential. *Tao* existed before heaven and earth were separated. Lao Tzu is known internationally as the founder of Taoism due to the numerous English translations of his texts.

The beliefs of Taoism were developed in southern China, where the climate was warm and the major crop was rice. It was greatly different from the Confucianism generated against the background of the strict moralistic spirit of northern China. Taoism was born in the free and natural mental climate of southern China. Taoism basically affirmed the pleasures of human living and thus never negated the worldly desires of people, such as long life, sex and wealth. Traditionally, people held the dragon, a Taoist symbol, in high regard. Actually, there is a story according to which Confucius commented that Lao Tzu was "like a dragon" after seeing him, and it is well known that the Blue Dragon defends the east in the Taoist tradition. After 2,500 years, we still have in Asian countries so many paintings of dragons soaring dramatically through the winds and clouds, images suggesting the generative power of the Mother. Images of the dragon were used as the Emperor's symbol in feudal Vietnam and Ryukyu (now Okinawa) as well as in China.

The basic concept of Taoism is that there are two ambivalent but inextricably linked principles. Both are indispensable for the resumption of the initial totality. In other words, Being comes from Non-being and Two comes from One. Such unstable states can recover their stability again when the original state of Nothing or the connection between separated elements has been reestablished.

For example, *Yin* and *Yang* both require the other. *Yang* exists because of *Yin* and vice versa. If there is a dimple, it can store water. If water is stored, it can return to its original peaceful state.

Taoism showed a marked preference for a strongly maternal society. For example, the sun is female in Taoism. Taoists believe that the female sex is hidden in the male sex. Likewise, the womb that generates all matters is female.

Taoism does not have strong laws, unlike Buddhism; instead it has a magnanimity which affirms sexual intercourse and good fortune in the present world. Therefore, it is likely to be accepted by the common people. Immortality is another characteristic of Taoism. Since the early days of Taoism, people held the immortal mountain hermits in awe, and longed to attain the three major goals of life: happiness, wealth and long life. They admired not only mountain hermits but also their own ancestors. Taoism has two elements in common with Confucianism, namely ancestor worship and the affirmation of the body.

Taoism is individualistic and relativistic. Therefore, it has always shown a marked tendency toward anti-authoritarianism and anti-Confucianism. Taoism served as the driving force of the Yellow Turban Rebellion of the common people that destroyed the later Han dynasty of China. However, it gradually became a religion in the eyes of the government (4th-6th century), and became a national religion during the Tang dynasty (618-907). In Korea, the kingdom of Koguryo (37 B.C.-668 A.D.) adopted Taoism as the national religion. It is said that Japanese mythology (gods such as Izanagi, Izanami, Amaterasu, etc.) was strongly influenced by Taoism (according to Fukunaga).

The belief in supernatural beings who obtain immortality and magical powers and the belief in Mt. Horai, the immortal land, are typical of secularized Taoism in their pursuit of worldly benefit. These also induced people's desire for longevity. The folk belief associated with the *Ko-shin* vigil is derived from Taoism and is related to the desire for longevity. Here follows a brief description of the story of *sanshi*, which determine a person's demise.

In the Chinese astrological calendar, which combines ten calendar signs with twelve zodiac signs, the *Kanoe-saru* (庚申, *Ko-shin* in an *on* reading) day comes once every 60 days and the *Kanoe-saru* year comes once every 60 years. On the night of the *Ko-shin* day, the *sanshi* (three imaginary worms) living in the human body go to heaven and inform God of the conduct of the host, who is judged as fit to be punished or killed. The *Ko-shin* vigil (*Ko-shin-mori* in Japanese) is a gathering in which people eat and drink all night without sleeping to prevent the *sanshi* from going up to heaven. Concerning this popular Taoistic belief, there are descriptions of it already in 4th-century China, in the Koryo period (918-1392) in Korea and in the Heian period in Japan. In Japan, this custom was mentioned in the *Makura-no-soshi* ("The Pillow Book") of Sei Shonagon written in approximately 1000. Afterwards, *Ko-shin* mounds and *Ko-shin* pagodas which served as the material expression of the belief in the *Ko-shin* vigil became popular in Japan due to the syncretization of Taoism and Buddhism. Stone-made *Ko-shin* monuments were built at the roadside every Ko-shin year. The oldest *Ko-shin* house is on the grounds of Shitenno-ji (a Buddhist temple built by Prince Shotoku) in Osaka, and is a notable example of the syncretization of Buddhism and Taoism.

Taoism was popular among the common people because it was never abstinent but rather pursued worldly benefit (the ease of the body and mind, longevity and prosperity).

The nature of Taoism, with its firm anchor in reality, was easily understandable and its prescriptions easily performable in everyday life. Taoists actively performed special breathing methods and gymnastic exercises (*Qi-gong, Tai-ji-quan*), took hermit drugs ("golden tablets"), went on dietary therapies (not eating cereals), used magic talismans and held ceremonies to become hermits. All these actions derived from people's honest quest for a long life. People's hopes brought about myriad deities in Taoism, which is natural for this realistic and highly popular religion. The pantheon includes the deified Lao Tzu as the most important god, the Yellow Emperor, the Queen Mother of the West and other divinities emanating from *Tao*, as well as many gods of popular belief, including the deified Kuan-ti (関羽, *kan-u* in Japanese), who is a historical hero described in The History of the Three Kingdoms (三国志), and Ma-tzu (媽祖, *maso* in Japanese), who is still a popular goddess protecting travelers.

The thought of Lao Tzu, which is the basis of Taoism, includes the theory of Yin-Yang and the Five Elements, as described below. The theory was specific to China and was developed in ancient China (during the Yin and Chou dynasties). Therefore, we can say that the beliefs of Taoism appeared in the early stages of Chinese history.

The relativism of Taoism had a much greater impact on Zen Buddhism. Zen was generated in India as a sect of Buddhism. Daruma-daishi (Bodhidharma) brought it to southern China in the 6th century (southern Zen). Southern Zen became syncretized with Taoism, which was the main religion of southern China. According to Zen, people can reach Buddhahood internally, through inner reflection and meditation. Therefore, Zen is sometimes at odds with the rest of Buddhism, as Buddhists worship certain images and believe in Amida. Although Zen is a Buddhism sect, it does not pay too much attention on the rigorous interpretation of the *sutras*. Zen especially emphasizes meditation in the Lotus posture as part of the requisite ascetic training. Zen Buddhists perform ascetic training in order to reach the truth through independent effort in the form of repetitive philosophical meditation. Zen is in part similar to the theory of Yin-Yang and the Five Elements, because people meditate to reach philosophical enlightenment. The art of flower arrangement and the tea ceremony are cultural elements specific to Japan established in close connection with Zen, the doctrine of Yin-Yang and the Five Elements, Taoism, etc.

6. The doctrine of Yin-Yang and the Five Elements

The doctrine of Yin-Yang (陰陽) and Wu-Xing (五行, the Five Elements) is a philosophical theory developed in ancient China, a kind of ontology partially analogous to Greek natural philosophy. The Yin-Yang theory is dualistic, in that there are two types (*Yin* and *Yang*) of basic energy (気, *Chi*) from which all matter is generated. For example, the two types of energy manifest as females (yin) and males (yang), night (yin) and day (yang), the moon (yin) and the sun (yang), north (yin) and south (yang), and autumn (yin) and spring (yang). *Chi* (*Qi,* or *Ki* in Japanese) is ubiquitous, like *Tao*, and all objects in the world are formed according to the balance between the two types of *Chi*.

On the other hand, the Wu-Xing theory (五行説) is pluralistic, based on five elements (wood, fire, earth, metal and water), and appears to be incompatible with the dualism of Yin and Yang. However, both theories were complementarily linked to form the doctrine of Yin-Yang and Wu-Xing in ancient China. In this doctrine, the supervisor of the universe is Heaven. The concept of the Lord of Heaven (天帝) can be dated back to the Yin (殷) period (16th-11th century B.C.) of ancient China. Heaven was assumed to express its wishes (the dispositions of Providence) clearly by changing the balance of *Chi*. The constellation Ursa Major was thought to be sacred as the place where people could consult with the will of Heaven. The Wu-Xing theory is based on the Five Elements, which are used to interpret dynamic changes in the world. The Five Elements are intrinsic to every phenomenon and substance in the world, and they both generate and suppress these. These two old theories have become intermingled throughout China's long history.

The original state before earth and heaven were separated is called "*taikyoku*." Human beings are a part of nature, and human disease is also a part of nature. Health is the *Chi* before *Yin* and *Yang* are separated. The theory of Yin-Yang and the Five Elements prevailed from the 3rd century B.C. to the later Han period (25-220 A.D.). The Taoists adopted this theory without hesitation. It is presumed that the theory was originally an ontology meant to explain the universe and nature, or to deal with the relationship of the human being to her body and mind. It was thought that the universal resides in the particular. However, the theory was misapplied later, yielding superstitions, fortune-telling practices, etc. People tried to explain all substances and phenomena based on this theory, and the theory soon became complicated and irrational. In Japan, *On-yo-do*, which is an example of such a superstition, prevailed among people of the Heian period. Calendrical and directional taboos derived from *On-yo-do* are still observed by modern Japanese people as customs.

It is said that the doctrine of Yin-Yang and the Five Elements was imported to Japan in 513 via Baekje, Korea. The creation myth presented in Kojiki or "A Record of Ancient Matters" shows traces of influence by Chinese thought, including Taoism and the doctrine of Yin-Yang and the Five Elements. In the Heian period, the schedules, geographical directions, etc. of events were determined in accordance with the *On-yo-do* (the theory of Yin-Yang and the Five Elements in the Japanese style) as shown in The Pillow Book by Sei Shonagon, The Tale of Genji by Murasaki Shikibu and *Midokanpaku-ki* by Fujiwara-no-Michinaga.

The doctrine left an imprint on the cultures of Japan, China and other East Asian countries. In Japanese culture, the art of flower arrangement, the tea ceremony and the almanac are evident examples, to name a few. In China, both Confucianism and Taoism were generated and the doctrine of Ying-Yang and the Five Elements was adopted. Buddhism, which was imported to Japan via China, was already strongly influenced by the theory of Yin-Yang and the Five Elements when it reached Japan. Buddhism had undergone a substantial modification under the influence of Confucianism and Taoism.

On-yo-do, or *Onmyodo* (陰陽道, the Way of Yin and Yang), which pervaded the Heian period of Japan, was a folk belief in magic and took the form of vulgar superstition, although it was influenced by the original Chinese theories of Yin-Yang and Five Elements. Evidently, therefore, we should differentiate this *On-yo-do* from the doctrine of Yin-Yang and the Five Elements which arose in ancient China. *On-yo-do* was especially popular during the Heian period and many descriptions thereof are contained in "The Tale of Genji", which is the oldest novel in the world. Generally, the theory of Yin-Yang and the Five Elements became blended with Japanese native customs and vulgar superstitions, and remains to this day as habits and customs. For example, fortune-telling, *katatagae*, the Oriental Zodiac, the luckiest day and the unluckiest day of the year, *tomobiki*, etc., are all customs which determine people's schedules in accordance with the events in the traditional calendar. There are many modern Japanese words with the prefix "*ten*" (heaven), such as "*ten-i*" (the mind of Heaven), "*ten-sei*" (the voice of Heaven), "*ten-noh*" (emperor), "*ten-shi*" (the son of Heaven), "*ten-mei*" (the will of Heaven), "*ten-ri*" (natural law), "*ten-sei*" (instinctive), etc.

With regard to the art of flower arrangement, in the Sagagoryu Ikebana School, flowers are arranged according to the principle of concord between *Yin* and *Yang* and the concept of "*ten-en tsi-ho*" (heaven is circular and earth is square), both of which are aspects of traditional Chinese thought. The most fundamental flower composition is *sansaikaku*. In *sansaikaku*, a flower is symbolically arranged using three branches. It means that all matter is generated between heaven (天, *ten*) and earth (地, *tsi*), and human beings (人, *jin*) are positioned between these two lords of creation; thus, the ensemble symbolizes the combination of heaven, earth and human beings (Fig. 9). *Gogyokaku* in the same Ikebana School is a more formal flower composition than *sansaikaku*, and is in concert with the doctrine of Yin-Yang and the Five Elements.

Each branch plays the role of one of the Five Elements (wood, fire, earth, metal and water) and certain rules of arrangement are followed.

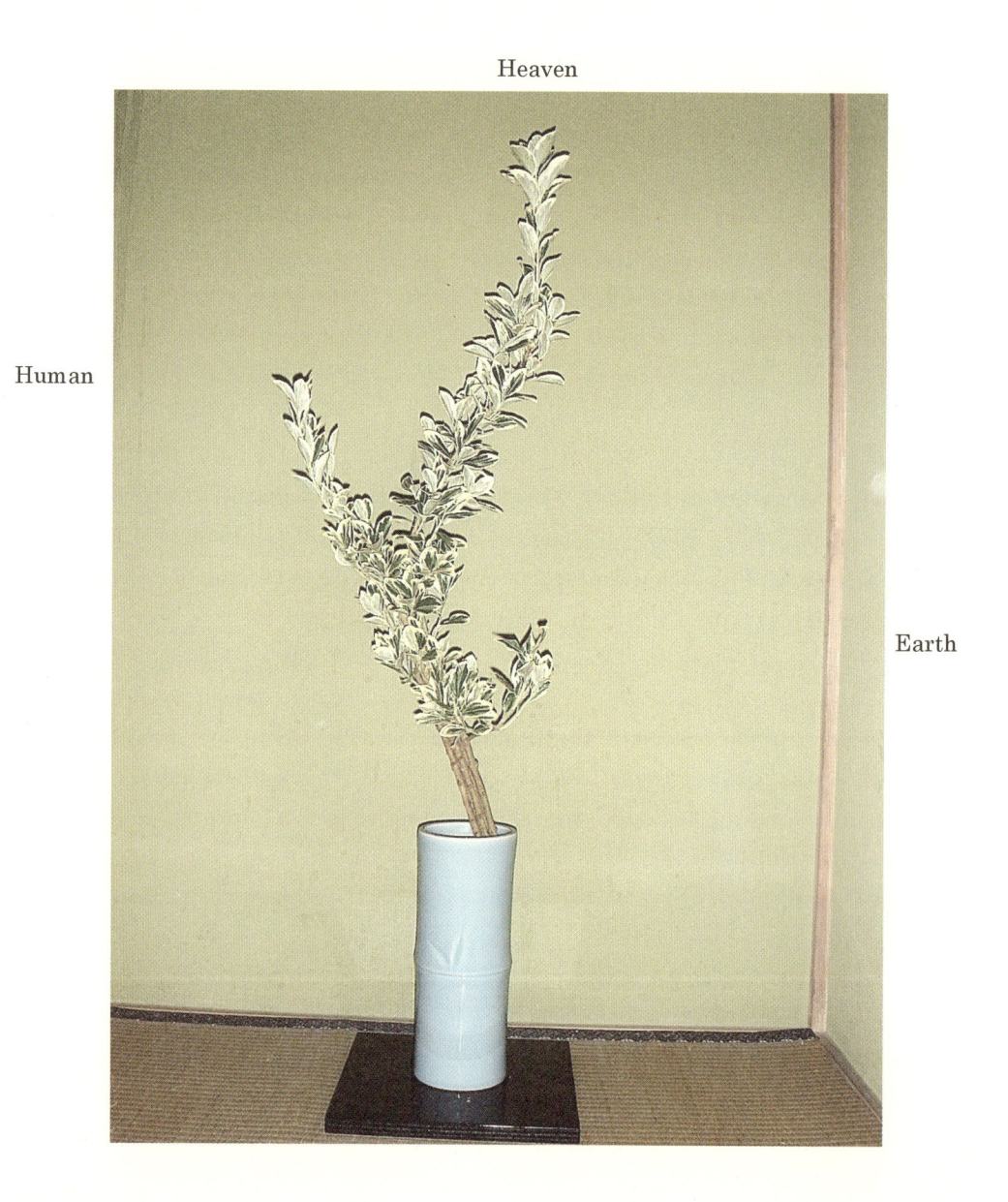

Fig. 9 A typical work of Ikebana.

Chapter IV: *Japanese Religion* 103

Table 3 Correspondences of the Five Elements.

	Wood	Fire	Earth	Metal	Water
Planets (five planets)	Jupiter	Mars	Saturn	Venus	Mercury
Directions (five directions)	East	South	Center	West	North
Seasons (five seasons)	Spring	Summer	Midsummer, Dog Days	Autumn	Winter
Tastes (five tastes)	Acid	Bitter	Sweet	Hot	Salty
Sentiments	Angry	Happy	Musing	Worrying	Scared
Colors	Blue	Red	Yellow	White	Black
Months	1, 2, 3	4, 5, 6		7, 8, 9	10, 11, 12
Virtues (the five cardinal virtues of Confucianism)	Benevolence	Decency	Faith	Gratitude	Wisdom
Five solid organs	Liver	Heart	Spleen	Lung	Kidney
Five hollow organs	Gallbladder	Small Intestine	Stomach	Colon	Bladder
Five crops	Oat	Millet	Japanese Millet	Rice	Beans
Five sense organs	Eye	Tongue	Mouth	Nose	Ear
Five gods	Blue Dragon	Red Phoenix	Kylin (Chinese Unicorn)	White Tiger	Black Turtle-Snake

<Restraint>   <Enhancement>

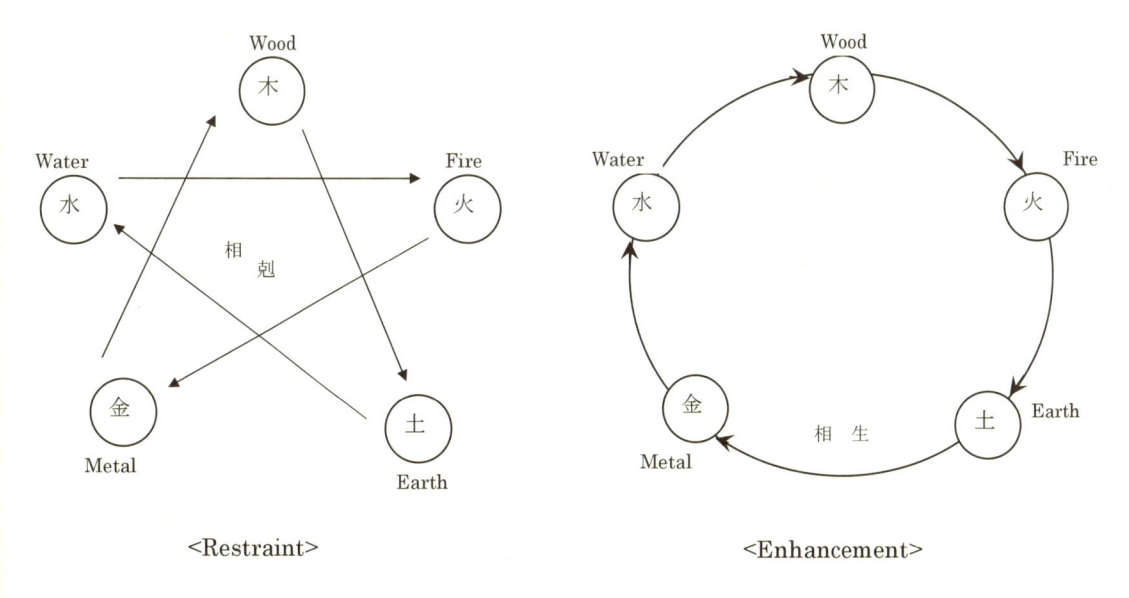

Fig.10 The Five Elements in their interrelationships characterized by Restraint (left) and Enhancement (right).

Shogonka is a flower composition placed on the Buddhist altar. The basic principle of this type of flower arrangement is the *Roku-dai* or the Six Major Elements: earth, water, fire, wind, air and spirit. These elements are derived from Shingon esoteric Buddhism.

Tea plants and the habit of drinking tea originated in China. Chinese people began to drink tea habitually early in the 4th and 5th centuries, knowing that it was good for the mind and body. Initially, they boiled tea leaves with rice, salt, milk and other food items. Their crude manner of drinking tea as a beverage improved to a kind of art in the 8th century (Tang dynasty), when Luwuh (Lu Wu, 陸羽), a poet and Buddhist priest, published a great book on tea entitled "*Chaking*" (*Cha Chin*, 茶経, The Holy Scripture of Tea) around 760. In this cutting-edge book, he describes the nature of tea plants, the preparation of tea leaves and the method of brewing tea. For instance, he tells us to put in salt when the water starts to boil, then to add the cake of tea leaves at the middle stage of boiling, and to finally add cooled hot water at the last stage of boiling. This was the manner of preparing tea described in the *Chaking*, and many such frameworks for tea-drinking were developed by priests in Tang China (618-907). Saicho (767-822) brought tea plants to Japan and planted them near Mt. Hiei in 805. Subsequently, during the Sung dynasty, the style of tea preparation in China evolved from boiled tea to whipped tea. To the ground tea whipped before drinking, no salt was to be added, and this new way of tea blossomed in Sung China, launching a new boom. During this period, in 1187, Eisai (1141-1215) who was primarily a Tendai priest educated on Mt. Hiei as a young man, went voluntarily to Sung China to study more about Buddhism, especially Nanpo (Southern) Zen. He was then 47 years of age and stayed there for four years. Eisai returned to Japan in 1191 and brought with him tea plants and popularized the way of tea as well as Zen Buddhism in Japan. The descendants of those tea plants imported by Eisai have been continuously cultivated in Japan; in fact, one of these plant types is sold today under the famous brand name of *Uji-cha*, and is produced in the Uji district near Kyoto. He wrote *Kissa Yojoki* ("Care of the Health Using Tea") in 1211 and revised it in 1214; it was the first book about tea written in Japan. In this book, Eisai describes the beneficial effects of tea on anorexia, decline in energy, drowsiness and thirst after alcohol intake. Cardiac and diuretic actions were also written. This book was dedicated to the Shogun of Kamakura, Minamoto-no-Sanetomo.

Apart from tea, Eisai is known as the man who introduced Rinzai-shu (a Zen sect) to Japan. Concentrated meditation in the seated position associated with the pursuit of intellectually insoluble themes (*koan*) is used as the method of ascetic practice in Rinzai-shu. Soto-shu is a type of Zen imported by Dogen (1200-1253), a student of

Eisai who went to Sung China after Eisai in 1223 at the age of 24 years. He returned to Japan in 1227 and settled down in Kosho-ji temple in Uji. *Shikantaza* (sitting in a meditative state, cultivating awareness of oneself in the depth of the mind and attaining Buddhahood) was the sole and most important religious practice imposed on his followers. Dogen wrote a very difficult philosophical work entitled "*Shobogenzo.*" Although he claimed to propound a pure form of Zen and fundamentally rejected the concept of authority, people in power as well as the masses gathered around him for instruction. In 1244, he founded the Eihei-ji temple as the main training center of Soto Zen in the Echizen district far from Kyoto and Kamakura. These two sects of Zen, despite their minor differences in practice, captured the minds of the Japanese people at that time and are still a substantial part of life in Japan.

The habit of drinking tea, which remained a mere religious practice in Sung China, evolved in Japan into a uniquely refined practice after Zen was brought to Japan in the Kamakura period and after passing through the Muromachi period (1392-1573). While the manner of preparing tea evolved in China from boiled tea using a tea-cake during the Tang dynasty to the powdered tea whipped in hot water with a bamboo-made whisk in the Sung, and subsequently to the steeped tea in the Ming, as we see in modern days, the Japanese tea ceremony branched out at the level of the whipped or powdered tea used in the Sung. Remaining there, it started to deepen and evolve into a specifically Japanese way of tea which pursues quietness, well-seasoned beauty and refined simplicity. *Wabicha*, or the Japanese tea ceremony, was initiated by Jyuko Murata (1423-1502) in the Muromachi period as a way of preparing powdered tea tinged with Zen. This led to the generation of a novel Japanese culture under the influence of Zen, Taoism and the doctrine of Yin-Yang and the Five Elements as well as intrinsic Shinto factors; the idea was to seek the beauty hidden in nature. The majority of *temae* (点前, the way of serving tea) and *cha-dogu* (utensils) used in the tea ceremony embody the doctrine of Yin-Yang and the Five Elements. Examples include the *hoen* (方円) table, in which the top part is round and the bottom part forms a square, the *hakke* (八卦), a tray with eight images on the surface composed of a triplet combination of *yin* and *yang* signs (*yin-yang-yin* symbolizing the north, and *yang-yin-yang* symbolizing the south), *gogyo* (五行) items in the fireplace (炉) made under a *tatami* floor in the tea room which comprise a wooden frame (木), charcoals (火), an earthenware vessel (土), an iron tea-kettle (金) and water (水), *gogyo* (五行) shelves, the lunar calendar (暦), and five seasonal celebrations (五節句) which include the 7th day of January (人日, *jinjitu*), the Dolls' Festival on March 3rd and the Iris Festival on May 5th as yearly events.

6. The hardiness of the religious and cultural elements of Japan

If we are asked what the religion of present-day Japanese people is, our answer would be that it is a religion resulting from the blending of various religions from China and original Japanese Shinto. It is a formless, as it were "amoebic," religion that has grown big and strong. This would be a correct answer. This is because, for many Japanese people, the prevailing religions cannot be bundled together into one thing.

Shinto, a religion native to Japan, accepted the influence of foreign religions (Buddhism, Confucianism and Taoism transferred via China and Korea) because these had overwhelmingly superior doctrines and cultural elements (construction technologies and governance systems as well as Chinese characters, *kanji*). Shinto could not resist changing itself to survive and developed dramatically as a result. Shinto and the three foreign religions are polytheistic (unlike Islam and Christianity), and so they did not annihilate each other. Naturally, there were small conflicts between these religions when they first came into contact. However, from a comprehensive standpoint, they imitated and complemented each other, improving in the process.

The main characteristic of East Asian religions (China, Korea and Japan) is this peaceful syncretization. It can be said that much of the current culture in Japan grew from the coexistence of these religions and their elements, as seen around us in shrines, temples, customs, calendar and other cultural elements, including the way of tea, the art of flower arrangement, the art of gardening and Zen. Just as the religions which arose in Asia have generally been tolerant of each other and have evolved by complementing one another, we Japanese find it easy to live with other religions in daily life, or, to put it more pointedly, people have an arbitrary attitude toward other religions.

In retrospect, Japanese people early in the Asuka period, which preceded the Nara period and was the age of active official dispatching of diplomatic delegations to China during the Sui and Tang dynasties, in the modern Meiji Restoration which shifted rapidly to an open-door policy to Western culture and civilization, and currently in the period of rapid postwar growth of the economy and the industry, have generally accepted foreign cultures as they were when they first encountered them. Japanese people have an arbitrary mode of living, in that they digest and assimilate foreign cultures gradually in accordance with basic Japanese traits. This mode seems to date back to the policy of Prince Shotoku (574-622), who employed it as a national policy, and remains to this day as an aspect of a profound layer of Japanese wisdom. In fact, shotokn was a great statesman who initiated the democratic rule of Japan by issuing a code of 17 articles of government in which the virtue of harmony or "*wa*" was emphasized.

For example, many Japanese have a Buddhist altar at home which is richly decorated for the *O-bon* festival in summer to welcome the souls of ancestors; therefore, they are Buddhists. But they also have a *kamidana* (a Shinto god shelf) at home. They stretch a *shimenawa* (sacred rope) and clap their hands (*kashiwade*) in the shrine to greet the New Year. In other words, people greet the New Year in the Shinto manner, celebrate the *O-bon* festival in the Buddhist manner and also celebrate Christmas in the Christian manner. They freely adopt multiple religions in their lifestyles. If this is pointed out to them, they easily reply, "It doesn't matter." This arbitrariness, or in a good sense, hardiness, is the expression of one side of the Japanese identity. It is almost incredible for non-Japanese people who believe in a single god.

There are regional differences among the Japanese which manifest as differences in ethical values.

There is a Kansai expression, "*Ikemahennoka?*" ("Do you object if...?"). Kansai people say, "Don't be so restrictive," and import foreign cultures without regard to principles. Kanto people, on the other hand, act based on rules. Seen in this light, they are rationalistic and much more like Westerners. A *bushi* (*samurai*), even when starving, behaves as if his stomach is full. This attitude is expressed in a famous Japanese phrase, "*Bushi wa kuwanedo takayoji,*" which refers to the façade which must be held up by the *bushi*; this also applies to the temperament of the Kanto people. Historically, Japanese people and Japanese culture have developed based on the traits of the Kansai people. This is quite understandable when considering the historical fact that the Nara and Heian cultures originated in the Kansai district. The traits of the Kansai people often make them popular and successful in business and international negotiations. It seems that nations or groups with traits similar to those of the Kansai people are more adept at surviving or succeeding in a difficult situation.

The beliefs of present-day Japanese people regarding the body are based on the traditional customs and habits resulting from the syncretization of multiple Asian religions. We can therefore understand that the decisions regarding organ transplants, for instance, are made, not by the individual in question as in Western countries, but by his or her family. As shown above, *wa* (conformity, harmony) was emphasized in the policies of Prince Shotoku when the country was founded. This moral view has been deeply embedded in the core feelings of the Japanese people. "*Wa*," as defined in dictionaries, means "unstrained" and "warm." Japanese people always consult each other in order to create a buffer zone between them. This is quite different from Western individualism, where the action of a person is approved of only if it is based on autonomous decision-making.

A culture or an ethos is formed over a long period of time. We should understand that we cannot homogenize the world all at once.

Buddhism, a religion developed in East Asia, is based on the monism of the physical (body) and spiritual (spirit and soul) aspects (mind-body unity). The body is handled with care in Buddhism. Dead bodies are treated with the highest respect in Confucianism, in which people hold their forefathers in great veneration in the ancestral flow of life. The situation is the same for current Taoism. These East Asian attitudes are apparently different from the mind-body dualism espoused by the ancient Greeks and modern Westerners. They consider dead bodies simply as inanimate matter.

7. The history and religion of Vietnam, and similarities to Japan

Vietnam, which is an agricultural country in the South East, has a long coastline that stretches from the north to the south of the South China Sea. Recent statistics (according to the homepage of the Vietnamese Embassy) reveal that Vietnam has a territory of 330,000 km^2 and a population of 82 million, with 2.74 million people in Hanoi and 5.23 million people in Ho Chi Minh (formerly known as Saigon), and that Vietnam ranks second in the world in terms of rice exports. As shown in the following chronology, the history of Vietnam until the middle of the 20th century was characterized by tenacious national resistance to invasions by armies from neighboring countries.

In describing the religion and ethics of Japan, it is very useful to draw comparisons with Vietnam, which has undergone circumstances similar to Japan in its political history and religious background. In their relationships with China during the establishment of the great Asian empires, both Japan and Vietnam were invaded by the Yuan dynasty (元, 1271-1368) founded by Genghis Khan. Further, both countries are remarkably similar in terms of mentality, religion, and ethics. Also, by a curious coincidence, both countries have at some stage adopted the policy of national isolation and the banning of Christianity, attitudes which reflect the rivalry between Asian traditional culture and Western logic.

History of Vietnam reveals strong influences from China, as in Japan.
111 B.C.: Emperor Wu (武帝) of the Earlier Han (前漢, 202 B.C.-8 A.D.) conquered Vietnam (南越; Nanyue) and established three commanderies (郡), namely Jiaozhi (交趾; now known as Tonkin), Jiuzhen (九真; now known as Thanh Hoa), and Rinan (日南; near present Hue) in the north. Sinicization, which involved the introduction of sinicized

rules of decorum, Confucian ethics, and plowing using cows and iron farming implements, was stepped up in these regions.

40 A.D.: Rebellion of the Trung (徵) sisters against the Han. This ethnic uprising was suppressed after a few years by the Han army, but the story of the heroic acts of the sisters has been handed down from generation to generation in Vietnam as a symbol of and a point of pride in ethnic resistance until now.

The 4th century: The Kingdom of Champa (founded in the 2nd century by the Cham people in central Vietnam along the southeastern coast of Indochina; a Sanskrit inscription on a monument, some Hindu temples, and some sculptures from that period remain in existence showing the influence of Indian culture) prospered as a location for marine trade in perfumes (such as *agalloch*), ivory, ceramics and slaves, and gradually became a power that confronted northern Vietnam (Dai Viet). The prosperity of Champa continued until the 15th century. From 1278 through 1284, Champa was invaded from the sea by Kublai Khan, who coveted the fortune to be made from trading (Mongol invasion).

679: The Tang (唐) dynasty in China established a Duhufu (都護府; 'protectorate'), which was called the Annan Duhufu (安南都護府), in Vietnam. The administrative system of Tang was introduced.

766: Abe-no-Nakamaro (阿倍仲麻呂; Chinese name: Chao-Heng), who was originally a student sent to the Tang from Japan in 717 and served Emperor Xuanzong without returning home, was dispatched to the Annan Duhufu in Vietnam by the Tang to act as a Governor General.

938: Ngo Quyen (呉権) defeated the Chinese military from the Southern Han, succeeding the Tang dynasty after its downfall at the Bach Dang River, to become the first independent king of Vietnam.

980: The Early Le (前黎) dynasty was founded and repelled the invasion of Sung (宋) China.

1009: The Ly (李) dynasty was founded, and in the following year its capital was moved to Thang Long (昇龍; now known as Hanoi). The Ly dynasty (1010-1225) gradually accepted Confucianism, but since all of its kings were worshippers of Buddhism, many pagodas and temples were constructed.

1225: The Tran (陳) dynasty was founded, with its capital in Hanoi. During this period, nationalism peaked as invasions by the Yuan were repeatedly repulsed. This dynasty succeeded in the centralization of power through active land reclamation in the Red River Delta in the north, the development of paddy fields, and the introduction of the Chinese legal system. Buddhism, as well as Confucianism and Taoism, prospered due to the influence of Chinese culture. Thai Tong (太宗; reign: 1225-1258), the first king of the Tran dynasty, was a pious Buddhist who contributed to the fusion of the three religions in Vietnam.

1428: The Le (黎) dynasty was founded and Confucianism prospered. Le Loy, who won the war of liberation against Ming (明) China, founded the Le dynasty (country name: Dai Viet). He became king under the name of Le Thai To (太祖; reign: 1428-1433) and brought the equal land allocation system into effect (capital: Hanoi).

End of the 15th century: Le Thanh Tong (黎聖宗; reign: 1460-1497), the fifth king of the Le dynasty, actively introduced Confucianism and the civil service examination (科挙) system to build up a centralized bureaucratic state that was more stable than either the Ly dynasty or Tran dynasty. The Chinese civil service examination system became entrenched in Vietnam. In addition, Le Thanh Tong was active in developing external policies. He virtually conquered the Kingdom of Champa and assumed hegemony of Indochina through ingenious diplomacy that persuaded the Ming to abandon the invasion.

The 16th and 17th centuries: "Japan Town" in Hoi An (central Vietnam) prospered [Age of Discovery; in Japan, it was the era of trade using Red Seal ships before national isolation]. The numerous pagodas constructed in Hue (central Vietnam) during this period bear testimony to the cultural influences of both ancient Vietnam and Champa.

1802: The Nguyen (阮) dynasty was founded and its capital was moved from Hanoi to Hue (central Vietnam). Gia Long (嘉隆), the first emperor of the Nguyen Dynasty, founded the dynasty under the patronage of local Chinese merchants and colonialists, and, as a matter of course, reigned over the country based on reactionary feudalism, which reflected the intention of the French colonialists.

1820: Upon accession to the throne, Minh Mang (明命), the second emperor of the Nguyen dynasty, changed the general Vietnamese attitude towards Western aggressors and adopted a policy of national isolation. The emperor was a devout Confucian who established a centralized system of government modeled after the system of Qing (清). He treated local Chinese merchants well, and on the whole he attempted to convert the country into a miniature version of China, exploiting the local Chinese merchants. The palace in Hue, modeled after the Forbidden Palace in Beijing, was constructed during this period. The vast mausoleum intended for the emperors of the Nguyen dynasty was Chinese in style, in that it was decorated with carved dragons and phoenixes. The emperor was a devout protector of Buddhism, and numerous pagodas were constructed and restored during his reign.

1833: Emperor Minh Mang prohibited the propagation of Christianity with the aim of preventing the invasion of the country by French colonialists. The relationship between France and the Nguyen dynasty gradually deteriorated.

1874: France forced the dynasty to approve French sovereignty over Cochinchina (southern Vietnam) and governed it as its crown colony. Furthermore, with regard to northern Vietnam, France forced the dynasty to approve the opening of ports and to allow free navigation of the Red River.

1884: All of Vietnam became a French colony. The Sino-French War broke out.

1885: The Qing Empire gave up suzerainty over Vietnam (a result of the Sino-French War).

1887: France established the Government-General of Indochina (French Indochina).

1930: The Communist Party of Vietnam was established.

Vietnam is a country with similarities to Japan in terms of history and religion. The two countries are similar in that they have long been Buddhist countries and, as small countries, have belonged to the cultural sphere using Chinese characters. The life of Abe-no-Nakamaro (阿倍仲麻呂, 698-770), who was a government-sponsored student sent from Japan to Tang China in the Nara Period, depicts faithfully the relationship between China and its neighboring countries during the Tang period (618-907). Abe stayed in Tang for some 50 years, and was dispatched to Vietnam (known to the Chinese as 'Annan') as a public servant of the Tang by Emperor Xuanzong (玄宗皇帝). "*Amanohara furisakemireba kasuganaru mikasa-no-yamani ideshi tsukikamo*" (translation: "Looking up at the night sky; there is a moon; oh, it is indeed the same moon; as I have seen it in my home in Japan; it was afloat like this beyond Mt. Mikasa in Kasuga.") is a *waka* (a 31-syllable Japanese poem) composed by Abe, who longed for a glimpse of his home in Nara, which at that time was the capital of Japan. Mt. Mikasa lies at the east to the Kasuga Shrine in Nara, and is adjacent to Mt. Wakakusa. After retiring from public service in Vietnam, Abe returned to Chang'an (長安), the capital of Tang China, and died there at the age of 73 years.

Abe left Japan primarily to study the advanced culture of the Tang, mastered the Chinese characters there, and was dispatched to Vietnam as an excellent public servant of the Tang. This story of Abe lends credence to the notion that both Vietnam and Japan were tributaries to the Tang during that era and constituted peripheral regions of the vast cultural sphere relying on Chinese characters.

Other examples of similarities between Japan and Vietnam include diligence as a national trait, the attachment of great importance to the Confucian family system and social ethics as evidently seen in the popularity of *Oshin* (a Japanese TV program) in

Vietnam, and national efforts towards industrialization with a striking resemblance between the current modernization process in Vietnam and Japan's post-war reconstruction.

Vietnam, which is a long and narrow country extending to the north and south, comprises some 50 ethnic groups, among which the Kinh group accounts for some 90%. The Kinh people live in granaries, such as the basin of the Red River in northern Vietnam, coastal plains, which include Hue and Hoi An in central Vietnam, and the Mekong delta in southern Vietnam, and hold pivotal positions in the politics, economy, and culture of Vietnam. The word "Kinh" (京) means "metropolis," which is reminiscent of how the people of Vietnam were obliged for long periods to live under the tutelage of the highly advanced Chinese civilization. In this respect also, Vietnam is similar to Japan, which has evolved by embracing Chinese civilization since the remote ages of the Imperial embassies to the Sui (遣隋使) and the Tang (遣唐使).

However, a decisive difference between the two countries would be that Vietnam has long survived by relying on its own ethnic wisdom even under incessant meddling by foreign countries including China, French, Japan and more recently the U.S.A.

Religion in Vietnam

Eighty percent of Vietnamese people are Buddhists. Every village has a temple and a pagoda that support the spiritual lives of the people. Over 2000 years have passed since the introduction of Buddhism into Vietnam, and Buddhism lives on in the people without change. There is a proverb that says: "The land belongs to the king, the pagoda belongs to the village, and the scenery belongs to the Buddha." This shows that Buddhism has long dwelt in the hearts of all villagers.

Gautama Buddha (566-468 B.C.) founded Buddhism at the basin of the Ganges river in India in the 5th century B.C. The doctrines of the Buddha preached a breakaway from the anguish of life through the practice of benevolence and the resulting attainment of spiritual enlightenment (*nirvana*). One hundred years after the death of the Buddha, Buddhism split into various small sects; roughly speaking, Buddhism split into conservative Theravada Buddhism, which is faithful and true to the words, deeds, and precepts of the Buddha, and Mahayana Buddhism, which propagates the doctrines of Buddha via the *sutras*.

Early on, Hinayana or Theravada Buddhism was propagated from India to neighboring countries, including Sri Lanka, Myanmar, Thailand, and south Vietnam. In contrast, Mahayana Buddhism was propagated to distant Xiyu (西域; 'the Western Regions'), Tibet, China, Korea, Japan and north Vietnam. Buddhism found its way into

China in the era of the Earlier Han (202 B.C.-8 A.D.). Thereafter, the fusion of three thought systems, Buddhism, Confucianism and Taoism, occurred. Following the translation of the Sanskrit Buddhist scriptures into classical Chinese by Kumarajiva (344-413), Buddhism attracted a large number of followers among the Chinese population and the peoples of adjacent countries controlled by China. In approximate terms, the era of Han (漢), which comprises the Earlier Han (202 B.C.-8 A.D.) and the Later Han (25-220 A.D.), was the era of Confucianism, and the eras of Sui (隋, 581-619) and Tang (唐, 618-907) were the eras of prosperity for Buddhism.

Buddhism in the northern and middle parts of Vietnam is the same as the Mahayana Buddhism which spread into China, Korea and Japan. Buddhism was first introduced into Vietnam in the 1st or 2nd century by way of the southeastern sea route. Later, Buddhism, which had been introduced into China by way of Xiyu (西域; 'the Western Regions') and prospered therein, was fully introduced into Vietnam by land. Since Vietnam has been a small country under the constant influence of China since the dawn of its history until the invasions by modern European colonialists, its politics, culture and religion bear strong resemblances to those of Japan. For example, the peaceful and smooth fusion of the three religions (Confucianism, Taoism, and Buddhism) is commonly observed in Vietnam and Japan as well as in China. In Vietnam, there are numerous Buddhist temples complete with pagodas, and Chinese characters are used therein. It is an ethical principle that parents live under the same roof as the families of their children, and children attach great importance to the intentions or views of their parents.

Since Confucianism is a religion that espouses social order, it has been historically exploited by various rulers for political purposes in China, Korea, Japan and Vietnam.

Ironically, after Vietnam achieved independence with the victory at the battle of the Bach Dang River in 938 A.D. as the turning point, the rulers of Vietnam implemented a policy of attaching greater emphasis to Confucianism than previous rulers, who were under the domination of China for about 1,000 years beginning with the conquest of Vietnam by Emperor Wu (武帝) of the Earlier Han in 111 B.C., as described next:

The Ly (李) dynasty (founded in 1009): The Chinese civil service examination (科挙) system was introduced, and the Chinese system of government was introduced in order to centralize the power.

The Tran (陳) dynasty (founded in 1225): The Chinese civil service examination system was refined, Confucian culture prospered, and Chinese poems were popular among people of high birth. Regarding Buddhism, the Zen sect was favored.

The Le (黎) dynasty (founded in 1428): The Chinese civil service examination system was inherited from the Ly and Tran dynasties, and the centralized system was consolidated further. Le Thanh Tong (黎聖宗; reign: 1460-1497), the fifth king, read and understood the Four Books and Five Classics (四書五経), as he was a distinguished Confucian. He was also an eminent composer of Chinese poems. It was during his reign that the Vietnamese people exerted their ethnic power to the maximum.

The Nguyen (阮) dynasty (founded in 1802) adopted the systems of the Le dynasty. Minh Mang (明命), the second emperor of the Nguyen dynasty, was a devout Confucian. He governed the country, drawing on the model of governance in Beijing. He also implemented the Chinese civil service examination system, exploited the people, and invaded Cambodia and Laos.

As shown above, Confucianism represents a highly sophisticated system of government that was used by the Vietnamese kings more as a system to maintain social stability and governance than as a religion. Confucianism and Taoism were introduced by the Chinese, who conquered and dominated Vietnam for as long as 1,000 years. In comparison with these two religions, Buddhism, which originated in India and was introduced into Vietnam first by sea and later by land, appears to have been a genuine religion that dwelt in the hearts of the Vietnamese people, as evidenced by the numerous pagodas constructed in ancient times.

A characteristic of Asian religion is the peaceful and smooth fusion of three major religions, Confucianism, Taoism, and Buddhism. It should be noted that this characteristic is commonly observed in the cultural sphere relying on Chinese characters, which includes Vietnam, Japan, Korea and China. However, the ethnic history of Vietnam clearly shows that Confucianism and Buddhism have played the main role in governance and religious faith, respectively. The religious mindset of the Vietnamese is characterized by the three religions, but always with Buddhism as the nucleus. This religious mindset was also shared by the kings of Vietnam. While both the Ly dynasty (李朝, founded in the 11th century) and the Tran dynasty (陳朝, founded in the 13th century) gradually adopted Confucianism with the aim of establishing a centralized state, the kings were devout Buddhists. The kings themselves practiced asceticism in the manner of Buddhist monks and willingly offered their treasures for the construction of numerous pagodas. In examining the significance of Buddhism for the Vietnamese people, it is noteworthy that this type of piety was adopted even by the rulers of the Le dynasty (黎朝) and the Nguyen dynasty (阮朝), at a time when Buddhism was in decline.

Usually, village pagodas are located in places that command an excellent view, and people gather for festivals at the pagodas. Layered pagodas, gates, ornamental flowers, and images of the Buddha together generate much solemnity. People offer prayers to the Buddha. At the pagodas, people find spiritual release in the scent of incense. As described above, the pagodas are vital to the villages and the people.

Regarding Buddhist sects, the Ch'an (Zen) school of Buddhism which prospered in southern China, and especially the Linchi (臨済, *rinzai* in Japanese) school of Buddhism based on the *koan*, or Zen texts, was the main school of Buddhism introduced into Vietnam. The Bodhidharma school of Buddhism (達磨宗) was introduced into Vietnam from China by an Indian priest in 580, and in the Tang era (820), the Southern school of Ch'an (南宗禅) Buddhism was introduced into Vietnam by Vo Ngon Thong (無言通). These two schools of Zen Buddhism gained popularity among the people of high birth in Vietnam, together with Chinese poetry, etc. During the Ly dynasty (李朝), policies were adopted which ensured the prosperity of Buddhism, and Zen monks were frequently promoted to important positions in the government.

Vietnam and the dragons

In Vietnam, there exists an old folk story about the birth of the country, in which the son of a dragon and the daughter of an immortal wizard fell in love. Dragons are frequently depicted on monuments in Vietnam. Although this appears to reflect the long-term domination by China, numerous legends, the designation of the capital (actual Hanoi) of the first Vietnamese state (the Ly dynasty) as Thang Long (昇龍; 'ascending dragon'), and the dragon worship by the Vietnamese people can be traced back to remote antiquity. Ly Thai To (太祖, 1009-1025), the first king of the Ly Dynasty, is well-known for his efforts to propagate Buddhism, and he skillfully used folklore, legends, religions and customs in the governance of the country. The literature of the Ly dynasty refers repeatedly to the appearance of dragons, including the story of the renaming of the capital to Thang Long. When Vietnam became independent from China, Ly Thai To encouraged Vietnamese nationalism by skillfully mixing the dragon worship indigenous to Vietnam (whether dragon worship originated in Vietnam or was imported from China or India is a subject that requires further investigation) with feudalism and the Buddhist culture imported from China. According to the legends of Vietnam, the Vietnamese (Kinh) people are the descendents of a dragon. The Ly dynasty used the dragon as the symbol of royal authority based on legends with the aim of governing the country, and in the Tran dynasty (陳朝), the dragon was used to enhance the legitimacy of the dynasty.

It is interesting to note that legends and folk stories about dragons, which are imaginary animals, persist worldwide. Most of these tales involve water or rain. Regarding the roots of the dragon legend, the Chinese dragon originates in the innermost depths of Mongolia. The Chinese dragon has four feet with sharp claws, two tusks, a beard, scales, etc. The dragon that was transmitted to Japan is identical to that described above. In the Han era, this image of the dragon was already accepted. In the Five-Element philosophy (五行思想), the Blue Dragon (青龍) protects the East, the Red Phoenix (朱雀) protects the South, the White Tiger (白虎) protects the West, and the Black Turtle-Snake (玄武) protects the North. On a bronze-ware piece dating back to the Yin era (殷; 16th-11th century B.C.), which is an ancient Chinese dynasty, there is a dragon-like image. On the other hand, the dragon in India is drawn as a *naga* (snake), which resembles a cobra, and is a guardian god of the Buddha. It lacks feet and nails, unlike the Chinese dragon. Cambodia is a landlocked country contiguous to Vietnam. This country, known for the Angkor Wat, came under strong Indian cultural influence. These circumstances are reminiscent of the Kingdom of Champa, which was once a prosperous place in central Vietnam but which eventually collapsed. The Cambodian people also have legends in which their ancestors are described as dragons. While the Cambodian dragon looks like a *naga*, the Vietnamese dragon has four feet like the Chinese dragon. It is very interesting to discover in Southeast Asia an isolated cultural sphere with a depiction of the dragon that is different from that found in neighboring Vietnam. In the future, our study of history, culture and ethics in Asian countries needs to encompass these profound aspects.

References
1) Michihiro Ishihara: Gishi Wajin Den. Iwanami Shoten, Tokyo, 1951
2) Keiji Nishitani: Shukyo To Wa Nanika (What is religion?). Sobunsha, Tokyo, 1961
3) Mannen Ueda, Masayuki Okada, Tadao Ihjima, Takeo Sakaeda, Denichi Iida: Daijiten. Kodansha, Tokyo, 1965
4) Genmyo Murase: Chazen Ichimai. Kyoikushintyosha, Tokyo, 1966
5) Keiji Nishitani: Shukyo To Bunka (Religion and Culture). Kokusai Nihon Kenkyusho, Nishinomiya, Japan, 1969
6) Yukei Matsunaga: Mikkyo No Rekishi. Heirakuji Shoten, Kyoto, 1969
7) Masaaki Ueda: Nihon No Genzo~Kunitsukami No Inochi~. Bungeishunjyu, Tokyo, 1970
8) Mitsuji Fukunaga: Dohkyo To NIhonbunka (Taoism and Japanese Culture). Jinbun Shoin, Kyoto, 1982
9) Yoshinori Takeuchi; edited and translated by James W. Heisig: The Heart of

Buddhism. The Crossroad Publishing Company, New York, 1983
10) Mitsuji Fukunaga: Dohkyo To Kodainihon (Taoism and Ancient Japan). Jinbun Shoin, Kyoto, 1987
11) Tetsuro Watsuji, Yoshinori Takeuchi: "Shamon Dogen", "Kyogyoshinsho No Tetsugaku". Ryubunkan, Tokyo, 1987
12) Mitsuji Fukunaga: Chugoku No Tetsugaku・Shukyo・Geijyutsu (Chinese Philosophy, Religion and Art). Jinbun Shoin, Kyoto, 1988
13) Minoru Sonoda: Shinto. Kobundo, Tokyo, 1988
14) Daisetsu Suzuki: Zen To Wa Nanika (What is Zen?). Shunjyusha, Tokyo, 1991
15) Yoshikazu Ishida: Nihon No Shukyotetsugaku, Sobunsha, Tokyo, 1993
16) Kaji: Silent Religion-Confucianism. Chikuma Shobo, Tokyo, 1994
17) Kohtaro Shima: Kukai No Hukei. Tyuohkoronnsha, Tokyo, 1995
18) Shuzo Ikeda: Shizenshukyo No Chikara (Power of Natural Religions). Iwanami Shoten, Tokyo, 1998
19) Yoshinori Takeuchi in association with James W. Heisig, Paul L. Swanson, and Joseph S. O'Leary: Buddhist Spirituality Ⅰ & Ⅱ. A Herder & Herder Book, 1999
20) Yoshinori Takeuchi: Takeuchi Yoshinori Tyosakushu Vols 1~5. Hozokan, Kyoto, 1999
21) Lao Tzu; translated by David Hinton: Tao Te Ching. Counterpoint, New York, 2000
22) Yasuhiro Ono, Sekiyo Shimode, Shigetugu Sugiyama, Norihisa Suzuki, Minoru Sonoda, Yasuaki Nara, Masahide Bitoh, Masao Hujii, Hitoshi Miyake, Noboru Miyata: Nihonshukyo Jiten. Kobundo, Tokyo, 2001
23) Hajime Nakamura, Mitsuji Fukunaga, Yoshiroh Tamura, Tohru Konno, Fumihiko Sueki (Editors): Iwanami Bukkyo Jiten. Iwanami Shoten, Tokyo, 2002
24) Kakuzo Okakura; translated by Hiroshi Muraoka: The Book of Tea (Tya No Hon).. Iwanami Shoten, Tokyo, 2002
25) Jennifer Oldstone-Moore: Taoism. Oxford University Press, Oxford, 2003
26) Dogen: Syobogenzo 1~4. Iwanami Shoten, Tokyo, 2006

Chapter Ⅴ: *Culture and Ethics*

1. Cultural relativity

Cultures are generated wherever humans live. A culture is an "atmosphere" surrounding humans, more specifically, a "human-smelled atmosphere at the very surface of the earth. As the physical atmosphere including expired gasses such as O_2, CO_2 and many organic gases deriving from humans become accumulated and blended to be brewed in the long interval of history ranging over centuries, cultures are formed over many generations in interrelation of humans with their surroundings. Cultures are what humans create or are conscious of and the behaviors of humans, and further, they are the nourishment on which humans thrive and grow. The English word "culture" originates from the Latin term "*cultura*," a word whose original meanings include "cultivation," "cultivated land" and "lifestyle habits" (Latin-Japanese Dictionary, 1974, Kenkyu-sha).

We are right in the midst of prosperity of natural science today. More appropriately, we are destined to be in the modernized life whether we like it or not. Actually, we cannot stop thinking in a rational way everyday and pursuing modernization or contributing toward scientific advance as a result. We are buried like a habit in an ordinary life with so rich convenience provided by profuse products of modern science and industrial technology. However, it is also true that real relief of mind or relax from mental tightness is indispensable for human existence or healthy mentality of humans, as is clear from the past. We are composed of two parts as shown in many ways of dichotomy as, emotional and rational, passion and reason, ideal and materialistic, metaphysical and physical. Accordingly, even if we are increasingly placed more and more from now on in a milieu of substance or causality, we need of necessity to get a time of relief of mind to maintain the totality of human. A well-mellowed and loose world which is spiritually fertile or the world in which complete humanity can be feasible exists independently of the world of causality. As shown above, culture is the whole of historical accumulation of all the customs, habits, regimes, religions, creations, developments, modifications, human actions and thoughts which are generated at the front of mutually transformative interactions between humans or between humans and their environments.

Humans make cultures. Cultures foster and change humans like incubators.

Suppose that a community (society, family, village, city, nation, etc.) is geographically isolated from other regions. The culture will be specific to that community, its climate and its atmospheric phenomena. Seen in this light, cultures have geographical and regional specificity. Cultures also change historically and temporally through various types of interactions. Therefore, it is natural that cultures have historical specificity as well.

The four major factors which determine the regional characteristics of cultures are as follows:

① **Isolation from or interaction with other cultures**
② **The ethos and the religious characteristics prevalent in the society**
③ **Ethnicity**
④ **Climate and geography**

With regard to the interaction of a culture with other ones designated as ①, in some cases, the regional characteristics are lost because transportation facilities or means of communication are made available. Cultures sometimes decline or perish due to wars or invasions. These examples are too many to list in the history and actually in progress currently in many areas around the globe.

Here is one example from the past. The Incan civilization initiated in the 13th century in South America was at the height of its specific prosperity isolated from the affects of other continents until the early 1530s when the Spanish conquistador, Francisco Pizarro destroyed the Incan Empire. The Empire had the capital at Cusco locating as high as 3500 meters above the sea level and controlled over a wide range of geographical areas in the Andes Mountains extending from the present Ecuador to Chili. The Incan people had a high level civilization attained enormously in the technology as seen in the construction of roads and irrigation systems as well as the architecture of palaces and temples but unfortunately they did not possess their own writing system. They worshipped in the sun god as state religion and magnificent facilities for rituals were left. Their proper religion was removed from the earth by a foreign monotheistic "steamroller" when their domestic culture came into contact with the one of conquering Europeans.

As an ongoing example of cultural interaction, we could take up the Internet. Its rapid spread is now enhancing the process in which the regional characteristics of various cultures are being wiped out. A great wave of cultural globalization is presently underway with an advanced technology of the Internet just in association with unipolarization of the world ideology around the United States and its colleagues after the disintegration of the Soviet Union. The one-way movement called "Americanization" or globalization brought about by the IT revolution is now destroying the wall causing the regionality of many cultures. In People's Republic of China which is another big country of socialism, industries related to IT are acutely rising and the prevalence of cellular phones among the people has been outstanding in a couple of years after 2000. How fast does the world-wide liberalization of information as such brought about by the IT revolution annihilate the conventional regionality and uniqueness of a culture or religion that has thus far been strictly preserved during history? This "experiment" has just started.

The ethos and the religious characteristics of a culture designated as ② are expressions of the religious feelings specific to the community in question. Religious feelings are indispensable elements of human existence as both archaeology and cultural anthropology have clearly revealed everywhere of the world. When we look at the establishment of any communities in the history, the religious feelings of all people there were generally the same and their worship was directed to a common object. Once a religious ethos is formed as such, the people react to the ethos and adapt themselves to take it in order to live on in the community. Cultures and communities grow in such mutual reflection. The ethos and the human are thus interdependent and cultures develop in a spiral cycle of the two.

The brewing of specific cultures in their own ethos is seen all over the world and throughout history.

For example, in China, which occupies a vast geographical area, there are cultural differences between northern China, which espouses Confucianism, and southern China, which espouses Taoism. Also, to outline the cultural differences between China and Japan, Chinese culture is principally based on Chinese thoughts (the doctrine of Yin-Yang and the Five Elements, the philosophy of Lao Tzu and Chuan Tzu, the concepts of Taoism and Confucianism), whereas Japanese culture is largely based on Buddhism. Additionally, when we look at Japan itself, Kyoto-Osaka districts called *Kamigata* or *Kansai* have traditionally different cultures from those of Tokyo-centered districts called *Kanto*, for instance in dialects, accents, wits appealing to the mentality, morals and business.

Ethnicity as ③ above is the largest factor which determines the regionality of cultures. This can be concluded from the fact that the first human beings were born in Africa, according to the studies on the human genome. Human beings then migrated to Europe, Asia and America by land. The various races and ethnic groups observed today were generated as a result of the need to adapt to the various natural environments in the places where these migratory humans settled.

Racial or ethnic diversification was inevitable for human beings in the world history, because wherever they settled they have always composed a regional part of the global ecosystem there. Dark skin was developed to protect the human body from ultraviolet rays causing dermal cancer and death. Dense body hairs and a robust physique were necessary for life of humans in cold climates and for their survival through hunting and defending themselves against carnivorous animals in a harsh environment. Seen in this light, it is very natural that each race or ethnic group has its specific cultural traits depending on the place where it relates. What is to become of this cultural diversity in the recent wave of globalization potently proceeding with information technology (IT), an acute process which started not more than two decades ago?

With regard to the climate and geography as ④, Hippocrates (460-377 B.C.), an illustrious physician of ancient Greece, discussed the effects of climate on the disposition of the human organism. Aristotle (384-322 B.C.) who was a great discipline of Platon (427-347 B.C.) made similar observations. In Japan, Tetsuro Watsuji (1889-1960) published a famous Japanese work, *"Hudo"* or "The Climate" concerning the influence of the climate on the racial mentality in 1935.

In the "On Airs, Waters, and Places" included in the "*Corpus Hippocraticum*", Hippocrates, an outstanding scientist in the ancient Greek, mentioned that differences in human disposition were due to differences in the climate. Asia has a warm climate and good water; therefore, grasses and trees grow well there, and the human temperament is generally warm and soft. However, he also described that the people living in such bounteous natural conditions are rather not gifted with courage, patience and spiritual energy:

And with regard to the pusillanimity and cowardice of the inhabitants, the principal reason the Asiatic are more unwarlike and of gentler disposition than the Europeans is the nature of the seasons, which do not undergo any great changes either to heat or cold, or the like; for there is neither excitement of the understanding nor any strong change of the body whereby the temper might be ruffled and they be roused to inconsiderate emotion and passion, rather than living as they do always in the state. (Part 16, *On Airs, Waters, and Places*)

A Japanese philosopher, Tetsuro Watsuji, who was a leading ethicist as wrote "Ethics as a study on humans", established ethics as a separate field of study in Japan. In his another book named *"Hudo"* or "The Climate", he described his thoughts about the affect of climates on human character. In this context, he separated the pattern of climates into three categories, based on the landscapes, seascapes and weather which he observed during his long voyage to Europe via the coast of the South East, the Indian

Ocean and the Arabian Gulf by steam ship.

Japan, China, India and many other countries in Asia fall under the category of the monsoon climate, which is characterized by "high humidity" according to Watsuji. He said that the monsoon causes humans to become receptive and submissive and to lose motivation and firmness of intent.

He characterized the desert climate using the word "constant dryness" In such a difficult climate; nature does not bestow any blessings on humans, who become militant and resistant. In his view, it is best for humans to develop because they have to endure the trials of life through fighting hard in a milieu of the desert. He described about humans and climates which he observed in the Gulf of Aden, Mt. Sinai, and Arabian deserts.

The third is the climate related to pastures, as observed in the large grassy areas of Europe. Watsuji thought that this climate typified Europe. It is neither too moist nor too dry. There is dryness in summer and moisture in winter, and the pastures yield rich grass without weeds. Nature shows in this climate both its "rationality" and "submissiveness". This is the theory of Watsuji as it was expounded in "The Climate". Although we note today that his theory at the time should be something discounted considering his heightened feelings as an enthusiastic traveler going so far on ship to Europe to learn, there are surely acute and important factual observations in his book as shown in differential affects among the climates of the "tropical monsoons" seen in South Asia and the Indian Ocean, the "deserts" of the Arabian Peninsula and the "wide pastures and grasslands" of Europe on the mentality of habitants in each region. Yet, it is inevitable that he is to be criticized for having the preconceived notion that the cultures of ancient Greece and modern Europe are ideal and worthy of aspiring to. Also, he placed the "monsoons" and "deserts" on the same level with the "European grasslands," which I think is incorrect. Because, the latter is an artificial condition induced and employed by the hunting and cattle-raising people in a long history of the land.

2. On ethos

The Greek word "*ethos*" means custom, habit or habituation. According to the anthropological definition, it is a configuration of customs specific to a culture (Dictionary of Philosophy, 1998, Heibonsha).

Cultures change over time, across societies and regions, and throughout history. The ethos which constitutes a core of culture has naturally the same characteristics in a community. The extent and volume of an ethos are always vague at first. However, when the same ethos repeatedly appears, an essence or something like that emerges for the ethos to be appreciated as jellied broth is formed in a pot. The unwritten rules, orders, regulations and tendencies that are gradually formed in a long history comprise altogether the ethics and morals of a group or community (family, village, nation, etc.). At the center of an ethos, there is usually a religious factor or faith in a charismatic figure. Therefore, the influence exerted by religion is overwhelming in a morality that can be said the sublimation of an ethos.

For example, to a Buddhist, the killing of any animals is basically an evil. There is a Kansai dialect in Japanese, "*Sonna sessho-na!*", which could be directly translated as "so murderous!" is so often used in everyday conversation in Osaka, especially among merchants, as a light and immediate response to convey reproach to "heartless" behaviors given. There is also a well-known work of *haiku* (Japanese short poetry composed of three lines of the 5-7-5 syllables) by *Issa*, a noted haiku poet in the later Edo period lived in 1763-1827, "*Yare utsu-na, hae ga te wo suri, ashi wo suru,*" roughly translated as "Look, don't kill that fly! It is praying to you by rubbing its hands and feet." Or, to mention a more practical example, *Dogen* (1200-1253), who was the founder of Soto Zen Buddhism in Japan and erected Eihei-ji temple in the mountain of Echizen, did not kill the mosquitoes that bit him during Zen practice. Both *Issa* and *Dogen* were Buddhists, of course, and it is an essential thought of Buddhism that all animate beings possess potential Buddhahood as is typically described in the *Nirvana sutra*. It seems that the Japanese have an inherent modest morality according to which living things are not to be killed except it is absolutely necessary. "Never kill!" is one of the five precepts of the Buddha (the other four are: do not tell untruths, do not steal, do not commit adultery and do not drink alcohol). We, Japanese, have this moral rule of not killing because we have been brought up in an ethos which prohibits killing, and the moral education has been carried out by parents and ancestors in a community which is tightly knit both historically and racially. Some people think that we have this kind of morality naturally or *a priori*. I think that our morality has been formed as our racial history moved forward, and lies in the deepness of mind like the "collective unconscious" postulated by C.G. Jung (1875-1961).

Here, I want to refer to another example of ethos of which Japanese people are never aware in their ordinary lives. Modern Japanese people are fostered in the Japanese tradition of Buddhism, which is certainly a result of religious syncretism among Buddhism and Asian religions including Shinto. However, when we are asked "What is your religion?" we are usually somewhat restless and bewildered a while, and especially younger generations may be apt to answer at once "I have no religion". In other words, we cannot respond immediately as "I am a Buddhist." This unawareness is alike to the situation discussed above: the moral rule of "never kill all that lives" has been a part of our lives without our consciously noticing it, and it has continued to be embedded in the national ethos since the importation of Buddhism to Japan in the sixth century. In this sense, it is perhaps more appropriate to state that the moral rule concerning "Never killing" in this case looks as it were being equipped *a priori* for Japanese people but correctly it has existed as an ethos in the deepness of Japanese culture. This notion becomes especially apparent when it is lightened from outside. I could show here an example. When I was living in Kyoto, I took a young European man and woman to *Koke-dera* (*Saiho-ji*) which is a so famous Rinzai Zen temple for its well-kept garden buried with moist moss (*koke*) as it is commonly known as "*Koke* temple". We walked along a path in the quiet garden and came to a small stone bridge over a small pond. Then, a carp rose up to the surface and slowly approached us just crossing the bridge. The young German man arranged his fingers in the shape of a gun, pointed to the carp, and said "Boom!" This in a Buddhist temple! I was quite amazed and shocked by this cultural difference. This experience remains still fresh in my memory.

3. Factors related to the formation of ethics, morals and ethos in Japan
① Religions

Buddhism has the Five Commandments since the very beginning by the Buddha; they prohibit people from taking lives, telling untruths, stealing, committing adultery and drinking alcohol.

In countries in which Hinayana Buddhism is prevalent, for example, Thailand, these precepts are still observed in strict ascetic training. In Thailand, adult men must perform ascetic practices for a certain period, and Thais do not even kill wild dogs. Naturally therefore, industries in which humans kill animals and even feed them to other hervivorous animals never grow in Hinayanist countries, because such activities go against the basic mentality of the nation. In Japan, where Mahayana Buddhism is prevalent, the principle of *ahimsa* ("non-injury") is still relatively intact. However, self-regulations concerning drinking alcohol and sexual conduct became rather loose today. When we look back early days of Buddhism in the Nara period (710-794) in Japan, Emperor Shomu (reign: 724-749) who was a devout Buddhist constructed the Todai-ji in 745 as the head temple of the Kegon sect and a huge bronze statue of the Buddha Rushana (*Vairocana, Rushana-butsu*) as high as over 16 meters in the Todai-ji in 752. Todai-ji functioned both politically and religiously as it became the highest of many national temples already built in every province (*kokubunji*) since the decree of

Shomu in 741. As Shomu was deeply impressed by the *Kegon Sutra* (*Avatamsaka Sutra*) holding the shining *Rushanabutsu* as the central Buddha surrounded by many Buddhas like a wreath, he placed the Todai-ji at the core of Japanese Buddhism based on the thought. Besides, Shomu called the visit of Ganjin (Chien Chen, 688-763), a high-ranked monk of the Ritsu Buddhism in the Tang who was expected to perform in Japan a full-scale ceremony of Buddhism on the *kaidan* (precept platform) prepared in the Todai-ji temple. It was the purpose of Shomu to control centrally or rectify Japanese Buddhism which was rather randomly imported and in a sort of decadence at the time through performing the original procedure for the Buddhists by a monk of great sanctity after the style in the continent. Responding the request of Shomu, conveyed in 733 by Yoei and Fusho who reached the Tang as Japanese students of Buddhism, Ganjin tried to voyage all the way to Japan six times in all over 12 years at the risk of his life and finally at the sixth trial, he was successful to land at Kyushu in the end of 753 when he became blind caused by the sickness during hard attempts for long years. Next year (754), Ganjin gave Shomu and other more than 400 persons the authoritative ceremony of becoming a discipline of the Buddha (*jukai*) for the first time in Japan. *Jukai* with dual meanings of giving and accepting the Buddhist's cardinal precepts was performed using a solemn platform (*kaidan*) in the Todai-ji at the attendance of Ganjin and other high ranked monks associated with him. In the *jukai* ceremony, Ganjin preached and made swear the participants first to respect the three Buddhist treasures composed of the Buddhas, Sutras and Monks (仏法僧), and second to be strict to the Five Buddhist Commandments against murder, lust, theft, lying and intemperance. Of six Nara Buddhism sects (so called Nanto-roku-shu) as Kegon, Ritsu, Kusha, Jojitsu, Sanron and Hosso, all of which were formally imported for the elite people, the Ritsu (*Vinaya*) sect emphasizing in particular the Buddhist's precepts was founded by Ganjin and the Toshodai-ji temple was built in 759 in Nara as the head temple of the sect which has perpetuated until today. Thus, it can be verified that we Japanese have been familiar with Buddhist's precepts since the days of Shotoku in the Asuka period (593-710) when Buddhism was first introduced into Japan. Further, so-called "the Great Buddha of Nara" or *Rushana-butsu* in the Todai-ji is unchanged and sits before us with gentle and noble smile as it was in the Nara period when the first regular ceremony of Buddhist's Commandments was performed by Ganjin coming across the sea from the Tang.

Confucianism has many sorts of virtues. Among them, a set of five principal moral rules is composed of filial piety, loyalty, matrimonial bonding, respect for one's elders and friendship. These rules are designed to harmonize the members of society into a coherent and functional whole. Other virtues of Confucianism include benevolence, faith, courtesy, wisdom and piety. Benevolence is a moral virtue especially emphasized by Confucius. It is the foundation of all other virtues. It is the tender love or compassion which should be manifested by persons in high positions. As Confucianism has so many virtues, it is sometimes called a moral philosophy. Communities such as families, societies, villages and nations are stabilized by the incorporation of these inner principles or rules. In a good many Asian countries including Vietnam, Korea, Japan and China where, the rulers in the feudal age positively adopted Confucianism into politics to stabilize their reigns. Actually, Confucianism was the national religion of the Han dynasty (the Earlier Han, 202 B.C.-8 A.C.; the Later Han, 25-220 A.C.) before moving later to the periods of the Three Kingdoms (220-280) through Sui (581-619) and Tang (618-907) in which a return to free thoughts of the philosophy of Lao-Tzu and Chuang-Tzu and an introduction of Mahayana Buddhism from India occurred.

Both Confucianism and Taoism are traditional thoughts passing long history in China. Buddhism was transplanted on them afterwards to be mixed with these native religions. The Sung period is of note in that an old style of Confucianism was innovated through reinforcement of the philosophical system which was a traditionally weak point in the religion with the aid of the theories in Taoism and Buddhism under the name of syncretism. Thus, the doctrine of Chu Hsi arose as a school of Confucianism under the leadership of Chu Hsi or Zhu Xi (1130-1200) in the Southern Sung, while Buddhism in China subsequently faded away except Chan (Zen) in Sung. The doctrine of Chu Hsi or the refurbished Confucianism was further potently applied for the inner control of the people by political leaders in China, Korea, and Japan. In fact, Tokugawa government in the Edo period (1600-1867) adopted the doctrine as the official education system for the people and this predominance held until the end of World War II in Japan. This is one reason why we Japanese are still deeply immersed in moral virtues of Confucianism.

② **The teachings of nations or communities passed down in nonlinear or anonymous ways**

This is morality internalized without positive or conscious effort, and includes moral rules that are called "innate", "*a priori*" or "intuitive."

Not telling a lie, keeping a promise and performing good works are the basic teaching of most communities. Most of these basic rules of conduct are generally held to be common-sense for the people living in those communities. It is beyond the scope here to discuss whether humans are born good or not.

③ **The impact of philosophical theories dominating the age**

Philosophical theories on human morality usually have a strong effect on society. The assumption is that a theory penetrates a community fully through education and propagandas based on dialogue in a common language. The "benevolence" of Buddhism, "virtue" as understood by Aristotle and the "categorical imperative" as understood by Immanuel Kant are concepts deeply ingrained in the Japanese consciousness.

The Kantian ethics has exerted a strong influence on the development of moral philosophy in Japan.

German idealistic philosophies, from the Kantian to the Hegelian, had a great impact on the process of westernization and modernization of Japanese philosophy after the Meiji Restoration. They greatly influenced the formation of moral theories and rules in Japanese society. The strict dogmatism of these philosophies meshed well with the self-sacrificing nature and an idealism to indigenous teachings of the Japanese people.

For example, in the *Grundlegung zur Metaphysik der Sitten* (1785), Kant describes "Act only in accordance with the maxim through which you can will at the same time that it become a universal law". This was translated from German to Japanese by Yoshishige Abe, a former Minister of Education, and Tadashi Fujiwara in 1920 (Iwanami Shoten, p.71).

This is the universalizability formulation called FUL (the Formula of Universal Law) giving the first of three formulations in the Categorical Imperative. Kant enabled as such the definition of a moral law which is directly linked to reason inherent everybody *a priori*. We have to hear reason if our action or practice be ethical or not. The terms used by Kant are strictly defined and accordingly sometimes difficult to interpret immediately, but we can imagine now how his thoughts as exemplified above have penetrated into the educators in Japan in the 20th centuries covering the Meiji, Taisho and Showa periods.

④ **A theory tentatively put into practice in a community in order to materialize an ideal through a social movement**

Two movements as "*Atarashiki Mura*" and "*Ittoh-en*" are examples. "The "*Atarashiki Mura*" or "A New Village" movement was initiated by Saneatsu Musha-no-koji (1885-1976), a famed painter and writer who advocated an affirmative trust in human ability by starting his ideal community on his private fund in a local region of Kyushu in 1918. "*Ittoh-en*" or "The Garden with a Single Light" is a religious movement initiated in 1905 in Yamashina located at the suburb of Kyoto by a lay Buddhist, Tenkoh Nishida, who advocated to the followers their voluntary social services such as cleaning the toilet of others through which each could pray for the light of the Buddha. "*Atarashiki Mura*" faded out in the history, while a social movement of "*Ittoh-en*" is still going on as a religious practice of modern people.

In the United States, many specific communities were formed around respective Christian churches in the places where planters lived in pioneer days. Such communities remain to specifically continue to this day. They include many towns with German, French, Italian, Chinese and Japanese immigrants. Usually, they gathered under a similar ethos or have shared symbolic religious buildings from the beginning. So, in a sense, they may be defensive and exclusive to new comers. Again, it could be said that ethos is important as a centripetal force of the community when it functions and survives.

⑤ **Past examples of ethos that has captured the spirit of an entire generation in Japan**
These include as follows.
- The spirit of the *samurai (bushi)*
- The aesthetics of *hara-kiri (seppuku)*
- Self-immolation
- Male chauvinism
- The family system, and so on

Some of these aspects of life have not been eliminated completely. They are hidden in our subconscious and sometimes rise into the conscious mind.

4. Factors stipulating Japanese culture

Japanese people have molded Japan's inherent cultures throughout its long history, starting from the Jomon and Yayoi periods. These cultures are different from the Chinese, Indian and European cultures. Some factors in Japanese culture have already perished and others are still alive and expected to have a large impact in the future. It seems important to sort out here several important factors that have contributed to the formation of Japanese cultures in order to understand the necessities of alteration of them in the present and future.

The past determines the future. This is an important point when we take thought of cultures. We should not focus only on the present, which is being so easily affected by globalization and internationalization as we are aware of currently. In order to cope with an acute extend of this influence rightly, it is important for us to correctly understand the present based firmly on the past history and to observe the present as an extension of the past. We should not dismiss the past as irrelevant or old. It must be a "frivolous present" if the present is freed from the past.

① **A country of agricultural culture**

In Japan, rice farming established itself as the main economic activity during the Yayoi period (from the 3rd century B.C. to the 3rd century A.D.), after the Jomon period (from the 10th century B.C. to the 4th century B.C.). The Yoshinogari ruins (unearthed since 1986 in Saga Prefecture in Northern Kyushu) was announced in 1989 as the largest colony in Japan with a big surrounding moat which thrived in the latter half of the Yayoi period (from the 2nd to the 3rd centuries A.D.); one of their salient features is the arrangement of ritual structures near to a cluster of burial mounds. It is now established that there were at least three major places in ancient Japan where agrarian civilization established itself: Izumo (in Shimane Prefecture), Northern Kyushu and Kinki districts; this conclusion is based on the distribution of bronze wares, such as swords, pikes, and the bell-shaped vessels excavated from the ruins in the Yayoi through the Kofun (Tumulus) Ages, discovered by archaeological researches. Since then, agrarian civilization has long been the basis of Japanese culture until industrial civilization was superimposed onto it after the Meiji Restoration in 1867. With this westernization or cultural enlightenment, rapid modernization of Japan has begun in both culture and industry. As a result, Japan is now established as one of the most developed industrial countries. However, it is so important to keep a viewpoint that Japanese are essentially a people raised on agriculture as clearly shown in their long history, when we consider the present ethics and religion in Japan.

In the Japanese agrarian civilization, people lived in harmony with nature - its rain, wind, mountains, grass, trees and animals. They saw gods in nature (animism) and made them the object of their religious faith. In other words, the people were an integral part of nature. In agrarian civilizations, people plant seeds, cultivate crops and harvest them, appreciating the blessings bestowed by nature at every step. People mold their lives to fit nature. Nature is not a thing to be destroyed or controlled, but an entity to live with. People in agrarian civilizations generally lack individuality; they are passive and their thoughts, feelings and actions form generally groupism.

Civilization based on hunting and a cattle breeding is very different from agrarian civilization, and is the foundation of Western cultures. People in this civilization are aggressive toward nature and believe that it is natural for them to control it. They believe that animals are a part of nature, and that it is therefore natural for people to keep cattle as livestock. They believe that humans are at the summit of a natural hierarchy. This has not changed since Aristotle. It is necessary for humans to be combative in a civilization based on hunting and livestock breeding; otherwise, they will be killed. An individual must always be alert in this environment, and people are generally aggressive, positive and individualistic.

② **A moderate mixture of domestic and foreign religions in particular among animism, Shinto and Buddhism; a specific characteristics to Japan**

We should note the existence of a moderate mixture of many religions in Japanese culture. This "moderate mixture or syncretism" deserves special mention, when we go back and review the history of varied religions in Japan. I will focus here on intertwining of animism, Shinto and Buddhism in earlier Japan where they mix each other rather mildly.

Animism is a primitive religion that can be observed in all races in the world. The ancient Japanese believed that there were gods or spirits in mountains, rivers, rocks, water, trees, seas, fields, rice paddies and crops. They considered extraordinary phenomena in heaven and earth and disasters to be a curse or an expression of anger of these gods or spirits, and they worshipped them in order to calm down their anger. Of these, there were many objects of worship, including sacred trees, uncommonly large rocks and springs. People considered the spirit of a newly dead person to be unstable and this harmful spirit causing harm to this world. Naturally, religious rituals for the repose of a dead person's soul were so important. People believed that the soul of the dead became stable as the times went by eventually to grow up to a level of the ancestral spirits which protected living people; they worshipped their dead ancestors as well as the newly dead. Magical formulas and religious rituals dedicated to the spirits of a dead person and his ancestor gradually became the custom of praying for the welfare and safety of living people in the community. Many of such customs, habits and cultures can be traced back to animism and are still observed in modern Japan. In this sense, we may say that the mentality of contemporary Japanese is still in part intimate to animism.

Shinto developed from primitive animism specific to Japan. Shinto has a long history which stretches from the Yamato period (from the 3rd century to the 7th century) through to the Meiji, Taisho, Showa and present Heisei periods. During this long period, Shinto has all the time been fostered and managed by leading political figures in Japan. Since the introduction of Buddhism, Taoism and Confucianism from the continent to Japan, abundant foreign cultures associated with them have also been brought about. As is clear today, Shinto which remains living intact, has well incorporated these foreign cultures and doctrines by obtaining a good balance with them. As Shinto is the sole religion originating in Japan, it might have been fated to live on like an undertone in Japanese history. It is like an undercurrent in mentality of the Japanese showing itself to an outburst on occasion. The word "*Shinto*" was first used in the "*Nihonshoki*" or "The Chronicles of Japan" written in 720, in which the Japanese myths of *Izanami-no-mikoto* (Godess) and *Izanagi-no-mikoto* (God) were told. As the Shinto doctrine has provided the moral and cultural foundation of governance exerted by the Imperial Regime in Japan, it still has a great influence on the Japanese concept of divinity or *kami* (*kamigami* in the plural).

There are still many traditional Shinto customs observed in daily lives of modern Japanese. For instance, people pray for divine help (*kami-danomi*) in times of recession to *kamigami* (gods) of Shinto in the shrines or in front of the *kami-dana* (a Shinto altar in each house or a household shrine). Also, people so often say a set phrase of "Kami-sama, Hotoke-sama, ...",which means "Dear Kami (God), Dear Buddha," as the top words of making a wish, which is also an example of syncretism of Shinto and Buddhism. In the New Year holidays called *syogatsu*, Japanese people have various events of Shinto-style. As the biggest, the majority of people visit a shrine or a temple with shrine during the first three days (*sanganichi*) of New Year to pray *kami* for prosperity, health, marriage, enrollment and any desires in the year. Among many shrines, Meiji-jingu is the most famous because of its biggest collection of prayers. Besides events in the New Year's *shogatsu,* a Shinto-style festival called *matsuri* is also popular all over the country, which is usually held in the autumn to thank *kami* for harvest.

The animism in early Shinto was pure in its original religiousness. However, Shinto has been rather commercialized and popularized among contemporary Japanese, and the emphasis is now on its religious function as a site accepting any sorts of desire of ordinary people who pray for the welfare of the household, for safe driving, for passing examinations, for prosperity in business and so on. Seen in this light, Shinto is still in full flourish, having broadly penetrated into the daily lives of ordinary people in Japan, presumably due to a highly life-affirmative conception.

Buddhism developed uniquely in Japan since it was first imported from Korea and China in the Asuka (593-710) through Nara (710-784) periods. It was marvelously new at the time and had a substantial impact on Japanese culture and politics.

For instance, the equality of all human beings (the rejection of the idea of castes and untouchables) and the virtues like benevolence and tolerance were what the Buddha preached in India in the 5th century B.C. and have been hold since then in all sects of Buddhism. Religiously, he stated that the life is inevitably associated with existential sufferings (*dukkha*). The four such sufferings include: birth, old age, illness and death. The salvation or liberation from these sufferings or earthly bonds was the central aim of the Buddha and his disciples. For this purpose, early Buddhists usually retreated from mundane life in order to concentrate themselves in contemplation and rigorous precepts towards eventual appreciation of the eternal eternity or Buddhahood where alls should arise and vanish according to *Engi*. It is, therefore, of note that original Buddhism in India was rather negative to this mundane world, which was so contrasting to the classical Chinese thoughts as Taoism and Confucianism which were both affirmative to the secular world.

The outline of transmission of Buddhism from India to China and Japan. Buddhism was established in ancient India early in the 6th-5th century B.C. with the life of Shakyamuni or historical Buddha (566-486 B.C.), incorporating all of the traditional beliefs existing there which were majorly contemplatory, mythic and tantric. It gradually split into Hinayana and Mahayana after the death of the Buddha, although a meditation-based approach to an enlightened state of mind of the Buddha has been common to the both schools.

In Hinayana, the words of the Buddha and the traditions associated with his life were emphasized; this branch of Buddhism prospered mainly in Burma, Thailand, southern Vietnam, etc. In general, Hinayanists withdraw into a life of religious contemplation and devote themselves to ascetic practices as prior Indian thoughts before the appearance of Buddhism were traditionally so; Hinayana is a conservative form of Buddhism, in which the ascetic monk seeks his own personal enlightenment by mimicking the life of the Buddha and therefore lay persons are excluded from the enlightenment. Hinayana could be said self-seeking as it is characterized by the pursuit of personal benefit of a monk.

The other branch of Buddhism, Mahayana, prospered in China, Korea and Japan after passing several centuries since the death of the Buddha. This is a more inclusive form of Buddhism, attaching importance to the dependence on the sutras or scriptures and a variety of Buddhas (*butsu, nyorai*). Mahayana, therefore, had a time lag to develop until the formation of varied sutras in India. The *Wisdom Sutra* (*Prajna-sutra, Hannya-kyo* in Japanese) is the earliest scripture of Mahayana Buddhism written between the 1st century B.C. and the 1st century A.D. in India. *Prajna* or *Hannya* in Japanese is the highest wisdom aware of enlightenment. The *Vimalakirti-nirdesa Sutra*

(*Yuima-kyo* in Japanese) which expounds on *sunyata* (emptiness) is the second earliest sutra formed almost at the same time to the *Prajna*. Other earlier Buddhism sutras created between the 1st and 3rd century in India include the *Lotus Sutra* (*Hoke-kyo* in Japanese) and the *Avatamasaka Sutra* (*Hua-yen Sutra, Kegon Sutra* or *Kegon-kyo* in Japanese); the *Lotus Sutra* is a big and profound complex giving the basis to the birth of several Chinese Buddhism sects such as the Tendai and Pure Land, while the *Kegon Sutra* which was translated to Chinese around 400 gave rise to the Kegon and Zen sects in China. Such a unique and central philosophical concept as the "emptiness" (*sunyata, kuh* in Japanese), which is neither Being nor Non-being, was extensively explored by Nagarjuna between the 2nd and 3rd century although the concept had already existed from the first in the *Prajna* and *Vimalakirti-nirdesa Sutras* when they were written. In the historical process of transmitting Mahayana Buddhism outside India, excellent translation of the scriptures from Sanskrit to Chinese by Kumarajiva (344-413) contributed enormously and made it possible for varied Buddhism sects to rise in China and then in Japan. He actually translated the *Prajna, Vimalakirti-nirdesa,* and *Lotus Sutras* into the Chinese. Thus in the 4th and 5th centuries, important scriptures of Buddhism were one after another brought into China to cause gradually the birth of Chinese Buddhism sects during the time passing from the late 6th century to the Sui and Tang. These China-specific Buddhisms include the San-lun (Sanron) which was largely derived from the Madhyamika or Middle Way philosophy of Nagarjuna, Tien-tai (Tendai), Hua-yen (Kegon), Pure Land (Jyodo), and Chan (Zen).

Rather later in the Tang period, Xuan-zang (602-664), a famed Chinese monk or translator for the name of Genjo or "Sanzo-hoshi" in Japan, made a long trip to India by land from 629 to learn new trends of Buddhism including a unique idealism of the consciousness-only theory which was best translated by him to Chinese. When he came back to Changan (the capital of the Tang) after a long stay in India in 645, he brought with him many images of Buddha, Buddha's ashes and Buddhism scriptures. Consciousness-only theory which was established in the 5th century in India by the brothers Asanga and Vasubandhu (4th to 5th centuries) as an idealism opposing to the previous emptiness (*sunyata*) theory was thus transmitted to China and caused the birth of the Hosso-shu (Hosso Buddhism sect) in the Tang which was subsequently passed over to Japan in the Nara period (710-794) and composed one of Six Great Buddhism Sects (Nanto-Roku-shu) in officially imported Buddhism at the time. Kofuku-ji temple, which was built in the early 8th century in Nara with a financial support by the Fujiwara clan, has a long history until now to be a head temple of the Hosso-shu.

Esoteric Buddhism or *mikkyo* in Japanese has its root in ancient India and shares the basis with Hinduism. Primitive forms of esoteric Buddhism were seen in the 5th to 6th centuries but systematized only in the 7th century when two central sutras, the *Great Sun Sutra* (*Dainichi-kyo* in Japanese) and *Vajrasekhara Sutra* (*Kongocho-kyo* in Japanese) were completed in India as the final stage sutras of Mahayana Buddhism. Esoteric Buddhism was characterized by a modification of Hinduistic culture by Buddhism and made importance on performing three religious practices including the gesture of a Buddha's hands (*mudra*), chanting of sacred formulas (*darhani* or *mantra*, *shingon* in Japanese) and mental concentration on diagrams representing the universe (*mandala*). With the aid of these practices, one could attain enlightenment in this world which means the unification of the universe (macrocosmos) and an ascetic (microcosmos) or the awareness of the equality of the supreme Buddha (the Great Sun, *Vairocana*, Dainichi in *mikkyo*) and existential human. It was transmitted to China as a later Mahayana in the 8th century, and rapidly introduced into Japan of the Heian period by two monks, Saicho (767-822) and Kukai (774-835). They founded the Tendai and Shingon sects after coming back to Japan respectively; while the Tendai was with a taste of mikkyo at the first, the Shingon was a pure *mikkyo* from the first. Today, the inheritance of esoteric Buddhism is few in China but in contrast abundant in Japan and Tibetan countries. Shingon Buddhism has thereafter evolved extensively by Kukai in Mt. Koya in Japan.

Zen as *samadhi* (meditative concentration) existed from the very beginning of Buddhism with the Buddha, as it constituted an important praxis of the Buddha himself at attaining enlightenment. Zen was originally performed by incorporating yoga which was traditionally a physical practice for mental concentration dating back to ancient India. Zen in India was therefore rather static and simply employed as a means to attain enlightenment (*satori* in Japanese) of a monk who withdrew from ordinary life. Such Zen was transformed outside India to a more dynamic and profound form of religion placing importance on an intercommunication between *satori* and ordinary life as well as on self-reliance rather than learning scriptures or performing formal issues. Thus, Zen Buddhism sect was established in China in the 9th century attaching the ordinariness. After the tradition of Chinese mind, Zen Buddhism was transformed to a Chinese religion which was affirmative to the reality of this world. Zen was no more an ascetic practice but for enjoying life. People enjoyed solitude gained with Zen as a supreme state of mind. There are several famed poets including Li Bai (701-762) in the Tang period who left poems composing such supreme world. Zen Buddhism prospered to become a major Buddhism sect in the Tang through Sung in syncretization with Chinese thoughts. It was introduced into Japan by Eisai (1141-1215) and Dogen (1200-253) who both went overseas to the Sung.

In Mahayana Buddhism, even the laity is taught to be capable of achieving enlightenment through religious training. The major aim of Mahayana is to benefit others and to contribute to the common goal of emancipation before benefiting monks themselves. Actually, the *Bodhisattva* or *Bosatsu* in Japanese is an enlightened character remaining in this world just for alleviation of sufferings of ordinary people. Accordingly, Mahayana Buddhism could be said an altruistic religion. The great split between Hinayana, which was old and classical, and Mahayana started approximately 100 years after the historical Buddha passed away. Mahayana Buddhism was obviously brought to Japan in 538 and has flourished ever since. The spirits of egalitarianism, benevolence and generosity proposed by Buddhism were so fresh in the minds of the Japanese people at the time that they contributed to the elimination of the old clan system and became consecrated in the Constitution of Seventeen Articles promulgated by Prince Regent, Shotoku in 604. Thereafter, earlier political leaders in Japan followed Shotoku in governing successfully the people through Buddhism, and Buddhism itself also developed under the protection of leading politicians during the Nara and Heian periods.

Thus, a good volume of cultures, ranging widely from the Buddhist arts, technologies of constructing temples and irrigation works, Chinese literatures with Chinese characters, and varied high-grade craftworks which are still preserved as the imperial properties in the Shosoin treasure house were imported from China, Korea and the continent in the Nara period (710-784). As the importation was at the peak in the reign of Emperor Shomu (729-749) with an era name of Tenpyo, we could call the Nara period by the name of the Tenpyo from the view point of art history.

Shinto, in which native gods had been worshipped since long ago, was of necessity mixed with Buddhism under such situation. For instance, large rocks, waterfalls and springs originally worshiped in Shinto were actually transformed to the holy places related to Buddhism, respectively. The most popular was Buddhist's Kan-non worship in which the figures of Kan-non (*Kuan-Yin* in Chinese) in every holy places implied the "Bodhisattva of Compassion" or Goddess of Mercy, being a result of syncretism between Shinto and Buddhism. Kan-non, also called Kan-non-Bosatsu, Kan-ze-on-Bosatsu or Kan-jizai-Bosatsu, is the name of a symbolized saint who has already attained Buddhahood but remains in this world to observe and hear people everywhere (this is the meaning of "Kan-non") particularly for the purpose of aiding salvation of them; Kan-non has been broadly worshipped until now among physical sufferers ever since

Buddhism arrived at Japan.

Syncretism between Shinto and Buddhism was primarily observed in the construction of the *Jingu-ji* which is a temple attached to a Shinto shrine and the prevalence of the belief in vengeful spirits originally derived from Shinto. The syncretism between the Shinto's belief in the power of the mountains and the esoteric practice in Buddhism, most notably the Shingon, yielded the "Shugen-do" (mountaineering asceticism), in which practitioners wearing sumptuous clothing and accessories perform their religious training in the deep mountains.

Japanese transfiguration of Buddhism afterwards has been radical and multipolar by passing through the Kamakura period (1185-1333). The Kamakura was an age of unrest and innovation as known by transition of the political leadership from the nobility to the warrior (*bushi, samurai*) class, frequent domestic wars, arising of important new sects of Buddhism including Zen (Rinzai and Soto), Jyodo-shu, Jyodo-shin-shu and Nichiren-shu against the established sects of Buddhism as Tendai and Shingon in the Heian, the prevalence of pessimism due to the belief in the latter days of Buddhism (*mappo* concept), and repeated Mongolian invasions against Japan in 1274 and 1281 by Kublai Khan. In such a background, a variety of cultures unique to Japan have of necessity arose in the Kamakura. These include several effervescent forms of Buddhism appealing to the common people in the turbulent period, development of Zen and tea-related cultures including painting and preparing powdered tea, later developing to *cha-no-yu* (the tea ceremony), a sense of value attached to simpleness, and so on.

Although creative evolution in Japan of Buddhism itself was enormous in the Kamakura as was seen, wide-viewed effects of Buddhism (more accurately, Chinese Buddhism) on Japanese culture may be summarized by the following tenets:
- Dainichi Nyorai or *Mahavairocana* was ranked at the highest of Buddhas (esoteric Buddhism or *mikkyo*, with influences from the *Kegon Sutra*).
- All humans, and even grass and trees, can become Buddhas or possess potential Buddhahood (esoteric Buddhism and Kamakura Buddhism).
- *Sokushin-jobutsu*: Every person has the potential Buddhahood to become a Buddha or to attain enlightenment in his own body (esoteric Buddhism, especially the Shingon).
- Popular faith in the Pure Land and salvation by Amitabha Buddha (the *Jodo* sect of Buddhism or *Jodo-shu* founded by Honen, the *Jodo-shin* sect of Buddhism or

Jodo-shin-shu founded by Shinran, and the Ji sect of Buddhism or *Ji-shu* founded by Ippen).

According to the statistics disclosed in 2005 by the Government in its official home page, the differential number of temples among sects in Japan is 21,000 for *Jodo-shin-shu* at the top and 15,000 for *Soto-shu* at the second. Both belong to Kamakura Buddhism which appealed to the masses for an easy accessibility.

- When people die, they could become Buddhas (all sects of Buddhism in Japan).

This conception is due to the syncretism between Shinto and Buddhism. In Primitive Shinto, people believed that the spirits of a dead person and ancestors are living around us as was typical to animism. These concepts developed later to the notion that when a person dies, his soul becomes a Shinto god. Buddhism was then superimposed on this notion; the historical Buddha or Shakyamuni did not teach any such concept.

- Funeral Buddhism

The *Jodo* (Pure-Land) sects adopted the practice of allowing priests to accept fees for conducting funerals instead of conventional fees for performing incantations. This was followed by the Shingon, the Tendai and the Zen, which gives a general state of Japanese Buddhism today.

- The substantial development of Zen Buddhism

Zen Buddhism was transmitted to Japan at the end of the 12th century. Zen sects focus on philosophical training through meditation on the cross-legged position (*zazen*). Zen monks seek to realize themselves what they are through introspection, and the purport of Zen is to train participants with the aid of Zen practice to attain enlightenment. The process to it is transcendental. Purely speaking, neither difficult scriptures nor religious instruments including Buddha figures are needed for Zen Buddhism, but only excellent masters and quiet space to meditate on *zazen* are sufficient for this sect. Zen matched the mentality of the *samurai* in regard to self-help and standing apart. Aristocratic opulence in the Heian was avoided in Zen arts as calligraphy and calligraphic paintings and in the architecture of Zen temples; Zen assumes both simplicity and rigidness in its religious character. The Rinzai-shu and Soto-shu which were two great sects of Zen imported around 1200 as a new Buddhism from China were first expelled from Kyoto because of their innovative ideas and had to spread its roots in Kanto where the Kamakura Shogunate or the military government gradually gaining political power. As a result, Zen was accepted and became popular among the warrior or *samurai* class, residing gradually at the heart of their spirit. Actually, the martial arts of *the samurai* were formed basing on Zen thought. As the time passed from the Kamakura to the Muromachi period (1338-1573), the hegemony moved almost entirely from the nobility to the *samurai* and many zen temples were built and several Zen priests of great sanctity were invited from China to spread Zen in a close relationship with the Shogunate. The status of Gozan (five major temples of Zen) was authorized for Rinzai temples in Kamakura (Kentyo-ji, Engaku-ji, Jufuku-ji, Jochi-ji and Jomyo-ji) and Kyoto (Tenryu-ji, Shokoku-ji, Kennin-ji, Tofuku-ji and Manju-ji with an especially higher level for Nanzen-ji) by Yoshimitsu Ashikaga (1358-1408), the 3rd Shogun of the Muromachi Shogunate. These Zen temples played a role as the center of culture so variously sprouted in the Muromachi period. *Shoin-zukuri* or a residential architecture of Japanese style with a built-in *tokonoma* appeared and *Gozan* literature of Zen-related Chinese descriptions and poetries flourished in the Muromachi. Yoshimitu built Kinkaku-ji at the north hill of Kyoto as his villa in which Muso-soseki (later Muso-kokushi) founded Rinzai sect, setting up "Kitayama (north hill) culture", while Yoshimasa Ashikaga (1436-1490), the 8th Shogun of the Muromachi Shogunate built Ginkaku-ji at the east hill of Kyoto as his villa, thereby raising "Higashiyama (east hill) culture".

③ **The influences of Confucianism and Taoism**

Confucianism did not have as strong a doctrine as Buddhism. However, Confucianism was imported to Japan earlier than Buddhism, and was actively assimilated by Japanese culture because it conformed to the requirements of the governing mechanism (families, villages, nations, etc.); political leaders found it convenient as a governance tool, because it had a clear system of concepts which emphasized hierarchically organized social relationships. In addition, the constitutional Japanese predisposition, which placed great weight on the worship of ancestors and on the notion of continuation of their lives in the lives of their descendants, cannot be ignored. This virtue in particular bound Japanese families tightly until World War II. Even now, some people are re-evaluating Confucianism because they have witnessed the ravages of excessive freedom and the disintegration of proper education in the home. In other words, virtues such as doing one's duty both to one's lord and to one's parents, showing filial piety and good manners in general, and observing the five moral rules of Confucianism, have survived deep in the hearts of the Japanese people even in modern times, inducing in them a sense constant of urgency. The core of Confucianism is ancestor worship. Original Buddhism had metempsychosis as its inner nature; when Buddhism was superimposed on Confucianism, the Bon Festival of ancestor worship and the ritual of tomb building were created, and they survive to this day as folk festivities.

Taoism which is symbolized by the philosophy of Lao Tzu and Chuang Tzu had a profound effect on Shinto. Mitsuji Fukunaga maintained that the word "*ten-noh*" (emperor) belongs to Taoism and the theory of Yin-Yang and Five elements, and that this can easily be seen, for example, in the belief in using mirrors and swords as sacred emblems. While human conduct is regulated by Confucianism, nature is explained by Taoism. And while Buddhism (Indian Buddhism) seeks deliverance from earthly bondage, Taoism affirms this world and enhances its meaning, as exemplified by the worshipping a supernatural being like a mountain hermit and the belief in Koshin vigils. The desirable things of this world, such as perpetual youth and longevity, are actively sought in Taoism. However, they never seek these solely for their individual benefits but rather it is from devotion to the family, and in their desired religious images, their parents, ancestors and tribes would appear as enchanted hermits who are immortal. Perpetual youth and longevity represent the fusion of life and death. They are believed to be obtained through special diets, drugs, exercises, habitats and magic, which is indeed a distinguishing feature of secular or world-affirmative Taoism in that the methods ensuring never-ending life and ever-lasting youth are firmly anchored in mundane reality. While corporeality is an obstacle to enlightenment in Buddhism (Indian Buddhism), Taoism teaches that we should not be ashamed of, but rather esteem, our bodies, with their appetites for food and sex as they both ensure proliferation of bodies.

④ **The influence of Zen on Japanese culture**
   Of many Buddhism sects introduced into Japan, Zen Buddhism or simply Zen has been particular concerning the pivotal influence on Japanese culture. Eisai (1141-1215), originally a Tendai monk in Enryaku-ji temple on Mt. Hiei locating at the north back of Kyoto, left there hating the deterioration of the established sect, traveled twice to China in search of real Buddhism, and eventually brought Zen, a new Buddhism, to Japan. When he visited Southern Sung China for the second time, he was already at the age of 47 and even minding to travel by land to India pursuing true Buddhism. After he stayed in China for 5 years to study Zen, he returned to Japan in 1191 with Rinzai Zen. Comparing to the discipline in other sects of Buddhism, Zen was new in that it did not adhere too much to specific sutras, although the *Lotus Sutra* was deemed as the most important and basic in many Buddhist schools including Tendai, Nichiren and Zen, but attached entirely to the seated meditation just as the Buddha performed. Indeed, "*Fu-ryu-moji*" or "No reliance on words" is a very characteristic feature of Zen. In this

sense, Zen involves a tint of Hinayana Buddhism. As a natural course, Eisai was not welcome in Kyoto regarded as opposing to the established Tendai and at first forbidden to make religious activity there. It was only in 1195 that he started to build the first Japanese Zen temple, the Syofuku-ji, in Hakata (now Fukuoka) of northern Kyushu under the support of the warrior class getting political power in Kamakura. Hakata was a memorable place for Eisai as he first stepped on land there when he came back to Japan from Sung in 1191 after learning Zen and Sung culture. He is the founder of Rinzai Zen (*Rinzai-shu*) in Japan.

Dogen (1200-1253), who was a genius of aristocratic birth, entered young into the religious life with strong motivation at the death of his mother at his age of eight as well as of his father at his age of two. His mother was a beautiful daughter of the aristocratic Fujiwara family which was the clan eligible for regents or advisors to the emperor but was forced to be a wife of rustic Yoshinaka Kiso in the disturbances of war, who was a powerful warrior taking up arms from Kiso in the Shinano mountain district, acutely rose to the top, ruled Kyoto transiently, and killed in 1184. After Kiso's early downfall, she was made marry again with a scheming old politician, Michichika Koga, who became the Minister of the Right in the Imperial court in Kyoto and the father of Dogen. His father and his elder brother were notable poets of *waka* (Japanese poetry) at the time as their poetries were recorded in *Shin-kokin-waka-shu* ("New Collection of Ancient and Modern Japanese Poetry") compiled in 1205. Naturally, gifted Dogen was raised in these surroundings of a high-classed society very near to the authority in the Court and had abundant opportunities to access to Buddhist's texts, Chinese literature, Chinese poetry and *waka* (Japanese poetry). However, his drastic experience of separation from both parents in particular from his mother at his impressive days was so strong as to make him realize that the impermanence is the essence of life and decisively enter the way of Buddha instead of going up in the world as expected. In his religious career, Dogen entered Senkobo at Yokawa in Mt. Hiei at 13 years of age and next year get his head shaved under the care of the abbot of Enryaku-ji. Therefore, Dogen and Eisai were both Tendaists at the start of religious career. However, Dogen had to leave there soon because of fundamental contradiction he felt in religious practices of the established Tendai and became a pupil of Eisai in Kennin-ji which was the third Zen temple built by Eisai in 1202 in Kyoto for the common use of esoteric Buddhism (Tendai and Shingon) and Rinzai Zen. After the death of Eisai in 1215, Dogen was taught by Myozen, a disciple of Eisai, and they together went over to Sung China to study more of Zen in 1223, when Dogen was at 24 years old. After deep experience obtained through strict training under great-virtue Ju-ching (Nyojo, 1163-1228) in

China, he brought Soto Zen (*Soto-shu*) back to Japan in 1227 at his age of 28. Although Myozen was unfortunately dead in China and carried back in ashes by Dogen, Dogen himself was satisfied to meet and intimately learn much from Ju-ching, because he was so fresh to Dogen and actually so strict in religious training and in his life as no monk comparable to him was present in Japan. He preferred poverty and indicated to Dogen that true Buddhists should be off from the authority, political affairs, wealth and the like. Indeed, these teachings of Ju-ching impressed Dogen so deeply that Dogen lived definitely according to them throughout his life thereon. After returning to Japan, he stayed in or around Kyoto and described early parts of a big life-work of *Shobo-genzo or* "Corpus of the Essence of Genuine Dharma of Buddhism". However, Dogen was the same to Eisai in that the Tendai at Mt. Hiei and the Imperial Court in Kyoto were both unwilling to accept a new trend of Buddhism of Zen. After spending several years for his religious praxis and preaching in Kennin-ji temple, Dogen had to retreat to Fukakusa at southern suburb of Kyoto where he founded Kosho-horin-ji (Kosho-ji) at his 34 years and stayed for over 10 years until the age of 44 when he moved to Echizen, a mountain region remote from Kyoto. However, during these over 10 years in Fukakusa following his return from Sung, Dogen was the most energetic both physically and spiritually in his life. His religious deepening was prominent and many writings including earlier volumes of *Shobo-genzo* were written. There are minor difference between Rinzai and Soto. Whereas Rinzai emphasizes spiritual training through both the contemplation and the efforts for un-intellectual solution of metaphysical problems given (*koan*), Soto is characterized by only concentration in meditation in the cross-legged position (*zazen*). *Shikan-taza* meaning "Just concentration on meditation with all else shut out from one's mind" is a noted phrase of Dogen expressing his strict practice of Zen. Solely mediating this extensive *zazen*, one can attain Buddhahood or in Dogen's term, "*Shinjin-datsuraku*" meaning "to cast body and mind off". Dogen developed Soto into a highly abstruse philosophy as expressed in his most extensive work, "*Shobo-genzo*". This difficult book of religious philosophy of Buddhism was composed of 95 volumes, encompassing his metaphysical view of impermanence and Buddhahood ubiquitous in the world, and even the minutest details of *zazen,* was halfway completed during his stay in Kosho-ji temple in Fukakusa before moving to Echizen at his age of 44. Dogen at Echizen further concentrated himself in *zazen* (*shikan-taza*) and described on the rests of *Shobo-genzo* which was eventually left uncompleted as he died rather young at the age of 54. Soto Zen became another Japanese Zen sect, and is considered now almost synonymous to Dogen. In other words, Japanese Soto Zen developed in a specifically Japanese manner under Dogen.

Eisai, who was the first person to introduce Zen to Japan and a predecessor of Dogen in that sense, was greatly different from Dogen in character. Eisai was a man of passion and ambition who moved politically or outwards apart from being a monk of Zen, while Dogen was a pure-religious man solely aiming at the Buddhahood and always moved inwards and inwards rather hating a contact with the politics or the authority considering it as a hindrance of his religious practice. Although it is not surprising that Eisai and Dogen were both persecuted by the Tendai Buddhists at Mt. Hiei who were the central authorities on Buddhism in Japan at that time, Eisai took the position emphasizing the importance of religious precepts in Buddhism and was radical enough to stress a need of the independence of Zen from other established sects of Buddhism including Tendai and Shingon. He wrote the "*Kozen-gokoku-ron*" meaning "Defensing the Country by Enhancing Zen" in 1198, in which he asserted that Zen should be energized in order to protect Japan from its enemies. Because of his proactive stance, Zen quickly became popular among the *samurai* (*bushi*) increasing in power in the region of Kamakura which is located at the eastern Japan called *Kanto*. After proceeding to construct the first magnificent Zen-styled temple in Japan named Shofuku-ji in Kyushu in 1195 as the first job after he returned from China, Eisai founded the Jufuku-ji temple (Kamakura) in 1200 and the Kennin-ji temple (Kyoto) in 1202, respectively, demonstrating increasing supports by the *bushi* class. In fact, Minamoto-no-Yoriie who was the first son of Minamoto-no-Yoritomo, the founder and first Shogun of the Kamakura Shogunate, embraced in Rinzai and supported the general spread of Zen. Later, many Zen temples including *Gozan* (Five Authorized Rinzai Temples) in Kamakura and Kyoto were erected over the country.

Eisai is known as having introduced the tea to Japanese culture as well. He was a pioneer of the way of tea (tea ceremony); he brought home from China not only the rituals of tea drinking but also tea plants and planted them at Mt. Seburi in Kyushu and in Uji located at the suburb of Kyoto. He wrote the *Kissa-yojoki* meaning "The Effects of the Tea as Medicine" in 1211, four years before his death. In this book, he described beneficial effects of the tea on spiritual uplift and harmony of organs based on the doctrine of Five Elements in China referring to "*Chaking*" (*Cha Chin*, Tea Classic) by Luwuh (Lu Wu) and what he heard during his stay in the Sung. In the light of the present scientific knowledge, caffeine as an active ingredient of the tea possesses pharmaceutical effects to induce diuresis, activate cardiac contraction and sweep away drowsiness. However, it is interesting to note that Eisai referred in his book to Chinese doctrine of *Wu Xing* (Five Elements: Wood, Fire, Earth, Metal, and Water) for the explanation of the tea effect on the heart. In *Wu Xing*, the bitterness in the Five Tastes and the heart in the Five Solid Organs are similarly included in the group of Fire. Accordingly, by Eisai' view based on the Doctrine of *Wu Xing*, the bitterness due to the tea can enforce the imbalance of the Five Tastes (Acid, Bitter, Sweet, Hot, and Salty) in the food of Japanese people of his days, thereby restraining them from cardiac diseases. We could learn in this story that the tea culture had already incorporated the doctrine of *Wu Xing* at the time of its introduction into Japan by Eisai). This energetic book was dedicated to the young Shogun in the Kamakura Shogunate, Minamoto-no-Sanetomo (1192-1219) who was the second son of Minamoto-no-Yoritomo and became the third Shogun of the Kamakura. Sanetomo was an excellent poet of *waka (tanka)* as described later but politically ill-fated as to be assassinated at the age of 28 by his late brother's son. His tomb is in Jufuku-ji temple where Eisai died.

In fact, the tea of Eisai was absolutely new in an impact on life and thought at the time. As Zen and tea were eagerly accepted by the Kamakura Shogunate established by the samurai class, they were both appropriate symbols of the new Japanese culture emerging at those periods from the later Heian to the Kamakura.

Thus, Zen had a great impact on the evolution of the way of tea in Japan. Furthermore, Zen offered a strong support to the spirits of the *bushi*, and gave ordinary Japanese people a chance to participate in religious activity through Zen meditation which could be performed by everyone and everywhere. Zen allowed Japanese people to reflect on their own existence and to realize individually true reality of life. It played an important role in establishing Japanese culture as we know it today when we look back that the way of tea with metaphysical implication, the art of calligraphy, the Zen meditation, and traditional values on simplicity and poverty are all the foundations of the current Japanese culture.

⑤ **A religion by the name of "the amalgamation of many religions"**

As shown above, Japan is a polytheistic society. Religions contended with one another when they encountered each other for the first time, but they did not destroy each other in the end. They survived and rooted themselves deeply into each other. Thus, such vague boundaries and deeply rooted co-existences observed in religious matters form the very characteristics of Japanese culture in general. It would be most appropriate to call the Japanese religion, if the definition of it is absolutely required, by the name of "the tolerant amalgamation of varied domestic and foreign religions".

We should note carefully that "foreign" religions were already intertwined or syncretized for centuries in China and Korea before their advent to Japan. They came into contact with Japanese culture and changed themselves by acquiring specifically

Japanese issues. This is the state of the religions observed today in Japan. The following list shows examples of the mixture of religious notions observed in current Japanese individuals:

- **Animism**: faith in mountain gods, water gods, thunder gods, wind gods and so on.
- **Shinto**: visits to the Inari shrine, Tenman-gu, the Nogi shrine, etc., for respective divine favors, the New Year's Day celebrations, festivals for 3-year-old boys and girls and for 5-year-old boys and 7-year-old girls, New Year's visits to shrines, *jichinsai* (ceremonies for hallowing the ground), autumn festivals, *ikebana* (the art of flower arrangement), the concepts of *wabi* (simplicity) and *sabi* (tranquillity), the art of calligraphy, the fine arts, *haiku* poetry
- **Confucianism**: ancestor worship, tombs, paternalistic family system
- **Taoism, Yin-Yang, Five Elements and *On-yo-do***: We could see considerable influence of the Five Elements' doctrine on contemporary *chado* (*wabi-cha*, the way of tea) and *ikebana* (the art of flower arrangement). *Kimon* (the unlucky or northeastern direction), *katatagae* (directional taboos), and *uranai* or *eki* (fortune-telling) are from the doctrine of Five Elements. However, *On-yo-do* is a superstitious belief generated in the Heian period in Japan under the influence of Taoism. *Tomo-biki* (the day on which one's luck or lack thereof can be transferred to others; hence, a good day for weddings and a bad day for funerals) in the traditional calendar is a well-known example from On-yo-do. Other examples include *tai-an* (the luckiest day) and *butsu-metsu* (a very unlucky day).

⑥ **The absence of a monotheistic religion and the diversification of the moral code**

Monotheistic religions (Christianity, Islam, etc.) have strong commandments which form the foundation of an ethos. If a person is brought up from infancy in an environment pervaded by a monotheistic religion, he or she will internalize the relevant moral code, which will then guide his or her daily life after adolescence. In Christianity, God is a unique, absolute and omnipotent being.

Japan has no monotheistic religion. Instead, many authority figures have together offered moral guidance throughout its history, and accordingly the identity of these authority figures is likely to change in the time. Here are some conceptual systems or nexuses which have exerted a part of moral authority in Japanese culture:

- The virtues of Confucianism (decency, faith, loyalty, etc. taught in the community)
- Buddhist concepts (the concept of transmigration in the six lower worlds has penetrated into daily life in the form of imaged Hell and omens, and morality was also innerly appreciated in Zen practice)

- State Shinto (from the Meiji Restoration to the end of World War II) and general Shinto
- Animistic faith (*Yaoyorozu-no-kami,* myriad gods)

⑦ **Racial uniformity**

Japan is isolated by the sea and for this reason has not been easily conquered by other countries or races as was the case in other Asian countries. Therefore, Japanese people have seldom been coerced by foreigners through the force of weapons as seen in European countries and the American Continent where native people have experienced foreign threats on their soils, subsequent racial mixing and acute cultural change as well. In this context, Japanese culture has been allowed continuous and changed comparatively slowly and mildly.

Because Japanese people have such racial uniformity, they can collaborate domestically with ease and effectiveness. They are especially likely to cooperate to prevent foreign invasion, and are prone to slide into nationalism, as demonstrated by the nationalistic fervor in the face of the Mongol invasion attempts in 1274 and 1281, and more recently during World War II. Basically, Japanese people do not take to individualism; the individual is ensconced in the group mentality.

⑧ **A temperate and rainy climate bringing up diverse natural habitats and varied species of living matter**

Japan enjoys a large amount of rainfall each year, which is a godsend. The nation's land is rich in plants and other natural products during all four seasons, and because of the plentiful rainfall, Japanese people can take baths every day. In Japan, there is the expression "Spend money like water" because water is thought to be free of charge. In countries with small amounts of rainfall, people avoid taking baths and take showers instead; in restaurants across Europe, guests even have to pay for the water they consume at the table.

Because Japanese people live in a country rich in resources, they are generally peaceful and tend to avoid disputes. Hippocrates and Tetsuro Watsuji have pointed this out.

⑨ **Japanese people have shown tolerance to cultures imported from abroad; or rather, they have digested these cultures actively and quickly.**

This is a significant characteristic. Japanese people are broad-minded about the acceptance of foreign cultures in a good sense. However, sometimes it is a blind imitation lacking principles, or they show no independence of style or thought. Yet, they feel no shame in doing so; on the contrary, they carry on with their imitations in a positive frame of mind. But we should add that, in most cases, the imitations are not simply indiscriminate; as evidenced prodigiously in recent decades, Japanese people borrow advanced technologies and rapidly make them their own. This is the way Japanese people have managed to create so many valuable concepts and objects, and it is not a stretch to state that these things are the original creations of Japan. These are several examples as follows:

- The Shingon School of esoteric Buddhism was founded by Kukai (774-835) at Mt. Koya in Japan. *Sokushin-jobutsu* meaning "Attaining Buddhahood in one's own body" is the most remarkable feature of the Shingon of Kukai. This type of Buddhism is unique to Japan, not an imitation of Chinese Buddhism. We can say the same for Kamakura Buddhism sects founded by Honen, Shinran and Nichiren, and the Japanese Zen sects founded by Eisai and Dogen.

- Eisai imported the tea and the manner of drinking tea from Sung China, and the Japanese way of tea called *wabi-cha*, *cha-no-yu*, or recently *cha-do* was specifically developed in Japan to its style possessing distinctive Japanese "flavor." It is now an important expression of Japanese culture.

- The Chinese characters or *kanji* imported from China were modified into *kana* or Japanese syllabaries in the Heian period. *Kanji* characters are both ideographic and phonogramic as appeared in the Chinese literature imported in the Asuka (593-710) and Nara (710-784) periods. Therefore, it was fundamentally necessary for Japanese people at the time to establish an easy writing system of their own to express freely their spoken or poetic language. *Kana* characters are a modification of *kanji* in the way to employ only its phonogramic aspect to express spoken Japanese. While in the *Manyo-shu*, the oldest collection of Japanese poetry compiled in the 8th century, Chinese characters were used as a temporary measure to express the sound of Japanese, later in the *Tosa Nikki* or *Tosa Diary* written in 935 by Ki-no-Tsurayuki, newly invented *kana* syllabaries for Japanese were employed for the first time. Subsequently, at the middle of the Heian period, the *Makura-no-soshi* or "The Pillow Book" (in ca. 1001) and the *Genji-monogatari* or "The Tale of Genji" (in 1007) were written by female writers in *kana* characters. The Tale of Genji is the first known full-length novel in the world, while The Pillow Book is an excellent essay on seasonal changes of nature and affairs in the nobility.

- As Japan is a country isolated by the sea, the priority of some political regimes in

Japanese history was to import foreign cultures. For example, even official Japanese diplomatic delegations were sent to China during the Sui and Tang dynasties. On this extension, cultural aspects of the Sung dynasty were also imported into Japan including an original form of the tea ceremony performed in Chinese temples and Zen Buddhism, which developed today into the Japanese way of tea, Japanese-style Zen and Japanese mind as expressed in chivalry (*bushido*).

- By the Meiji Restoration, Japan emerged from its period of isolation and became rapidly modernized and westernized. As a result, Japan became a modern industrial nation and has succeeded in becoming an economic powerhouse after World War II.

⑩ The structure of the Japanese language appropriate to Japanese poetry and cadenced expression

The oldest known Japanese full-length literary works are A Record of Ancient Matters or *Kojiki formed in* 712, Chronicles of Japan or *Nihon-shoki* formed in 720 and A Collection of Myriad Leaves or *Manyo-shu* compiled in c. 760 at the end of the Nara period (710-784). Prior to these, no literary record is found, as there was no writing system to express spoken language of native Japanese. Ohno Yasumaro wrote *Kojiki* in *kanji*, Chinese characters, taking dictation on aspects of National history from Hieda-no-Are, who was an official dictator at court. Metrical songs passed down orally were also collected and contained within its pages. It consists of three volumes, and the first volume includes tales about early gods who created the country, especially, descriptions of the Izumo gods.

One of poetical description in it reads:

Yakumo tatsu izumo yaegaki	(5 and 7 syllables)
Tsuma gomi ni yaegaki tsukuru	(5 and 7 syllables)
Sono yaegaki wo	(7 syllables)

This is a short rhyming poem which means:
Izumo, my blue mountains surrounded <u>by layer upon layer of clouds</u> (yakumo tatsu)
I create a lot of hedges<u> to conceal my wife</u> within (tsuma gomi ni)
<u>The multifold hedges</u> (yaegaki), I make them!

This beautiful verse put between the narrative compositions of the *Kojiki* ("A Record of Ancient Matters") is apparently in the 5-7 syllabic style which is so popular to Japanese mentality still currently and possesses the same root with later-developed *waka* or *tanka*. "*Yakumo-tatsu*" is a pillow word of "*Izumo*" which is a name of the rural mountainous country located in the San-in district of Japan. However, this pillow word at the top is not solely decorative here but has a meaning linking to the latter part of the verse either. It is natural to consider that oral communications with this sort of rhyme were prevalent among old habitants in Japan before *kanji or Chinese characters as* a mean to write down spoken contents was transmitted from China.

Manyo-shu, the earliest collection of Japanese poems by a wide range of people from the emperors at the highest to the unknown populace, consists of twelve volumes and 4516 poems. They include the 31-syllable verses (*waka* or *tanka* poems: *wa* meaning Japanese and *tan* the shortness) and other longer verses such as *tyoka* poems which are typical for a long repeat of the 5-7 syllables like 5-7-5-7-5-7- and *sedoka* poems, a variation of *waka, which are composed of six phrases of 5-7-7, 5-7-7*. Usually, *tyoka* was placed in front of *waka* to describe the poetic background for *waka* to be composed.

These verses are unique to Japan, or not derived from China. Importantly, they were not recorded in the style of Chinese poems or *kanshi* in *Manyo-shu*, but people at that time for the first time recorded their oral expression of innate rhythm in the written language through borrowing the "*on*" sound from Chinese characters or *kanji*. It must have been exiting for people then, because domestic verses composed in people's spoken languages which were communicated only orally until then because there was no writing system for the Japanese. Indeed, they managed to utilize *kanji* for the expression of spoken Japanese. In the assimilation process of Chinese character (*kanji*) to Japanese, two readings appeared as an "*on*" expressing only the sound of Japanese and a "*kun*" for implying the Japanese meaning. Of these, the "*on*" sound of kanji was utilized as a phonetic symbol without any meaning in Manyo-shu and thus this pattern of expression was later called *manyo-kana* which was used only to transmit the sound of spoken Japanese and no meaning at all. Well-known Japanese verse reads:

Yamato niha murayama aredo	*(5 and 7 syllables)*
Toriyorohu ame no kaguyama	*(5 and 7)*
Noboritachi kunimi wo sureba	*(5 and 7)*
Kunihara ha kemuri tatsu miyu	*(5 and 7)*
Unahara ha kamame tachitatsu	*(5 and 7)*
Umasi kuni zo akitsusima	*(6 and 5)*

Yamato no kuni ha   (7)

These mean as follows:
There are many mountains in Yamato (Yamato is an old name of Japan)
Especially, is best Ame-no-kaguyama (Kaguyama is the name of a mountain in Nara)
I climb the mountain and see my reign
There are smokes coming up from the hearths
Seagulls are flying above the sea
Good country, is my Akitsushima Yamato! (Akitsusima is a pillow word of Yamato)

We now have many *tanka (waka)* poems, *haiku* poems and modern popular songs, all of which are the descendants of the *Manyo-shu* poems in possessing a rhyming form of 5-7 syllables.

The cadence specific to these poems is appropriate and perfect for expressing Japanese feelings; or rather, the mood of the country has been cultivated by this cadence. Its rhythm is memorable to the mind and can be easily reproduced from memory. This structure of the Japanese language itself maybe raised a national character of the tendency to be easily moved, which has functioned as both an advantage and a weak point. For example, the Japanese language has no verb equivalent to "be" which refers to the existence, and so the Japanese people have not produced philosophical ontology or systems of philosophical logic, both of which have been matters of serious scholarly concern in Western countries.

5. Japanese feelings in literature

Literary works are creations into which the minds of writers are projected. They are the direct reflection of people's mentality at the time. When the mind of a writer reacts to the environment and the actual state of people's life at respective periods, he creates an artistic work unique to him. In this sense, literary works are precious historical documents which give us insight into the cultures, customs and traditions of the prior age in which the works were created. A work is deeply influenced by the background of its creation. For example, we can understand ancient Greek culture by reading the works of Plato and Hippocrates. Japanese people have left their own verses since the *Manyo-shu* which is the oldest collection of *waka* organized by Otomo-no-Yakamochi et al. in c. 760 and proses since the "*Tosa-nikki*" or "The Tosa Diary" which is a travelogue diary associated with *waka* poems recorded by

Ki-no-Tsurayuki (865?-946) during the voyage between the years of 934 and 935. This was written for the first time in *wabun* or Japanese language using *kana* (a native syllabary) characters modified from Chinese characters. Tsurayuki was a distinguished *waka* poet as he confiled the first anthology of *waka* collected by imperial command called *Kokin-waka-shu* or "A Collection of Ancient and Modern *Waka* Poems" and diplomat who were just on his return ship from the province of Tosa in Shikoku to Kyoto when he wrote down the Diary. In those days, Chinese literature and poetry were limited for the use of elite men and not permitted for ladies even in the Court. Importantly, it should be noted that any native literary works would be formed on the writing system capable of fully and properly expressing spoken language of the habitants. In another word, any creative works, if expressed in Chinese characters and syllabaries even made by Japanese people, it is after Chinese way of thinking and not genuine expression of Japanese mind. In this context, the invention of the *kana* writing system for easy expression of spoken Japanese was epoch-making. It made possible for people to easily write down their spoken language and further most importantly gave ladies the chance to create literary works as poetry, diary, and prose. It was rightly this time that any creative works by Japanese authors were rendered possible in Japanese history. Actually, the *Genji-monogatari* (a long novel) and the *Makura-no-soshi* (an essay) were written by female writers using *kana*. Since then, Japanese people have been unchanged in creating literary works using Japanese syllabaries, which are a mixture of *kanji* and *kana*. However, when we review a so long-lived *waka (tanka)*, we notice a kind of commonality of feeling throughout ages to exist. A long time has passed since the new genres of Western literature (novels and modern poetry) were introduced to Japan in the Meiji period. However, there is something primitive and commonly shared which has been continuous until now in the feelings recorded in Japanese literary works throughout the history. These original Japanese feelings will now be explained.

- *Manyo-shu* (a compilation of 4516 impressive songs created by people of various social classes including the masses, warriors, clerks, and emperors who lived during the period of Emperor Nintoku through to 759 A.D. ranging over about 350 years)

#48	*Hingashi no no ni kagirohi no tatsu miete*	(5, 7, 5 syllables)
	Kaerimi sureba	(7)
	Tsuki katabukinu	(7)

There is turbulent air above the east field.
Looking around,
I watch the moon setting　　(Composed by Kakinomoto-no-Hitomaro)

#351　　*Yononaka wo　nanini tatohemu　asabiraki*　　(5, 7, 5 syllables)
　　　　Kogiinishi fune no　　　　　　　　　　　　　(7)
　　　　Atonaki gotoshi　　　　　　　　　　　　　　(7)

　　　What is the world like?
　　　It is like a boat leaving the shore in a morning mist,
　　　Rowed away with a wake vanished out for ever.
　　　(Composed by Sami-Mansei)

#925　　*Nubatama no　yo no hukeyukeba　hisagi ohuru*　(5, 7, 5 syllables)
　　　　Kiyoki kahara ni　　　　　　　　　　　　　(7)
　　　　Chidori shiba-naku　　　　　　　　　　　　(7)

　　　As evening deepens into the night,
　　　I hear plovers to sing frequently in the clean river
　　　Where many *hisagi*-plants have grown.
　　　(Composed by Yamabe-no-Akahito)

#1071　*Yamano ha ni　isayohu tsuki wo　idemuka to*　(5, 7, 5 syllables)
　　　　Machitsutsu oru ni　　　　　　　　　　　　(7)
　　　　Yo zo fukenikeru　　　　　　　　　　　　　(7)

　　　I have passed waiting for the moon to rise comletely
　　　Which was long wandering along the edge of the mountain.
　　　I realize now it is far into the night already.　(Author unknown)

#1511　*Yuh sareba　ogura no yamani　naku shika no*　(5, 7, 5 syllables)
　　　　Koyohi ha nakazu　　　　　　　　　　　　　(7)
　　　　Ine ni kerashimo　　　　　　　　　　　　　(7)

　　　Deer, usually cry in Mt. Ogura at becoming dark,

Do not cry tonight.
They seem to be asleep.   (Composed by Emperor Okamoto)

Humans, deep in meditation as a part of nature, watch the simple flow of nature in these verses. They imagine the feelings of birds singing in mid-night and deer crying in mountains. People share feelings with nature. They realize that their lives are as transient as the phenomena of nature.

We should note that we can observe a sense of mortality already in the #351 poem. What is the world like? It is like a boat in the morning gliding along with a slender wake. Nothing is left there when it is gone out of the sight.

- *Sanka-shu* or "A Hut In the Mountain", an anthology of *waka* poems by Saigyo (1118-1190)

#64   *Oshinabete   hana no sakari ni   narinikeri*   (5, 7, 5 syllables)
    Yama no ha gotoni   (7)
    Kakaru shirayuki   (7)

    Full bloom all around!
    It's like white clouds
    Covering all the edges of the mountains with cherry blossoms.

#66   *Yoshino yama   kozue no hana wo   mishi hi yori*   (5, 7, 5 syllables)
    Kokoro ha mi nimo   (7)
    Sohazu nariniki   (7)

    I've gotten restless, mind out of body,
    Ever since I saw the cherry blossoms
    Full to the top of every tree on Mt. Yoshino.

#470 *Kokoro naki   minimo ahare ha   shirare keri*   (5, 7, 5 syllables)
    Shigi tatsu sawa no   (7)
    Aki no yuh-gure   (7)

    How pathetic this dusk
    At the swamp of a mountain stream,

A snipe flying off.
I feel deeply if mindless I have been.

Saigyo was of an age with Taira-no-Kiyomori who became later the top of the great warrior family named *Heike* or the *Taira* family and took power of the country. Saigyo and Kiyomori were both *hokumen-no-bushi* (bodyguards at the Imperial Palace) or members of the elite fighting force in their young days. His given name was Sato - Yoshikiyo, and he belonged to a famous samurai clan. Indeed, Sato is the name of history and one of the oldest in Japan. Never the less, Saigyo became a monk when he was 23 years old, abandoning his wife and children, and adopting a new name of monk. Concerning his motive for this decision, his personal history remains ambiguous about whether it was caused by his disappointment in love or his metaphysical insights into mortality. However, he did choose the life of a monk, living his only - one life like producing a creative art as if it were a play in theater, abandoning the quest for personal glory. It is of note that there was such active selection of life already at the time. His purpose was not to escape from the world, but to try to study immanence thoroughly and explore it in an active manner. In his monk's life, he lived in or around Mt. Koya but did not attained much religiously so long as we see in the record rather traveled about the provinces soliciting contributions for religious purposes for reconstruction of the temples in Mt. Koya. Thus, we feel from him an image of the intellectual adventurer to nihilism.

- *Hojoki or* "An Account from My Hut", essays written in literary Japanese mixed with Chinese words by Kamo-no-Chomei (1155-1216) in 1212
  It begins as follows:

"The flow of water in the river is incessant and water is never the same as it was. Foams on the pool of a river form and vanish, repeating without a moment delay, or never remain long as they are. Such is the fate of men in the world and of their dwellings as well."

- *Heike Monogatari* or "The Tale of the *Taira* Family"was written in the early 13th ceutury or at the early stage of the Kamakura period. The author is not known.

  It is an epic or military chronicle describing the rise and fall of the *Taira* family, read in Chinese characters as *Heike*. In the military struggle between two great families of the *Taira* and the *Minamoto* (*Heike* and *Genji* in Chinese characters, respectively), in the 12th century, *Heike* were first successful to get political hegemony with possession of the Imperial Palace in Kyoto under the leadership of Taira-no-Kiyomori (1118-1181). He placed his aughter as the Empress of Takakura Emperor and their son as the Emperor named Antoku in 1180. However, the prosperity of *Heike* did not last long. After the death of Kiyomori in 1181, *Heike* declined rapidly and fled from Kyoto in 1183 when Kiso Yoshinaka belonging to *Genji* moved up to Kyoto with a large army.

The Tale begins as follows:

"The bell of Gionshoja (the Jetavanavihara Monastery in India) sounds
In the echo like telling the impermanence of all things.
The hue of the flowers of the sal tree exhibits solemnly
The way of things that the prosperous must decay.
Yea, the proud ones are but for a moment,
Like a dream in the spring night."

The authors of the *Hojo-ki* and the *Heike Monogatari* understood that actuality was the flow of time and that all things were flowing or transient from the standpoint of the spiritually awake.

■ *Kinkai-waka-shu* : a collection of *waka* works by Minamoto-no-Sanetomo (1192-1219).
  This anthology must have been compiled after the young death of Sanetomo as *"Kinkai"* is a proud name indirectly meaning the minister of the Kamakura which he eagerly wanted to be appointed by the Court in Kyoto but not fulfilled while he lived.

#604   *Yononaka ha   tsunenimo gamona   nagisa kogu*   (5, 7, 5 syllables)
       Ama no obune no   (7)
       Tsunade kanashimo   (7)

   Oh, how I wish this world would be unchangeable!
   A fisherman is passing along the waterside in front of me,
   Drawing hard a small boat by a rope.
   I feel sad suddenly when gazing at his rope.

#639   *Hakone ji wo   ware koekureba   Izu no umi ya*   (5, 7, 5 syllables)

Oki no kojima ni (7)
Nami no yoru miyu (7)

    Walking up a winding path of Hakone Mountains,
    Such a wide and distant view of the sea of Izu I have!
    Ocean waves break into ripples,
    Upon the shore of small islands
    Dispersed off the Izu Peninsula.

#641 *Oh-umi no iso mo todoro ni yosuru nami* (5, 7, 5 syllables)
    Warete kudakete (7)
    Sakete chiru kamo (7)

    Ocean waves beat rocks in a roar;
    The wave is broken, crushed, and tore,
    And finally it goes away.
    I keep watching the waves as they go.

Minamoto-no-Sanetomo (1203-1219) was the second son between Minamoto-no-Yoritomo, the founder of the Kamakura Shogunate (Government), and his wife, Hojo Masako, who was from the Hojo clan getting power in the Kanto districts. Young Sanetomo who were a genius of *waka* on a good amount of learning about Chinese and Japanese literatures was a naïve and sensitive statesman. After the death of his father in 1199, his elder brother, Yoriie, succeeded the shogunate for a while but was confined in a temple in the Izu peninsula in a political strife between clans. Yoriie was killed in 1204 at the year of 23. In 1203, Sanetomo was appointed as the third Shogun of the Kamakura Shogunate at his 12 years and brought up in a favorable environment for over 15 years as Shogun until assassinated by a son of Yoriie at as early as 28 years of age. Sanetomo possessed a literary ability as his father, Yoritomo and left behind a good volume of excellent *waka* poems which were compiled as an anthology named *Kinkai-wakashu* after his death. He was gifted Manyo-shu at the year of 22 by Fujiwara-no-Teika (1162-1241), an outstanding poet from the Fujiwara clan, and strongly impressed by the book. His poems beat our mind as they were unaffected and included in the poem a large scaled landscape with highly skilled distribution of words to reflect sensitively the mind just as the poems in Manyo-shu had been. The tombs of Masako and her second son, Sanetomo are in Jufuku-ji, a Zen temple in Kamakura. Jufuku-ji was founded in 1200 by Eisai, who imported Rinzai Zen from Southern Sung China (1027-1279) with the support of Masako and her first child, Shogun Yoriie. It was the site where the house of Yoshitomo, the father of Yoritomo, had been. Masako and her child, Sanetomo, went to Jufuku-ji and experienced Zen and the way of tea, which had just been imported from Southern Sung by Eisai. Jyuhuku-ji where Eisai died in 1215 developed later to became one of *Gozan* (the five great temples of Rinzai) in Kamakura which were cores of the culture of the Kamakura and subsequent Muromachi (Ashikaga) periods (1333-1568). When we look back to *waka* (*tanka*) works of Sanetomo selected above, we could say that he is realistic in the expression of the world faithfully following the *Manyo*-style and cool and strong as a Zen mind.

Zen is a religion of solitude, in which one benefits oneself with his efforts. It has no fixed icon or imagery but weighs on praxis. Historically, it has a root in Yoga in ancient India where meditative praxis had been traditionally prevalent. It was incorporated into Buddhism by the Buddha from its beginning; hence it was an essential part of Buddhism. It was imported to Japan from Sung China, later than other Buddhist sects. Two priests went to China in succession to study and brought back this new from of Buddhism: Eisai (Rinzai Zen) and Dogen (Soto Zen). Japanese Zen includes these two schools and Obaku Zen, which was brought to Japan by a Chinese monk called Yin-yuan (Ingen) at the beginning of the Edo period. Obaku Zen is a derivation of Rinzai Zen. Ingen founded Manpuku-ji temple in Uji, a region south-east to Kyoto, for Obaku Zen sect with the support of Ietsuna Tokugawa, the fourth Shogunate of the Edo period. There is a bridge named after Ingen hung over the river of Uji still now and Ingen beans which he carried from the continent are well implanted in the life of Japanese. Concerning the tea, Eisai introduced the powdered tea to Japan in association with Rinzai Zen, while Ingen, an invited Zen monk, brought here the steeped tea which has become the most popular tea in the present Japanese life in association with Obaku Zen.

Zen sects exerted a considerable influence on the formation of Japanese spirituality, through concepts such as proud independence, quiet reflection, transparency, self-help and the awareness of Non-being. Zen also offered the basic structure and concept of the way of tea (*wabi-cha, cha-do*). Coming back to Sanetomo, a memorable Shogun who died young, leaving substantial amounts of *waka* for the age as seen in the *Kinkai-waka-shu,* recognized his sad fate in the surroundings of a power struggle and individually reached a deep soul state of Zen under the influence of Eisai, transforming his experience into sublimely beautiful poetry which appeals to present-day Japanese. Indeed, Zen culture brought about by Eisai from the continent was embodied at the earliest in Kamakura by young Sanetomo. Zen then contributed gradually to the establishment of loneliness as a feeling typical of the Japanese style and loneliness-related conception of the martial arts. Sanetomo, however, already at his twenties realized the world in Zen quietness and created beautiful poems about nature with his Zen-inspired clarity.

- *Oku-no-Hosomichi* or "The Narrow Road to the Interior", by Matsuo Basho (1644-1694)

Oku-no-Hosomichi is the 5th writing dealing with Basho's travel which is famed for exellent quality of poses and *haiku* included in it. The book has an introduction beginning with "Days and months are travelers of eternity. So are the years that pass by travelers."

Matsuo Basho created *haiku* poems by making further shorter the 5-7-5-7-7 syllable format of *waka* to the 5-7-5, which is the shortest form of Japanese poems. *Haiku* is thus composed of only three lines. As a result, *haiku* became highly symbolic, leaping and intuitive; it also became a central component of the Japanese ethos because it opened the gateway to poetic expression to every Japanese person; any Japanese person can make poems by simply stringing together 17 syllables in the 5-7-5 style. This literary movement had a large impact on the formation of Japanese feelings. Haiku owes substantially to Zen for the brevity and simplicity as well as the metaphoric way of communication. In general, a poem is a creation. Poetic invention implies a descent to the horizon of existence. If a *haiku* is a poem, any Japanese person can immerse himself or herself in the horizon of existence every day as through Zen practice. Therefore, it comes that the whole nation has a small instrument on which to play feelings easily. Three representative haiku poems by Basho are shown:

Furu-ike ya	(5 syllables)	A so old pond!
Kahazu tobi-komu	(7)	A frog took a dive into it.
Mizu no oto	(5)	Just a sound heard and it's ever tranquil.

Shizukasa ya	(5 syllables)	Tranquility!
Iwa ni shimi-iru	(7)	The rock is penetrated
Semi no koe	(5)	By the voice of a cicada.

| *Tabi ni yan de* | (5 syllables) | I am taken ill during the trip. |
| *Yume ha kare-no wo* | (7) | A bad dream is of a desolate field |

Kake-meguru	(5)	Where it runs around swiftly.

- The poetry of Ryokan (1758-1831)

    Ryokan was a monk of Soto Zen highly attained in discipline. Soto derived from Dogen (1200-1253) is known for its strictness as already described. He placed himself at the core of original Buddhism all the life. His rigor attitude in religious mind and praxis and life was second to Dogen in Japanese history of Soto. Naturally, he was unaffected for worldly affairs and always in a torn-out robe carrying a bowl for begging. However, he has highly achieved at least in three genres of art as calligraphy, Chinese poetry and *waka* and the like of Japanese poems. Further, he is distinguished in that he lived actually the life of his poetry or existentially with a strong faith in the truth which he appreciated by his hard and strict practice of *zazen*. As an enlightened Buddhist, he was benevolent to all the livings including small insects and plants. He was contentedly poor in his life-style of a beggar but enjoyed in reality a delight of priesthood, and shared cloths and food with other beggars or even robbers. He lived alone in a simple and shabby hut in the mountains and played innocently with children until dark in villages which was also the place where he begged food to keep his life as a Buddhist. In his behaviors, he was fulfilling a life of the Buddha and as a result became appreciated the Buddhahood everywhere in mountains, rivers, children and ultimately cosmos. He was absolutely indifferent to the humors of people because he lived out his belief that he was at the mind of the Buddha than anyone else. This is indeed the point of Ryokan who still gathers so much admiration from many contemporary Japanese who cannot escape from their worldly fetters if they want to live their lives unrestrainedly like Ryokan. Indeed, Ryokan is one of the most missed characters among Japanese, or most Japanese share the same at the deep mind with Ryokan. He is a spiritual home for many contemporary Japanese to come back for a rest to restore them when they are at a loss of their way.

A famous Chinese-style poem (*kanshi*) by him reads:

Syogai mi-wo tatsuru-ni monouku
Tohtoh tenshin-ni makasu
Nohtyu-ni sansyo-no kome
Rohen-ni issoku-no takigi

160

Tareka towan meigo-no ato
Nanzo shiran myohri-no chiri
Ya-u soh-an-no uchi
Soh-kyaku wo tohkan-ni nobasu

I have not cared to make my way in the worldly life.
I have left it to chance.
As my belongings in this tiny hut, only three *sho** of rice in my beggar's sack,
And a faggot of wood at the fireside, those are all and enough.
Who asks my trace of illusion and enlightenment?
Why do I know wealth and fame, since I am above such dusts?
Rain in the night comes into my grassy hut.
I stretch out both of my legs unrestrainedly.
(* One *sho* corresponds approximately to two quarts.)

Besides an excellent poet of Chinese poems, he was a *waka* poet and the best calligrapher as well. While Chinese poems or *kanshi* were made in the prime of his life, Japanese poems or *waka* (*tanka*) were made late in his life.

Three representatives of his *waka* poems are shown:

Awa-yuki no nakani tachitaru mi-chi-oh-chi*	(5, 7, 5 syllables)
Mata sono naka ni	(7)
Awa-yuki zo furu	(7)

It snows lightly around my hut in the mountain.
In each flake of snow falling like these,
There exist three thousands universes,
In each of which, such a light snowfall occurs,
Including again three thousands worlds in each flake,
So and so, Ah!
(*Mi-chi-oh-chi is a word of Ryokan's coinage to express a well known concept in the *Lotus Sutra* about the universe. Reading this poem, it is clearly shown that he was aware of Buddhahood in which he and the universe are one and the same.)

Ki-no-kuni no takano no oku no furu-dera no	(5, 7, 5 syllables)
Sugino shizuku wo	(7)

Kiki-akasi tsutsu (7)

Lodging in an old temple, deep in the mountains in Koya of Ki-province,
I hear all day raindrops dripping from giant cedar trees.
I have passed a night awake listening to the sound.

Ashibikino ihama wo tsutahu kokemizu no	(5, 7, 5 syllables)
Kasukani ware ha	(7)
Sumiwataru kamo	(7)

Like a thin and tiny water flowing along the moss on the rock,
I live faintly my life all the way,
But, I'm sure; it's truly limpid as the water.

    As is clear from the three waka poems as cited above, Ryokan was a thorough Zenist absorbed in Dogen for mental attitude weighing the simplicity, pureness, and sincerity to the truth. He was also influenced by Saigyo in the lifestyle of renouncing the world. Although he was born to the village head family in Izumozaki in the Echigo district (now Niigata prefecture), he ran away from home at the year of 18 for spiritual conflicts and entered the Buddhist priesthood at the age of 22 (in 1779) and devoted himself to the ascetic practices of Soto Zen at Entsu-ji temple in Tamashima, a town in the Bitchu district (now Okayama prefecture). In Soto Zen, monks mediate single-mindedly in the *Zazen* position which requires rigorous training and concentration. Although he was authorized as a Soto Zen monk at the age of 33, he chose wandering further in the country as a beggar monk with a black robe and a bowl to beg rice to learn more from higher monks. He visited Kyushu, Shikoku, and Chugoku for this purpose, and went up to Mt. Koya with the ashes of his father who died in Kyoto. He returned home in Echigo at the age of around 39. His life style there was simple and unaffected as begging food when necessary, playing with kids until dark, sitting and thinking in his humble hut in the mountains, and creating artistic works for calligraphy and poetry. Because of such eccentric behaviors, he was called the fool monk by nickname by children but highly respected by village people as they all realized that he was one of the best calligraphers and an excellent composer of Chinese poems as well as *waka*. In his fifties, a couple of collections of *waka* and Chinese poems were completed. In his later years of 68, Ryokan took a female disciple named Teishin of 29 years old. They exchanged *waka* poems for their communication and later for love. After his death at the age of 74 (1831), Teishin compiled her master's works including *waka*, *haiku*, calligraphy and Chinese poems into a book, which have been transferred to us today. He was fundamentally different from Saigyo in that Ryokan abandoned riches and fame completely. Ryokan was the first-born son of the venerable Yamamoto family of Izumozaki. He left home at the age of 18 and transferred responsibility for his family to his brother. He concentrated in Zen ascetic practices to realize himself or the essence of life as Dogen did for more than ten years, until he was 33 years old. He also created masterpieces in the fields of Japanese and Chinese poetries and artistic calligraphy. The Chinese poem shown above is one of the most famous works of Ryokan. It demonstrates that he was confident of his free spirit, his simple life and his intent, and also that he was above any worldly fame or wealth through abandoning everything except his life. This is the absolute freedom or Buddhahood which is ubiquitous in the mountains, flowers, children, cosmos and myself as Dogen extensively stated in *Shobo-genzo*. In this freedom, the differential dichotomies of subject and object, mind and body, self and non-self, rich and poor, man and animal, and so on are all cast off. Enlightenment of buddhahood or *Shinjin-datsuraku* in a famous Dogen's term is to appreciate such magnificent wisdom which exists in the deepness of all and is above any dichotomic differntiation.

Ryokan as such abandoned everything in the ordinary life as well as renounced the world, through which he spent his precious time in his limited life for acquisition of the truth or deepening the way of Buddha. His behavior was akin to that of Socrates, the ancient Greek philosopher who found "the wisdom of ignorance" for himself (He is reputed to have stated, "I know that I do not know".) and Confucius, the ancient Chinese teacher of wisdom credited to the dictum, "I can die in the evening if I am taught the way in the morning.", which is included in *Rongo* or "The Analects of Confucius". These three sages are similarly popular to this day in Japan, because they all lived their lives rightly at the essence of human, which is commonly shared by the present people unchanged in the long history.

■   *Kiribi* or "Flint Sparks", an anthology of *tanka* poems by Akahiko Shimaki (1876-1926)

Hito ni tsuguru kanashimi narazu akikusa ni	(5, 7, 5 syllables)
Iki wo shiro-jiro	(7)
Tsukini kerukamo	(7)

Chapter V : *Culture and Ethics* 163

This is not a sorrow to tell others.
I breathed out a deep breath over autumn wild grass.
My breath turned white in the chill air of highlands.

Yuh-yake zora   koge kihamareru   shita ni shite   (5, 7, 5 syllables)
Kohran to suru   (7)
Umi no shizukesa   (7)

The sky is aglow to its extreme burn,
At the sunset in a mountainous country.
The lake is going to be frozen,
And lies quiet in the dusk.

Yuki tokete   toh-arawa naru   chi no taira   (5, 7, 5 syllables)
Samuku chiisaku   (7)
Hi ha iran to su   (7)

On melting of snow cover in a mountainous country,
Figures of the ground are thus disclosed until far.
How bleak, how small the sun is sinking into the horizon!

- *Aratama* or "An Uncut Gemstone", an anthology of *tanka* poems by Mokichi Saitoh (1882-1953), who is one of the most distinguished poets of contemporary *tanka* (*waka*).

Yuh sareba   daikon no ha ni   furu shigure   (5, 7, 5 syllables)
Itaku sabishiku   (7)
Furi ni kerukamo   (7)

The day is declining.
Rain falls on the radish leaves,
So deeply and so helplessly.

Hisakatano   shigure furikuru   sora sabishi   (5, 7, 5 syllables)
Tsuchi ni oritachi   (7)

Karasu ha naku mo (7)

    I am in a shower of rain in late autumn.
    It's lonesome to watch in the sky where it comes.
    A crow comes down on the ground and cries.

Yama-kai ni asana yuhna ni hito ori te	(5, 7, 5 syllables)
Mono wo iu koso	(7)
Aware nari kere	(7)

    Morning and evening, I hear a few voices in a ravine!
    Some cultivate the height, exchanging words to each other.
    I am deeply moved to hear their brief talks,
    Which are tense and clear in the mountain air.

- *Sho-kei* meaning "A Path with Weak Sunlight", an anthology of *tanka* poems by Miyoji Ueda (1923-1989)

Yuhtsu hi no nokoru kozue no sayuragu ha	(5, 7, 5 syllables)
Wakaba no mori to	(7)
Ie do sabishiki	(7)

    A treetop shivers, with remaining light of the setting sun.
    I feel somewhat disconsolate,
    Even though it is a wood of young leaves.

Ameniyuku yuhsaka nishite hitokage ni	(5, 7, 5 syllables)
Awanu sabishisa	(7)
Aitemo sabishi	(7)

    On a walk up a path of the suburb in the rain,
    I meet quite nobody this evening!
    I feel lonely, but perhaps the same even if I meet someone.

Chi ha kurete sora yuku kumo ni hikari ari   (5, 7, 5 syllables)

Toki no hazama wo   (7)
Fukare te ayumu   (7)

    The sun went down under the earth.
    A cloud going in the sky reflects light.
    I realize now walking between the times, blown by the wind.

    When we read the poems of these three modern-day *waka* poets, we understand that the 31-syllable verse is the most appropriate for expressing the feelings typical of Japanese people. And we realize rightly that this rhythm has been shared by our ancient people dating back to the period when *Kojiki* and *Manyo-syu* were written and by people today.

    Akahiko was a teacher in the education-minded Nagano prefecture (a rural country in the mountains with an old name of Shinano). Both Mokichi Saitoh and Miyoji Ueda were *tanka* (*waka*) poets and medical doctors. They left abundant works of literary critics too. The major achievement of Mokichi was to restore *Manyo-shu* to his contemporaries. The three poets had in common their delicate feelings for nature. They had lucid powers of observation like Zen monks, and they found the essence of life which was beautifully sublimated in each work of art.

    Their verses were inspired by the rhythm appeared in the *Kojiki* which is the first record of spoken Japanese in written form as it was and the *Manyo-shu* which is a big collection of verses of ancient people, or the rhythm has been continuously passed down since the historical period of Prince Shotoku. The poetic rhythm taken out from traditional verses is as it were imprinted in the gene of Japanese, like a small instrument playing the feelings of the people. Indeed, *tanka* (*waka*) is used still today to create poems expressing Japanese feelings.

6. Notions regarding the human body: a comparison between the East and the West

① The East Asian concept

    Human beings are part of nature and the universe. The concept is that there is a microcosm in the human body; the human being is a total existence in free communication with the universe. Such concept was previously shown in part in Ryokan's *waka* saying that in each falling snow, a number of cosmos are included; in each cosmos snow is falling; so and so in such telescopic relationship. This is more or less common among East Asian theories on the nature or world as seen in Taoism, the

Yin-Yang and the Wu Xing (Five Elements) as well as the Buddhist notion that the subject and the object are one and the same. Because the human being in her entirety is part of the universe, it has been described in the doctrine of Yin-Yang and Five Elements that there exists the basic law or principle governing not only the human body which is a constituent of natural world but also the human mind as an inner entity of the body. It has been believed that the disease is a state in which the human being and the universe interact abnormally (abnormal *qi* or *chi*), whereas health is the reverse. Concerning with Buddhism, *butsu-ga-ichinyo* (Unification of the World and I) is the ultimate aim of practice since the Buddha. In the concept of the fusion of consciousness and matter, the outer environment and our minds are not separable. In other words, nature is not an object independent of our objectifying mind.

In contrast to Western thoughts, East Asians thought generally that disease was caused by an imbalance among all organs, not by a single abnormal organ (the liver, heart, kidney, etc), although ancient Hippocratic physiology included "the four humors theory" composed of blood, phlegm, yellow bile, and black bile, which was later amplified as it was uncorrected by Galen (129-216). Therefore, they in Asia did not investigate out and out the causes of diseases through empirical observation or dissection of human corpses, as Westerners did. Rather, they simply relied on theories and speculations. They did not perform operations based on natural science, and used their skills mainly for magic. Empirical methods of surgery based on experience spread from person to person.

Japanese people were basically on the thought described above and further influenced in particular by Buddhism and native animism modified by Buddhism. Basically, Buddhists have not studied the human body analytically and generally did not dissect human corpses or damage the human body even it was dead. Rather than segmental observation of the body, they were inclined toward a varied concepts like an emancipation, a religious flight from the world, *sokushin-jobutsu* (attainment of Buddhahood in his own body), and a faith in the Pure Land.

② The Western concept

The foundation of the Western concept of body (shape) was established in the physics of ancient Greece. As shown above, ancient Greek physics was also a natural philosophy. The ancient Greeks understood natural phenomena and events through the prism of causality, and their overall view of the cosmos was mechanistic. The modern Western ego and rationality are based on this mechanistic worldview, as evidenced by the famous statement of Descartes, "Cogito, ergo sum." Ancient Greek physics was a basic driving force of the Western scientific culture and the development of natural science.

Dissections and operations on human bodies have been performed since Greek antiquity. People, such as the famed ancient Greek physician Hippocrates engaged himself or had interest in dissections to investigate the causes and effects of disease and made scientific observations of diseased organs, as is apparent by his right knowledge that epilepsy is caused by brain lesion and not due to Poseidon intrusion. From the viewpoint of Western traditional medicine, diseased organs can be removed and replaced with healthy ones without hesitation. In other words, organ transplantation is acceptable, and has now become routine.

7. On nature

The term "nature" can be used in two ways. One is to refer to external objects, such as mountains, rivers, grass, weather conditions, the universe, etc., and this is "the external nature" or the way in which "nature" is often used today. The other is to refer to the state or process of events which occur in our minds, in the world, and in the universe. So, this is the "internal nature" as opposed to the "external nature". In the second case, nature has been called from old "*jinen*" in Japan as notably appeared in the works of Shinran (1173-1262) who is the founder of the Jodo-shin-shu and a pupil of Honen who founded the Jodo-shu. Shinran used the word "*jinen honi*" in the second sense of nature, to describe that all are by nature endowed with dharma which is appreciated at casting off any human efforts. A Japanese word "自然" was for a long time read *jinen* until the Meiji Restoration, implying solely the "internal nature", and it was only after the Meiji Restoration when natural science was introduced from the West as a national policy that "自然" read "*shizen*" became popularly used. maintaining now the dual meanings of the "external nature" as well as the "internal nature".

A Greek word *physis* was translated into the Latin *natura*. Although the range of definition concerning *physis* which was an ancient Greek concept of nature was broad, the *physis* was basically employed to mean an essence or a state of being of all things from which the "internal nature" is derived. Hippocrates (c.460- c.377B.C) used the expression "natural healing power" as *vis medicatrix naturae* meaning a competitive strife between *physis* and illness leading to a crisis. As *physis* was metaphysically an original state at the time, it was considered to possess an almighty ability to recover normalcy from illness. Later, Galen (Galenus, 129-216) who fancied himself as the greatest successor of Hippocrates but in fact influenced erroneously the medicine throughout the medieval period from a historical viewpoint of today, stated that the growth of living organisms was caused by *physis* (nature) and that animals were differentiated from plants because of possessing souls (*psyche*). Anyway, in these old uses of *physis*, they both meant "internal nature" by it.

① External nature

"External nature" refers to the natural environment. Our bodies are also a part of external nature, as seen from the standpoint of the mind (spirit).

In the West, the attitude of humans toward nature initiated from Greek natural philosophy inquiring to the *arché* which was deemed the primary substance or underlying principle of all things. Traditionally in the Western knowledge, it was thought that nature was created by the Creator and that humans, existing next to the Creator at the summit of the hierarchy of all creatures, were permitted to control, modify and conquer all of nature. This is an attitude in which the vector of the subject (ego) to object (target) by humans is exerted over all living and non-living things in the world. This basic attitude was applied unchanged to the consideration of organs in the body and becomes a basis of modern Western scientific culture including medicine..

Meanwhile, in East Asian wisdom in general, nature is what we humans live with and not an object of control as we have traditionally grown up in Buddhism. Humans are only a component of all living things in nature where they live together in "coexistence". This concept is of old and symbolically appeared in the pictures of the Buddha immediately after his death (nirvana pictures). Also, as commonly observed in local religions in East Asia, animistic gods (spirits) are everywhere in nature. The primary importance in East Asian wisdom was getting general harmony among all things in nature and did not involve an establishment of the modern ego (the confrontation between human and nature, the conflict between the mind and body) which the Western thought remarkably dealt with. People in the Asia did not pursue nature thoroughly in the sharp contrast to an attitude of the Western people who tried to get answers to the inquiry of "What is the *arché* ?" People in the East accepted nature first as it was, and subsequently the harmony between all livings to share life within nature was figured out. This is best understood when we read Buddhism sutras, e.g. the *Mahaparinirvana Sutra* formed in India. This is the salient characteristic of East Asian wisdom.

We should note that this is not a question which of East Asian wisdom and Western wisdom is superior. An important fact is that we Japanese are living at and guided by a mixture of both types of wisdom.

② Internal nature

In modern life of the Japanese, the "internal nature" refers most often to all things "natural", "spontaneous" or "of itself". I will explain this using example from literature for easier understanding.

Internal nature is the essence of matter as best shown in the following two *tanka* in the usage of a Japanese term *"onozukara"*.

Onozukara *uragaruru no ni   tori ochite*
Nakazarisi kamo
Irihi akaki ni

   The field died **naturally** in wilting.
   A bird fell and did not warble,
   Though the sunset is red.   (composed by Akahiko Shimaki)

Kayoumono   sudeni taetaru   jujiro ni
Onozukara *narite*
Kawaru sigunaru

   There is no one in the intersection of the midnight.
   The road signal sounds **of itself** abruptly in this stillness,
   Followed by changing of the color of the signal-light.
                          (composed by Norihiko Aoki)

The words "naturally" and " of itself " appear in these poems. They relate to the second way of using the term "nature."

East Asian wisdom attaches as such a high value to natural or beyond-human power processes and their consequences which may be best expressed as an inner principle., which not causality but rather near to *engi*. This is employed for the sequence of events at back of Buddhism and beyond causality. Naturalness or freedom from all sorts of thoughts and ideas of humans has been a pivotal importance in Buddhism in particular Zen. More ordinarily, the expressions such as a "natural" attitude (a calm and relaxed manner) and a "natural" course or, in the most recent usage in Japanese life, a traffic jam in the highway due to a natural course refer to the processes of nature generally accepted among the Japanese. This implies a withdrawal from human efforts and to leave a matter to the process of the cosmos. In this mindset, people wait for nature to take its course. In this respect, nature in East Asian wisdom is different from nature in Western wisdom, which emphasizes causality and deliberate control.

8. Human attitudes toward nature: a comparison between the East and the West

East Asian people find out their minds (spirits) in nature and reflect their minds on nature as it is, feeling undividedly at one with nature. They show a passive or indecisive attitude toward nature in the subject-object relationship, because they are a part of nature physically and mentally. They get relaxed when they feel they are in harmony with other all livings in nature as taught in the ethos of Buddhism. In the contrast, Westerners thoroughly and actively objectify nature. They search for the hidden truth in nature using the so-called "scientific methods" including observation and reasoning traditionally derived from natural philosophy in ancient Greece and hereby obtained results are utilized to control nature further. That is, it is an attitude of insatiable objectification of nature. Nature is primarily a target of scientific investigation and modification by human.

The difference between the East and the West concerning the attitude to nature would be explained using the art of gardening as a best example.

① The Eastern-style garden

In Eastern-style gardens, beauty in nature is borrowed as miniature without modification. This is an imitation of nature. Nature has been of itself beautiful already before the work of humans is added. When Japanese people figure out to design landscape gardening, they usually try to reproduce the distribution of the beauty in nature as rivers, ponds, rocks, water falls and trees close to them. They generally possess artistic minds to find beauty in nature in its pristine state and want to bring it near him. Japanese people seek peace of mind in nature in its naturalness and simplicity, which might be related to animism and Zen. As they admire natural products, even small river stones and roots, they brought them into the house and garden in the desire of placing nature in their familiar environment. Expressions of Zen philosophy are naturally projected onto the art of landscaping, and they become infused with "Eastern thoughts." The philosophical thoughts and people's mind are reflected on nature and people exist in nature forming a perfect whole. It is a characteristic of Japanese-style garden that there exists an asymmetrical beauty. This is because nature has an asymmetrical beauty which appeals to Japanese mind (Fig. 11).

② The Western-style garden

Artificial streams and water works, geometric architectures, and arrangements of man-made objects are general characteristics seen in the gardens of ancient Greece and

Rome. It was a trend for people to pursue geometrical or perfect beauty including sphericalness, roundness, and symmetry using processed goods or their arrangement in their garden, which is basically still kept unchanged in modern European countries (Fig. 12).

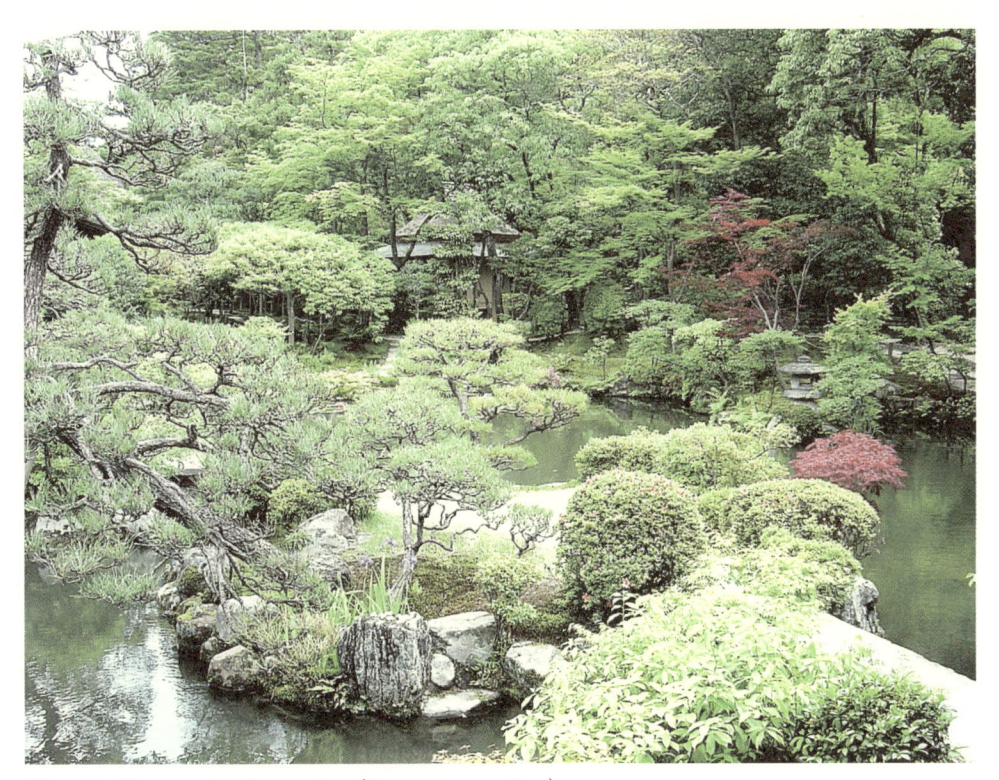

Fig. 11 Eastern-style garden (Japanese garden)

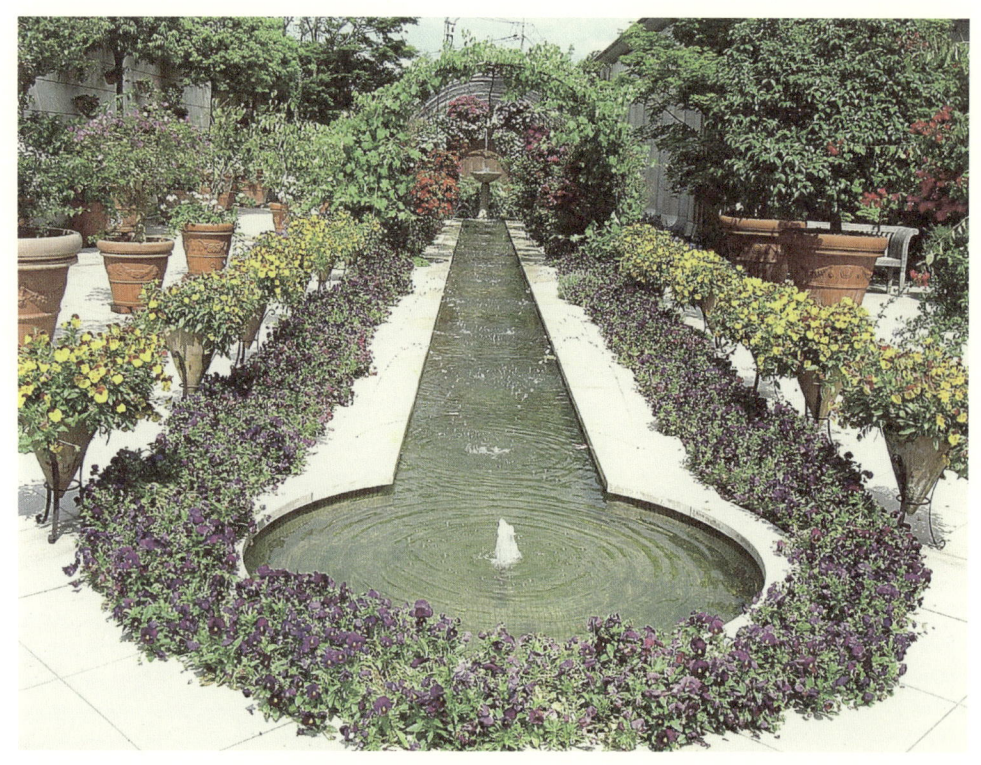

Fig. 12 Western-style garden

In Western-style garden, water flows down from a jug lifted on the shoulder of a woman figure. Alternatively, water comes out from the mouth of a lion. In the contrast, East Asian people hope that water should come out of natural settings to make them think of for instance deep mountains and dark valleys. The cultural difference between the West and East regarding beauty is thus evident. As we realize in Western －style gardens, nature is nothing but a material used to express the beauty contrived by humans. Actually, Pythagoras, Plato and Aristotle in ancient Greece, as well as people at the time believed that there should be a mathematical principle, which they regarded mystically divinity. The mathematical principle was the "*arché*" for Pythagoras which was hidden behind all of the secrets of the universe, the beauty in nature and the melodious music moving humans. To discover and interpret this mathematical principle or divinity was the primary concern of religious activity for the great philosophers and religious leaders then. This concept that supreme geometrical principles are at work in back of phenomenal beauty in the world is presumed to be carried on in the Western gardening tradition. Westerners think that nature should be objectified always by humans and controlled by them, and that the knowledge or objective facts discovered by humans should be reproduced or applied in an exaggerated manner in nature. For Western people, to arrange their garden beautifully is equal to devise and develop beauty as envisioned by humans, using nature freely as the raw material.

References
1) Inazo Nitobe: Bushido The Soul of Japan, G. P. Putnam's Sons, New York, 1905
2) Imanuel Kant; translated into Japanese by Yoshinari Abe and Tadashi Fujiwara: Grundlegung zur Metaphysik der Sitten. Iwanami Shoten, Tokyo, 1919
3) Kakuzo Okakura; translated into Japanese by Hiroshi Muraoka: The Book of Tea. Iwanami Shoten, Tokyo, 1929
4) Tetsuro Watsuji: Hudo (Climate). Iwanami Shoten, Tokyo, 1935
5) Daisetsu Suzuki; translated into Japanese by Momoo Kiagawa: Zen Buddhism and its Effects on Japanese Culture (Zen To Nihonbunka)). The Eastern Buddhist Society, Otani Buddhist College, Kyoto, 1938 and Iwanami Shoten, Tokyo, 1940
6) Kitaro Nishida: Nihonbunka No Mondai. Iwanami Shoten, Tokyo, 1940
7) Hideo Kobayashi: Mujyo To Iukoto (On Mujyo), Kadokawa Shoten, Tokyo, 1954
8) Shoko Watanabe: Nihon No Bukkyo (Japanese Buddhism), Iwanami Shoten, Tokyo, 1958
9) Hippocrates; translated into Japanese by Masakiyo Ogawa: On Ancient Medicine. Iwanami Shoten, 1963
10) Hideo Kanda, Yasuaki Nagazumi, Kosaku Yasuraoka: Hojoki, Tsurezuregusa, Shohogenzozuimonki, Tasnnisyo – Nihonkotenbungakuzenshu 27 -. Shogakukan, Tokyo, 1971
11) Jyunzo Karaki: Tyusei No Bungaku. Chikuma Shobo, Tokyo, 1972
12) Yoshinori Takeuchi: Shinran To Gendai. Tyuokoronsya, Tokyo, 1973
13) F. A. von Hayek and Kinji Imanishi: Shizen・Jinrui・Bunmei. NHK, Tokyo, 1979
14) Junzo Karaki: Zen To Shizen. Hozokan, Kyoto, 1981
15) William N. Porter:The Tosa Diary by Ki-No-Tsurayuki. Tuttle Publishing, 1981
16) Mitsuji Fukunaga: Dokyo To Nihonbunka (Taoism and Japanese Culture) Jinbun Shoin, Kyoto, 1982
17) Miyoji Ueda: Kono Yo, Kono Sei –Saigyo, Ryokan, Myoe, Dogen-. Shintyosya, Tokyo, 1982
18) Mitsuji Fukunaga: Shukyo To Kodainihon (Taoism and Ancient Japan). Jinbun Shoin, Kyoto, 1987
19) Mitsuji Fukunaga: Tyugoku No Tetsugaku・Shukyo・Geijyutu (Chinese Philosophy, Religion, and Art). Jinbun Shoin, Kyoto, 1988

20) Nobuyuki Kaji: Jyukyou To Wa Nanika? (What is Confucianism?). Tyuokoronsha, Tokyo, 1990
21) Keiji Nishitani: Nishitani Keiji Zenshu (Works of Keiji Nishitani) Vol. 16. Sobunsha, Tokyo, 1990
22) Junzo Karaki: Mujyo. Tsikumashobo, Tokyo, 1991
23) Keiji Iwata: Cosmos No Shiso. Iwanmi Shoten, Tokyo, 1993
24) Takeo Ashizu, Bin Kimura and Ryosuke Ohashi: Bunka Ni Okeru Shizen. Jinbunshoin, Kyoto, 1996
25) Akira Yoshie: Shinbutsu-Shugo. Iwanami Shoten, Tokyo, 1996
26) Shizuteru Ueda: Syukyo Heno Sisaku. Sobunsya, Tokyo, 1997
27) Galenus; translated into Japanese by Kyoko Taneyama: Function of Nature. In "Galenus II". Kyoto University Press, Kyoto, 1998
28) Koshiro Tamaki: Bukkyo No Kontei Ni Aru Mono. Kodansya, Tokyo, 2001
29) Imanuel Kant; translated into English by Allen W. Wood: Groundwork for the Metaphyisics of Morals. Yale University Press, New York, 2002
30) Daisetsu Suzuki; newly edited by Shizuteru Ueda: Toyoteki Na Mikata. Iwanami Shoten, Tokyo, 2002
31) Hajime Nakamura, Mitsuji Fukunaga, Yoshiro Tamura, Toru Konno, Fumihiko Sueki: Iwanami Bukkyo Jiten, Second Edition. Iwanami Shoten, 2002
32) Norihiko Aoki: Hito Wo Ikiru. Tyusekisya, Tokyo, 2003
33) Chofu Nunome: Chakyo-Shokai. Tankosha, Kyoto, 2003
34) Britanica Concise Encyclopedia, Encyclopedia Britanica Inc., 2004
35) Norihiko Aoki: Mikomokaru. Kindaibungeisya, Tokyo, 2005
36) Takeshi Umehara: Saityo To Kukai. Shogakukan, Tokyo, 2005
37) Dogen: Shobo-Genzo, Iwanami Shoten, Tokyo, 2006
38) Yuichi Kajiyama, Syunpei Ueyama: Bukkyo No Shiso 3 – Kuh No Ronri (Tyukan) -., Kadokawa Shoten, Tokyo, 2006
39) Seizan Yanagida, Takeshi Umehara: Bukkyo No Shiso 7 – Mu No Tankyu (Tyugoku-Zen)-. Kadokawa Shoten, Tokyo, 2006

Chapter VI: *Science and ethics for their proper orientation*

1. How far does natural science go?

In the previous chapters, I mentioned that natural science originated from ancient Greek physics which promoted the modernization of Western countries, and this modernization is spreading to all matters on Earth under the name of "globalization." Basically, science (natural science) and its by-products are created by humans. However, their proliferation is out of control. There is a concern that science and its products are invading humans both physically and mentally. With this concern as the background, bioethics and environmental ethics have appeared as independent branches of inquiry.

Humans are at the forefront, and this has remained unchanged throughout every age. However, there are many artificial things produced by modern science and industry, and they are invading the core (the mind, spirit and soul) of human beings without limit. This is the typical schematic of today's society.

With regard to the contraposition between humans and substances in this schematic, our bodies are included among the substances and are therefore targets of modern scientific wisdom. But how about the appeals rising from the inside of human beings, their basis of existence, their existential self-assertiveness?

Among contemporary ideas, there is that of the monism of science, the idea of science's absolute versatility. It is thought that science can explain all human mental activities (human thought, creativity, inspiration, religion, etc.). On the other hand, there is also an effort to orient science to its appropriate place by limiting the range of things that can be investigated by science when considering totality of things and the psyche. Causality, mechanistic theory, positivism and pragmatism are included in the former category of ideas. The humanities, which consider the human spirit and mind as existing outside causality (broadly speaking, "Romanticism"), are related to the latter category of ideas, whose underlying standpoint is to deny that the activities of the mind, such as thinking, creativity and inspiration, can be investigated by science. For example, it is thought from the latter standpoint that computers cannot perform mental activities no matter how far technology progresses. We should note, however, that this standpoint never denies the usefulness of science in general and accepts its results. However, it limits science to theoretical contributions in certain areas of inquiry. This trend originates from Socrates, Plato and Aristotle in ancient Greece, and it is especially important for people concerned with ethics, morality, philosophy, religion, truth, literature, the arts, etc. These areas of human endeavor belong to human science, in contraposition to natural science.

It is an historical reality that the quantum leap of modern science is now making the IT revolution possible, in the aftermath of the Industrial Revolution. Many people believe that robots with mechanical brains will be created by those who believe that science reigns supreme. Under these circumstances, a critical period is approaching for the mind and the spirit.

Modern science originated from ancient Greek natural science and philosophy. The scientific methods proposed by Francis Bacon (1561-1626) and the declaration of the independence of modern wisdom made by René Descartes (1596-1650) ("I think, therefore I am.") were also very important after the long period of religious focus (Academicism, Scholasticism and Hermetism) in the Middle Ages. They shared a common enthusiasm for the intellectual and cognitive abilities of humans. However, their epistemologies were different. Bacon and Descartes espoused empiricism and rationalism, respectively.

Bacon was the first to adopt the inductive method as a basic method of natural science. His inductive method included ① the correct observation of phenomena, ② the extraction of principles and laws from observed facts (the proposal of hypotheses through induction), and ③ the verification of hypotheses through experiments. The first two elements of Bacon's inductive method are the same as those of Hippocrates' method (Hippocrates was a physician in ancient Greece); Bacon added experimentation as the third. The advancements in scientific experimentation techniques and protocols that have become possible in the modern age have revealed many facts. We can now link together a series of scientific facts to arrive at deductions and generate new hypotheses to be demonstrated through new experiments.

Bacon emphasized sense experience and experimentation as cognitive methods. He became the founder of empiricism in England (in empiricism, all cognitions originate in actual experience). The empiricist first investigates facts, extracts the law of causality governing those facts, and then investigates the way in which that law manifests itself in other areas of nature. This is precisely the method being used in current science. The expression "modern natural science" is almost identical in meaning to the expression "modern rationalism." Empiricism can be included in modern rationalism if we consider the fact that to deduce is to think rationally. Hobbes (1588-1679) continued to develop the empiricism of Bacon. Hobbes denied the existence of final causes and formal causes, which were elements of Aristotle's theory adopted by Bacon; Hobbes extended the mechanistic view of nature to the human mind, abandoning the mind-substance dualism in favor of materialism, in which only matter exists and the mind is a certain pattern of material objects.

Rationalists, in contrast to empiricists, thought that human reason (mind) exists before the onset of sense experience and that reason forms ideas based on experimental facts. Descartes (1598-1650) was one of the major philosophers working in this direction. German idealists such as Kant (1724-1804) and Hegel (1770-1831) were also rationalists. For rationalists, the principle of human cognition exists *a priori*. If a human being considers a fact to be clear and obvious (e.g., a principle of mathematics) based on the principle of cognition, he considers it to be an indubitable truth.

Empiricism promoted the development of natural science by proposing new methods of observation, deduction and experimentation. Rationalism promoted the development of natural science by asking, "What is the truth?" Therefore, modern natural science has been promoted by the fusion of empiricism and rationalism resulting from the elimination of their differences in epistemology.

The development of modern science based on the establishment of modern wisdom (Descartes, Galileo and Newton) and the notion of causality is one of the two axes of the progression. The other axis is represented by the people who, while accepting science, limit its application in the sphere of human totality. The former is the genealogy of causality, mechanistic theory, positivism and pragmatism. The latter is the genealogy which values human autonomy, and includes the idealism typified by Kant and Hegel, the philosophy of life of Bergson, Heidegger and Jaspers, and the existentialism of Sartre. In the field of psychology, there is experimental psychology which is based on the scientific method, and there is another type of psychology, spearheaded by Jung in particular with his concept of "the unconscious," the part of the mind in which irrational cognitions are actively generated. This latter approach to the human mind is equivalent, broadly speaking, to the humanities, an antithesis to the rapid progress of modern science; it is the standpoint of Romanticism.

In order to simplify this chapter's question, "How far does natural science go?", I will explain modern science through the prism of Descartes, the symbol of modern science and the founder of the innovations of modern wisdom. I will also explain the thoughts of Jaspers from the standpoint of Romanticism. Jaspers tried to investigate human existence by reflecting on and limiting science while also valuing it. Then, I will explain the theory of Jung, a psychologist who strictly differentiated the regions of the psyche covered (consciousness) by scientific wisdom from those which are not (the unconscious). His is another example of a worldview according to which there is an irrational world not covered by reason. The opposition between Jaspers and Jung on one hand and

Descartes on the other seems to be analogous to the establishment of bioethics and environmental ethics against the rapid development of natural science.

2. The modern knowledge established by Descartes

The major achievement of Descartes (René Descartes, 1596-1650) was the establishment of subjectivity in contrast to objectivity. He also considered that the "cogito" was true. Through this newly established subjectivity, he tried to observe the world from the viewpoint of human wisdom for the first time. Therefore, he is called the founder of modern science and wisdom. His words "cogito, ergo sum" mean "I think, therefore, I am."

The philosophy of Descartes is characterized by the establishment of the mind as "cogito," the mechanistic rendering of the physical world, and the requirement that God exist as an absolute spirit.

"... and finally, when I considered that the very same thoughts (presentations) which we experience when awake may also be experienced when we are asleep, while there is at that time not one of them true, I supposed that all the objects (presentations) that had ever entered into my mind when awake had in them no more truth than the illusions of my dreams. But immediately upon this I observed that, whilst I thus wished to think that all was false, it was absolutely necessary that I, who thus thought, should be somewhat; and as I observed that this truth, "I think, therefore I am (COGITO, ERGO SUM)," was so certain and of such evidence that no ground of doubt, however extravagant, could be alleged by the skeptics capable of shaking it, I concluded that I might, without scruple, accept it as the first principle of the philosophy of which I was in search." (On pathos, *Discourse on Method*, translated by Yasuo Noda, Chuohkoronsha, p.43)

People in the Middle Ages did not clarify their attitudes toward existing objects because they were profoundly affected by theology. They emphasized faith. Descartes expressed strong doubts about the validity of this worldview. He declared the independence of human wisdom as an innovation. He investigated what really existed and tried to mathematically or logically reconstruct the world based on truth. Descartes was the precursor of existentialism because he investigated humans without the help of God. He started by doubting everything, and came to the conclusion that he existed because he could think; the statement that subjectivity exists was true, because subjectivity meant thinking. Descartes considered this to be the primary principle of philosophy. According to his method, various observations of facts in the world should be verified by subjectivity, now that the existence of subjectivity has been established. He used the qualifiers "clear and distinct" to describe the conditions of this mathematical verification. In other words, he adopted a dualistic theory, in which the universe consists of two types of substance: mind and matter.

According to Descartes, what is verified to be clear and distinct is the truth. Descartes considered this to be the second principle of philosophy.

Descartes valued the principles of mathematics and geometry as methods of recognizing the truth, as Pythagoras and Plato had done in Greek antiquity. This affected the introduction of his second principle of "clearness and distinctness." He considered the judgments of geometry, mathematics and mechanistic theory to be "clear and distinct."

Thus, by assuming that ① I exist as a thinking being and that ② whatever I (mind) consider to be clear and distinct is also true, I can expand the characteristics of objects and construct the truth. Descartes departed from the world of the Middle Ages controlled by the teleology of Aristotle. This was innovative because human thought was emphasized for the first time. In other words, it was the starting point of modern rationalism and natural science.

This pattern of thought was similar to that prevalent in ancient Greece. However, Descartes may be considered to be the founder of modern science, because he assimilated the scientific findings of Harvey and other discoveries made in England based on empiricism and actively integrated them into his theories. Descartes' first and second principles of philosophy are discussed in Part IV of his *Discourse on Method* (1637), where he also includes a lengthy quotation from *The Circulation of the Blood* by William Harvey published eight years earlier. Thus, modern science began when the teleology which had controlled the Middle Ages since the time of Aristotle was abolished and the mechanicism and concept of causality expounded by English empiricism (Bacon and Hobbes) became the preferred worldview.

We should note that, for Descartes, the world of nature, including animals, was naturally under the control of humans. Nature was cognized and controlled by reason based on the principle of "clearness and distinctness" which he had verified. Dualism meant that reason, also called the "I," controlled all of nature other than the "I". The essence of spirit was thought, and the essence of matter was extension. The mind was strictly differentiated from nature as the outer world. The principle of "clearness and distinctness" belonged to mechanicism and mathematical physics. Animals were assumed to be automatic machines with no divinity or mind (reason), and they were included in the part of nature controlled by humans. Thus, modern wisdom was applied to the world of nature without limit. It is interesting how Descartes understood divinity; however, he had little interest in divinity as compared to the clear contributions of natural science. God was for him simply a requirement for existence, because God as an absolute mind was required to ensure the existence of the finite and imperfect human mind.

3. Human understanding in the system of Jaspers

Karl Jaspers (1883-1969) was a scientist who began his career as a physician and psychopathologist. He sought to understand the totality of human existence, and found that it could not be revealed by science; he therefore abandoned science and developed his own existential philosophy. There are several terms which have originated from Jaspers, including "*das Umgreifende*" and its various aspects, "philosophical faith," "scientific superstition," "cipher," etc.

According to Jaspers, *Sein* (existence) is an open horizon without limits. He classified the various types of foundations or conditions that appear before us. He called these "*das Umgreifende*" ("the encompassing").

Das Umgreifende consists of seven types. He used a method to aggregate in a dialectic manner various types of *Umgreifende* that appeared to be superficially dispersed, in order to investigate the totality. His method was analytic because he was a physician, i.e. a scientist. His method shows signs of his beginnings as a physician (psychiatrist), even if he did pursue a new course as a philosopher. The various types of *Umgreifende* will now be explained according to his definitions.

1. The *Umgreifende* as the existence surrounding us (it exists even if we do not exist)
① *Die Welt*

We constitute a small part of the various existences of the world. The world is a totality that generates us. The world is not an object, but the location of the objects of cognition.

In this case, the physical world, which is an object of science, and the world of human relationships are both included in the "world" of Jaspers. As is apparent here, Jaspers' perspective on the "world" was philosophical, going beyond the perspective of scientists, even though he started as a scientist.

② *Die Transzendenz*

No *Transzendenz* is required if the world is everything there is. The thing which speaks to the natural existences of the world is the *Transzendenz*. An *Umgreifende* into which the system of the various *Umgreifende* ultimately converges is the *Transzendenz*. In other words, the *Umgreifende* of the *Umgreifende* is a *Transzendenz*.

2. The *Umgreifende* in us

① *Das Dasein*

Das Dasein includes the various types of our vital, physical, psychological and behavioral existences. We are the same *Dasein* as other living organisms with respect to the *Dasein* in the environmental world. Briefly, that is because we and other living orgasms are the target of research. However, humans are different from other *Dasein* because humans have communication with other *Umgreifende* (*Transzendenz*).

② *Das Bewußtsein überhaupt* (consciousness in general)

People are different in the consciousness of their experiences. However, there are some things common to all people, namely the intellectual function of consciousness in general. Human beings share this consciousness in general. The universal application is extracted as long as we are targeted by consciousness in general.

We think and recognize in the form of objectivity in this *Umgreifende*. The consciousness in general investigates scientifically, recognizes and shares logical demonstrations. In addition, this *Umgreifende* (consciousness in general) can think of the world, which includes the environmental world, as an object, a part of itself, and it can think beyond the world. In other words, the thing that enters our consciousness in general is the only existence for us.

③ *Der Geist*

The function of the mind is fantasy. A world penetrated by the mind is offered to the real world in the form of rich images such as art and poetry. In this *Umgreifende*, we can see ideas. We extract ideas from various events in the emerging world and possess these ideas. The idea guides us. There are practical ideas (for business, social actions, moral matters, and lifestyles) and theoretical ideas (society, politics, ethics, history, life, etc). One role of the mind is to read out the meanings of emerging events and to systematize the extracted ideas. The idea is the target of life for the *Geist*.

④ *Die Existenz*

We confront the *Transzendenz* in the *Existenz-Transzendenz* relationship as a possible *Existenz*. In this case, *Existenz* is superficial subjectivity, whereas *Transzendenz* is objectivity. However, one does not exist without the other. Each one requires the other as an opposite. *Existenz* is an existence that we are, with *Dasein*, consciousness in general (*Bewußtsein überhaupt*) and mind, as shown above. *Existenz* is the basic *Umgreifende* that exceeds the three others (or cannot be completed by the three). *Existenz* cannot be a target of science. If it is a target of wisdom, then a human is no longer *Existenz*. The human being is more than the wisdom that can be known objectively. *Existenz* is not a target of wisdom, but an awareness or conviction; it is required as an *Umgreifende* because of the dissatisfaction with oneself, the quest for freedom, the recollection of perfectibility, immortality, etc. In this case, *Transzendenz* as the extreme opposite of *Existenz* is called "sole existence," "complete thing", "Author of our being", "God", etc., all of which are expressions belonging to theism.

Die Vernunft (reason) connects and unifies all of these *Umgreifende* (*Welt*, *Transzendenz*, *Dasein*, *Bewußtsein überhaupt*, *Geist* and *Existenz*) without dissecting them. This is also an *Umgreifende* according to Jaspers. No *Umgreifende* should be lost, but all of them should be connected and unified to face *Transzendenz* as a single existence. Reason is an adhesive which prevents the various *Umgreifende* from becoming alienated from each other, keeping them in a coherent order. Thus, the *Umgreifende* is diversified, and we are and are not *Umgreifende*. We can understand the entire picture of existence only when each *Umgreifende* is positioned correctly inside of us. We understand our original existence not through scientific wisdom (consciousness in general), but through total wisdom. Our approach to total wisdom is an existence. Existence is opened to *Transzendenz*. Reason keeps each *Umgreifende* in its original relationship and makes the *Dasein* realize the existence-*Transzendenz* relationship in the ultimate sense. Therefore, reason does not allow scientific wisdom (consciousness in general) to be absolutized. To be "conscious" means to realize *Transzendenz* necessarily.

Table 4 *Das Umgreifende* (the encompassing) of Jaspers

Das Umgreifende, das wir sind (The encompassing that we are)	Subjectivity-Objectivity axis		*Das Umgreifende, das das Sein selbst ist* (The encompassing that is being itself)
	Subjective side	Objective side	
Dasein	Inner world	Environmental world	*Welt* (World)
Bewußtsein überhaupt (Consciousness in general)	Consciousness	Object	*Welt* (World)
Geist (Spirit)	Internal idea	Objective idea emerging from objects (art, poetry and science)	*Welt* (World)
Existenz	*Existenz*	*Transzendenz*	*Transzendenz*
Vernunft (Reason): It connects and prevents all *Umgreifende* from scattering within us.			

3. Subjectivity and objectivity

At this moment, *Transzendenz* is a target, from the viewpoint of existence (subjectivity). However, it may be inappropriate to consider it objective, because existence cannot reach nor objectify *Transzendenz* even if it can perceive it.

The vector from existence goes towards *Transzendenz* in a solid line. However, the vector from *Transzendenz* is sent in cipher in a broken line.

Existence knows that it was sent by *Transzendenz*. Existence (*Existenz*) understands the meaning of the message from Transzendenz through faith (philosophical faith). Therefore, objective wisdom, or the wisdom or definition of universal application, cannot enter the *Existenz - Transzendenz* axis.

4. *Subjekt-Objekt-Spaltung*

Subjectivity and objectivity are clearly differentiated when objectivity is an event in the world (including the body in the *Dasein*). Briefly put, all targets of Western modern science originating from the modern ego established by Descartes apply to the subjectivity-objectivity schematic.

However, a relationship such as the subjectivity-objectivity split is required in order to understand the *Existenz-Transzendenz* axis, which is not restricted to a one-way relationship (i.e., it is subjective and objective at the same time). We subjectivity consider ourselves to be objective, while this objectivity controls our subjectivity. The clarification of this axis is not the purpose of scientific investigation (generally, the intellect plays this role; *Verstand* is the ability to understand various targets by arranging the targets in accordance with its own form after receiving the targets through the sensibility; *Verstand* is narrower and lower than *Vernunft*) characterized by the pursuit of universal validity of objective knowledge. That is the role of philosophy. The subjectivity-objectivity split is the original horizon of Being. All *Umgreifende* are generated and have a relationship with each other. Scientific knowledge is a horizon that is opened to the entire wisdom. The truth in each *Umgreifende* is connected to the common truth in the horizon of being. No *Umgreifende* is lost in this common field. All *Umgreifende* should function towards the enrichment of totality. Reason integrates each *Umgreifende*. The role of reason as *Umgreifende*, as understood by Jaspers, is very large. It exceeds the dimensions of the world of objective knowledge (performed by *Verstand*).

The *Umgreifende* of all *Umgreifende* is *Transzendenz*. In order to obtain ultimate total wisdom, it is absolutely necessary to understand the relationship between *Existenz* and *Transzendenz*. According to Jaspers, the modes of *Umgreifende*, such as

Dasein, *Bewußtsein überhaupt*, *Geist* and *Existenz*, are destined to be in such a way that *Existenz* forms a relationship with *Transzendenz* in the end. Thus, in the total perspective of Jaspers' understanding of human beings, there is a clear limit to the scientific activities pursued by humans.

"Science enjoys enormous prestige in the modern age. People expect from science a penetrating knowledge of all things and salvation in times of trouble. **These wrong expectations are scientific superstition, and the ensuing disillusionment turns into a disdain of science.** If a person believes something to be self-evident without really knowing it, it is a superstition. The experience of a superstition's fall becomes a disregard of wisdom. Science does not occupy itself with superstitions or show disdain. Thus, scientists are surely the hallmarks of the age. However, science has changed into something other than itself.

This is how illusions are generated: **when performing a study, we start from the premise that the world can be cognized. If we did not have this premise, all studies would be meaningless.** In addition, this premise can be interpreted in two ways. One is to understand it as a premise of the probability of cognition of various things in the world. The second is the probability of cognition of the world as a totality. Only the first premise is valid. We cannot know how far cognition will advance in the world; in spite of this, however, the second premise is not valid, as illustrated by the basic problem discussed below. The problem does not limit the study of contents; however, it does reveal the limit of wisdom. In other words, **our cognition cannot approach the world as a totality, which is supposed to be the only thing which has boundaries. In addition, a world that can be thought of and experienced without contradictions can never exist for us.** This fact is a limit. These limits become clear when the invalid premise of the probability of cognizing the entire world conflicts with the actual state of all studies. It is very difficult to gain proper insight into errors. This error takes modern science for philosophy and has been repeated since Descartes. Therefore, it is still a daunting task to clearly understand the meaning and limit of modern science." (*The Origin and Goal of History*, translated into Japanese by Hideyo Shigeta, in *The World's Greatest Thoughts* II-12, p.93, Kawadeshobo Shinsha)

"**The plague of human existence starts when the knowledge obtained scientifically is considered to be the existence itself, or when all things that cannot be known scientifically are considered not to exist. Therefore, science becomes scientific superstition, and this superstition piles one folly onto another, cloaking itself in vestments which look superficially scientific. In these follies, there is no science, philosophy nor faith.** There has never been an age when science and philosophy are so clearly separated as today. There has never been an age when their differentiation is as crucial as today. However, scientific superstitions blossom in gray and philosophy seems to have disappeared.

This deceiving deviation from pure science and the root of philosophy ruins our consciousness of existence. As a result, our consciousness of existence becomes vacant as a function of the *Dasein*, which understands and experiences itself abstractly. Our consciousness of our existence has been released from the magic which once dictated our image of the world; we saw that things are limited in the universe. However, our consciousness of our existence has deformed our feeling of the basic deterioration of life, and has furthered scientific superstitions through which people finally lose sight of the objects themselves, though they communicate with objects. This deviation closes the door to philosophy. The purpose of philosophical speculation is to remove the blockage and return humans back to themselves." (*Small School of Philosophy*, translated into Japanese by Shinzaburo Matsunami, in *The World's Greatest Thoughts* II-12, p.389, Kawadeshobo Shinsha)

"We exist in the world. However, we never target the world as a whole. Various objectives appearing in the world must be studied without constraints.

The world is not integrated in our cognition. Or rather, it is ripped apart. A scientific study proceeds under the unifying idea that is appropriate in a certain region of the world. However, there have yet to be any scientific and fruitful unifying ideas which explain the whole world. The world should not be understood in isolation. In addition, the world should not be understood according to the objects, lives or spirits in it. **Existence that cannot be known precedes the possibility of cognition. In addition, existence cannot be reached by cognition. The world cannot be known by our cognition.**" (*Small School of Philosophy*, translated into Japanese by Shinzaburo Matsunami, in *The World's Greatest Thoughts* II-12, p.390, Kawadeshobo Shinsha)

Science is an indispensable condition of philosophical speculation. However, science is called on to satisfy certain requirements in the present age due to the spiritual condition generated by science. These requirements, shown below, have not been regarded as having much clarity and rigor.

(1) **Scientific knowledge should be obtained in a very pure form.** This is because unscientific assertions or behavior patterns penetrate science when it is expressed in real-life activities and average speculations. Pure and accurate scientific knowledge about all things existing in the world is still far too remote for our total spiritual reality today. It is acquired in the personality of each "scientist" as venerable as the degree of the remoteness.

(2) **Superstitions about science must be investigated and gotten rid of.** In this age of bewildering infidelity, people select a science that they consider to be solid and believe in the results of that science. They obey blindly the persons whom they suppose to be authorities and believe that science and planning can bring order to the world as a whole. They expect to gain insight into the purpose of life, an insight which science cannot really offer by itself. They also expect science to cognize existence, which cannot be reached by science.

(3) Philosophy itself must be investigated anew in accordance with a certain method.

Philosophy is a science called "speculation," which proceeds in accordance with a certain method in the oldest and permanent sense. However, it is not a science in a purely modern sense, i.e. in the sense of producing irrefutable cognitions through studies carried out on behalf of people.

The viewpoint that wrongly considers science to be the total wisdom was generated and philosophy was degraded because Descartes equated philosophy with modern science, and this error of Descartes has been highly valued over the last several centuries.

Today, we should strive for purity in philosophy as well as purity in science. Science and philosophy cannot be separated. However, they are not identical. Philosophy is not a specific science among sciences, or a science which synthesizes all other sciences, or the basic science which makes other sciences possible.

Philosophy is connected to science and speculates by way of all sciences. We cannot approach truth in philosophy without ensuring the purity of scientific truth first.

Each science exists in a harmonious universe of diverse sciences and guided by various ideas generated as a philosophy across all sciences, while this cannot be explained scientifically.

Consciousness of the truth is only possible based on the varied sciences of the 19th century. However, such consciousness has not yet been established. Engagement in the realization of this consciousness of the truth is one of the most urgent necessities at this historical moment.

By resisting the disorganization of science into disparate things which are not related to each other, by halting the onslaught of scientific superstition in laypeople and opposing the neglect and frivolity of philosophy caused by the conflict between science and philosophy, (scientific) studies and philosophy should cooperatively guide us on the path of actual truth. (Philosophy in the future, translated into Japanese by Shinji Hayashi, *What is Philosophy?*, p.198-200, Hakusuisha)

As shown above, it is natural that the criticism formulated by the existentialist Jaspers against Descartes, who was the founder of the now prospering modern science, is severe.

We should note that Jaspers was also a scientist. He became a philosopher because he realized the limitations or unsatisfactory methods of science. Jaspers thought that the speculation ("cogito") considered by Descartes to be the first principle departed from the totality of the *Umgreifende*. Jaspers' *Umgreifende* is always linked to the totality of human existence. The ego of Descartes is really required only for intellectual cognition. It is assumed that the ego was established as subjectivity. The ego established by Descartes as the first principle of the logic of subjectivity-objectivity is precisely the independent wisdom of modern science. It has departed from *Existenz* (*Umgreifende*). The method used by Descartes is intellect (*Verstand*). Intellect is the cognitive faculty applied only to scientific cognition (causality, mechanism); it is the ability to synthesize the things made available by sensibility. The world of Descartes constructed by ego and intellect does not reach the truth (totality). The objection of Jaspers is that the intellect only clarifies the world of objects scientifically. In other words, Descartes mistakenly thought that total wisdom is obtained through scientific wisdom.

We should note that Jaspers, who was originally a scientist, naturally emphasized scientific and objective wisdom based on intellect or consciousness in general. He mentioned that scientific wisdom should be integrated in the total wisdom by the power of reason, and philosophy should try to accrue scientific qualities. However, what was important for Jaspers was to give science the correct position (orientation) in the totality, to stop its absolutization. The absolutization of science generates new superstitions, which Jaspers called "*Wissenschaftsaberglaube.*"

4. The unconscious as Jung found it

It was Sigmund Freud (Vienna, 1856-1939) and Carl Gustav Jung (Switzerland, 1875-1961) who discovered something called the "unconscious" in the psyche and distinguished it from the conscious. They both began their careers as psychiatrists in German-speaking nations, and were invited to the U.S. to deliver a series of lectures on the world of the unconscious in 1909.

Freud thought that the unconscious is a dark world in which the *libido* (sexual appetite) is confined. Meanwhile, Jung thought that the unconscious has a productive and positive effect on consciousness. For both psychologists, the subjective intellect called the ego exists at the center of consciousness and controls all of it. They speculated that there must also be another world, that of the "unconscious". Freud introduced the concept of "*libido*". He thought that consciousness controlled the unconscious (centralized control by the ego) through the libido. Jung adopted a method in which the totality of the psyche is probed through the consenting participation of the patient and not through unidirectional analysis; he recorded the status of the patient's psyche phenomenologically. We can observe a substantial East Asian influence in this.

Consciousness is the world that can be reached by scientific cognition in the sense that subjective intellect is at its center. At least, Freud thought so, and adopted the view according to which a strong ego, which could also be called scientific cognizing intellect, investigates the world of the mind based on a scientific theory. This was one reason why Freud was popular in the U.S., a nation of pragmatists. Freud is known to have established the word "psychoanalysis." He thought that complexes suppressed in the unconscious can be analyzed using the scientific method and that the diseases of the mind can be cured in this way. He interpreted suppressed urges according to his theory of sexuality, and relied on a unified methodology and a simple causal mechanism. In other words, Freud tried to expand the scientific method to the sphere of the unconscious mind.

Jung was 19 years younger than Freud, yet they had in common a fascination for the unconscious. It was Jung who started to use the term "complex." They worked together for five years, from 1907 to 1912. Freud chose Jung as his successor. However, they became aware of a crucial difference in their understanding of the unconscious. Jung broke away from the suppressed-complex theory and the sexual-energy theory. After that, the theory of the unconscious (the world of the total mind) was developed by Jung to the state in which we know it today. It was Jung who defined the unconscious, a realm which cannot be understood by scientific intellect, and actively developed the theory. Jung was very different from Freud in that he esteemed East Asian thought, as it coincided with his own. He was impressed by mandalas, the *Tibetan Book of the Dead*, Eki (I Ching), etc., and integrated these into his practice. I will now outline Jungian psychology and describe how it contradicts natural science (causality) with regard to the unconscious.

① **Ego (*das Ich*) as the center of consciousness**

Consciousness is the part of the mind where the ego (subjective intellect) is in full control. Therefore, it is also the world of natural science. In general, the ego is very strongly formed in Westerners. Asian people, including the Japanese, have a weaker ego in some cases. Therefore, the ego does not always take the lead in consciousness (Hayao Kawai). The ethos, culture and history which have lasted for a longer period in East Asian countries, including Japan, have formed such weak egos. I do not want to imply that this is bad or that it is good.

Messages from the unconscious to consciousness appear in dreams. In addition, various complexes (deep-layer complexes formed in relation to prototypes such as the Anima/Animus, the Great Mother and the Wise Old Man, as well as the acquired complexes formed as a result of individual experiences and traumas) hidden in the unconscious sometimes rise into consciousness and interfere with normal behavior and activity.

Jung had a respect for the psychological energy of the unconscious and actively developed his theories on the unconscious. Freud thought that the complexes hidden in the unconscious were suppressed ideas. He analyzed them and tried to put them under the control of subjective intellect by giving interpretations integrated with his own sex theory. He tried to understand and control the unconscious in the light of consciousness. The world of Freud was really a world of analysis of the mind using the methods of modern intellect.

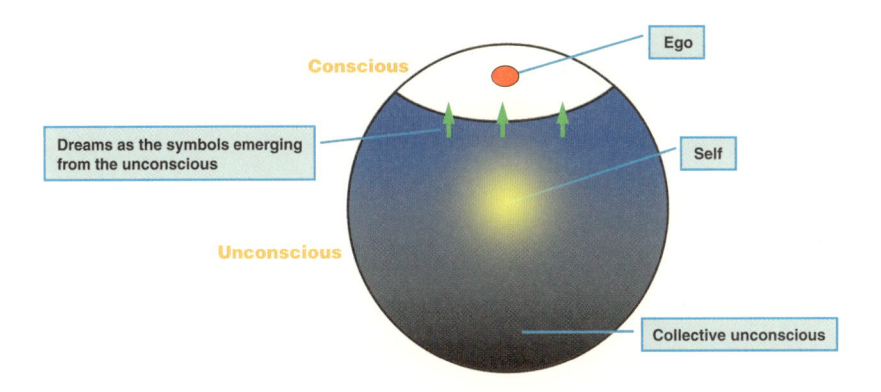

Fig.13: Consciousness and the unconscious in the psyche

② Self (*das Selbst*) as the center of the mind

The self is different from the ego.

The ego is the center of consciousness, while the self is the center of the mind (psyche) and also the totality of the mind. The mind falls under the psyche, which integrates the unconscious and consciousness. Figure 13 shows the mind (a modification of the work of Hayao Kawai). Consciousness is controlled by the ego to form the human personality. The world of causality and scientific cognition belongs to consciousness. The world that exists behind consciousness and cannot be controlled is the unconscious. Freud and Jung both discovered the unconscious, but it was Jung who differentiated between the personal unconscious and the collective unconscious. The personal unconscious is composed of the complexes formed as a result of personal experiences, family relationships, professional and social relationships, and trauma. The collective unconscious is more innate. It has been inherited by individuals and entire races since the beginning of time. It is preserved in the mythologies and folk tales of many countries. It appears in the dreams and obsessions of psychopaths in a transparent manner. Jung called these ancestral memories "archetypes."

As shown above, Jung made the unconscious account for much in the mind. This is a world that cannot be investigated by scientific wisdom. He thought that the mind is governed by a law different from causality. He developed the concept of synchronicity to explain this. Synchronicity is the meaningful psychological relationship between two events which apparently have nothing to do with each other. Jung understood the meaning of Eki, a type of Chinese fortune-telling based on Taoism. Eki is based on the dualistic theory according to which Yin and Yang both confront each other and also become fused (all things exist in pairs which are made of opposing elements). Synchronicity and Eki are generally laughed away by causality-based natural science. Jung showed that the scientific method has its limits when it comes to understanding the (conscious and unconscious) mind.

③ The mind (psyche) is originally composed of two opposing factors.

Jung showed that there were two psychic attitudes or directions in which the psychological energy flows: extroversion and introversion (these terms were invented by Jung). One of them is dominant in any given person. The other is the shadow responsible for the compensatory effects. The dichotomy between the two is also observed in the psyche's functions: thinking and feeling are rational, while sensation and intuition are irrational.

Modern intellect and modern science, which originated from Descartes, were conceived in such a way as to allow their self-propagation. However, we cannot find in science the ability to investigate the totality of human existence, as shown by Jaspers and Jung. Ethics is based on this very totality.

5. Theories on ethics linked to contemporary bioethics

I mentioned previously that Francis Bacon (1561-1626) and Thomas Hobbes (1588-1679) established empiricism (they rejected the worldview constructed by the non-empirical Middle Ages and believed that the source of all cognition was sensory experience). Empiricism adheres to objectivism, and is the basic principle that promotes the development of natural science. It is equipped with an ideatic innovation called "human autonomy," which was indispensable in the confrontation with the overwhelming history of medieval thought. Any cognition starts from experience, or depends only on facts obtained through scientific experiments. These are the ideas of empiricism, and they are very easy to understand for those of us who are at the center of a scientific civilization, partly because the methods of scientific analysis are used even in moral matters.

The system of empiricism was further developed by John Locke (1632-1704), George Berkeley (1685-1753) and David Hume (1711-1776). Empiricism became the womb which generated utilitarianism in England in the field of moral philosophy. In utilitarianism, usefulness is the sole standard of value. The human good is assumed to be the pursuit of pleasure. The first utilitarians adopted simple empiricism; for them, the amount of pleasure (happiness) could be quantified objectively by analyzing it through mathematical calculations.

Meanwhile, on the European continent, Descartes (1596-1650) established rationalism, which later acted in concert with empiricism to develop modern science in Western countries. This rationalism was succeeded by the pantheism (God is the only substance; God is nature) of Baruch Spinoza (Holland, 1632-1677) and the monadism (a fusion of mechanicism and teleology) of Gottfried Wilhelm Leibniz (Germany, 1646-1716). They all recognized that human beings are equipped with reason (the faculty of supraempirical cognition) as an *a priori* faculty of cognition and that the truth is not reached through sensory experience. They tried to obtain the universal truth through reason.

It was Immanuel Kant (Germany, 1724-1804) who unified empiricism and rationalism. Kant adopted a new type of clarity in thinking, as well as the innovative principles of Newtonian physics. He also valued reason and the metaphysics related to reason, as expounded by Descartes, Spinoza and Leibniz. Therefore, their scientific and metaphysical methods were unified and made compatible by Kant.

Kant called the cognitive faculty (scientific cognition) the "intellect" (*Verstand*). He also introduced the terms *Vernunft* (reason) and *Urteilskraft* (judgment) as technical terms in philosophy. These are faculties related to ultra-emotional or metaphysical representations (including concepts such as idea, reason, beauty, substance in itself, spirit, virtue, ethics, soul, absolute existence, etc.), which exceed the intellect (*Verstand*). He differentiated reason and judgment from intellect, and limited scientific cognition to the world of phenomena (the only source of truth recognized by empiricism), which are brought to the mind through the five senses in terms of time and space, because scientific cognition is the product of the intellect. He promoted the development of concepts which emphasize reason as viewed in rationalism. He established a philosophical theory characterized by scientific qualities and speculative reasoning.

With regard to morality and moral philosophy, Kant still exerts a considerable influence on the world because he established a system of deontological ethics (moral duty). Kant did not offer specific moral advice, such as "Do not kill," "Do not steal" or "Do not lie." He tried to show that there is a moral law inherent (given *a priori*, before any experience or education) in everyone as the source of specific moral rules. He introduced the concept of the "Categorical Imperative," which is unconditional and which enables people to recognize the beauty of morality inherent in human beings.

German Idealism was represented by Kant, Fichte, Schelling and Hegel, all of whom created innovative bodies of work from the 18th century to the beginning of the 19th century. They had a large influence on philosophers in Japan after the Meiji Restoration.

The major works of Kant are *Kritik der reinen Vernunft* (1781), *Kritik der praktischen Vernunft* (1788) and *Kritik der Urteilskraft* (1790), which are often referred to as "the three *Critiques*," and *Grundlegung zur Metaphysik der Sitten* (1785). He established a new theory of cognition by answering the question, "What can we know?" in his first critical work, *Kritik der reinen Vernunft*. He outlined the fundamental problems of moral philosophy by answering the question, "What should we do?" in *Grundlegung zur Metaphysik der Sitten* and *Kritik der praktischen Vernunft*. He explored the problems of beauty, art and teleology in *Kritik der Urteilskraft*.

We should first understand the major theories of moral philosophy in order to proceed with our discussion of bioethics, a historically new type of moral theory, from the viewpoint of the history and customs of East Asian people. It is easy for us to understand Kantianism, virtue-based theories and communitarianism, which stress the benefits of community life, because we experience these on a daily basis and they are close to our souls. Other major moral theories include utilitarianism, pragmatism and liberalism, which emphasize personal freedom, autonomy and human rights from a global viewpoint. They were imported to Japan after World War II. We confront many bioethical problems on a daily basis due to the rapid progress of science and the shift to a capitalistic industrial society. Ethical judgment is based on a combination of multiple theories, not a single theory. In the Western mindset, people understand the word "life" as referring only to biological or scientific life. However, for East Asians, the word "life" also means "spirit" as understood in Buddhism. This difference is important. Japanese people use the expressions "continuity of life," "considering life", "importance of life" and "as long as someone lives" in everyday speech. These expressions are do not have the usual Western meanings. The East Asian meaning should be included in bioethics. As shown in this example, it is clear that moral judgment based on a single theory does not have any beneficial effect in modern times. It is also clear that human conduct cannot be understood based on a single theory, such as mathematics or natural science, when we consider that moral laws govern associations of beings (communities). Meanwhile, emphasis on the individual is also required in today's bioethics.

For example, we are witnessing a casuistry renaissance. Casuistry is accepted in all religions as a source of gradual modification of the accepted doctrine. A famous instance of casuistry is the method of determinations and judgments applied in the Catholic Middle Ages. It consisted of legal reports issued according to the rules and principles of the strong Catholic dogma. Individual cases were judged according to the their specific conditions. The prioritization of the major virtues was determined based on a thorough consideration of each case. Those cases for which a consensus was reached were recorded in legal reports. People sought examples similar to their own moral difficulties in the casuistry, as a lawyer might look for legal precedents. This technique, which at first glance would appear to be antiquated, has come back in bioethics because people value moral viewpoints which emphasize the individual and resist moral dogmatism and uniform ethical theories. We also find examples of casuistry in ancient Greece; one of them is the confrontation between Socrates (strict deduction and induction) and the sophists (relativism). In general, Socrates, who sought strict reasoning ("Know thyself"), is better thought of than the sophists (Protagoras, Gorgias, etc.), who relied on sophistry to win arguments. From the viewpoint of casuistry, on the other hand, the sophists and their relativism (anti-dogmatism) are preferred in the sociological evaluation of ethics and morality.

Ethics is not a science; it is practical wisdom.

In general, ethics is a practical philosophy or one of the humanities. Ethics extracts subjective decisions from the mind and handles them according to the regulations that control individual conduct. The standards of conduct can be of two types. Standards of the first type are embedded in human nature *a priori* (inherent and absolute). Standards of the second type are formed empirically (*a posteriori* and relative). The former type is espoused by Plato and Kant, the latter by Locke and the other empiricists. Within the framework of the humanities and practical matters, we can easily understand moral relativity, since ethical theories are specific to each race and religion and are largely influenced by customs and habits (e.g., theories of virtue in Asia, utilitarianism in Anglo-Saxon countries). The relativity generated in this historical crucible is important for the mutual understanding and the acceptance of diverse ethical views in the global culture projected for the future. In fact, Kantianism and utilitarianism both have powerful principles and rules for handling any variety of moral theories. They have a lot to say in bioethics, which is a new type of moral theory developed mainly in the U.S. in the latter half of 1970s. In this sense, *Principles of Biomedical Ethics* by Beauchamp and Childress played a large role in this field.

I will now explain some major moral theories in reference to above issues.

5-1. Kantianism

Kant arranged the concepts of physics, metaphysics, etc. into systems by defining technical terms strictly. He remained single throughout his 80 years of life; his daily routine (going for walks, taking meals, working, etc.) was so controlled by strict rules that he was called "the clock of Königsberg"; he never lived anywhere outside of Königsberg, where he was born.

Kant learned much from British empiricism. He agreed that objective cognitions, such as those of general science and natural science, are based on sensory experience (observation, experience and induction) and that science is a system of various truths called laws. On the other hand, he was profoundly affected by the moral theories of Jean-Jacques Rousseau (France, 1712-1778). Kant believed that morality and religion cannot be approached or analyzed by empiricist wisdom. He lectured on geography (physics) by day and on philosophy by night at Königsberg University. His major work, *Kritik der reinen Vernunft*, is, in effect, reason put on trial. Pure reason is a human mental faculty completely independent of experience (*a priori*).

He praised highly the natural science fostered by empiricism in his *Kritik der reinen Vernunft*. Meanwhile, he also remarked that there is something (*etwas*) in human nature (the totality of human existence) which cannot be revealed even by the most thorough scientific investigation. Kant believed that the ability to cognize the metaphysical world is exclusive to reason. However, even this pure reason is not given unlimited power. He defined a limit beyond which reason cannot tread, a sanctuary that cannot be invaded by reason. This was the positioning of reason. In this book, Kant discriminated between sensibility, intellect and reason, and appointed sense perception to the first, scientific cognition to the second, and notional cognition to the third. Kantianism is characterized by the precise definition of terms, and rigorous analyses and constructions based on these terms.

Sensibility (*Sinnlichkeit*) and intellect (*Verstand*) are used for understanding and elucidating the facts and principles produced by British empiricism and natural science. Reason (*Vernunft*) is used to clarify the region that cannot be processed by the sensibility or the intellect. This region remains unknown even after repeated scientific probing into human nature. Reason is deductive; it applies to the metaphysical world to which the unknown region belongs.

We perceive the things outside ourselves through sensibility. They are offered to us in the forms of time and space (forms of intuition). Pure time and pure space are forms with which the human mind is equipped *a priori*. Kant differed from the empiricists in that he did not seek to extract everything from sensory experience. The intellect is triggered into action by the phenomenal material received via the sensibility; it arranges this material into scientific knowledge and cognizes it as concepts (concepts of the intellect). The intellect processes objects scientifically or analytically, using forms called categories, which we also have *a priori*. There are four classes of categories :

quantity (unity, plurality or totality), quality (reality, negation or limitation), relation (subsistence, causality or reciprocity) and modality (possibility, existence or necessity). Thus, intellect is the capacity to cognize objects (phenomena) in science and it works based on logic.

Kant distinguished the intellect from reason and positioned the intellect under reason. In other words, Kant limited intellectual cognition to scientific cognition. He also actively pursued anthropology and transcendental science (the world of metaphysics). He believed that the ability to deduce and systematize is specific to reason. The intellect recognizes the appropriateness of objects in the relationship between subjectivity and objectivity. The world that reason relates to is not an object targeted by the intellect. Reason illuminates the intellect wherever the intellect reaches its natural boundaries. The world of reason is an idea and cannot be objectified. If we want the intellect to objectify, then reason becomes intellect at that moment.

The world around us is a world of scientific objective wisdom and a world of phenomena. Kant affirmed that if the phenomenal world is a world of things (*Dinge*), there must also be a world of things in themselves (*Dinge an sich*) behind it. Intellect is the cognitive ability employed in the world of things. Meanwhile, the world of things in themselves cannot be understood by scientific methods. This is the limit of the intellect. This means that the intellect can only think about the world of things in themselves. However, the intellect with its analytical methods is impotent by nature. Only reason can speculate and cognize the things in themselves or the metaphysical world. The cognitive faculty called "reason" is far broader than the intellect. Broadly speaking, it contains the intellect. The worlds clarified by reason through deduction and positioning include metaphysical concepts such as things in themselves, ideas, reason in itself, the transcent, freedom, immortality, psyche, ethics, and the good. Sensibility and intellect target objects. Reason targets the ideas. Modern people are accustomed to the thinking method of the intellect; in other words, many of us are trapped by causal thinking and living habits related thereto, and may not understand this world as it really is. However, everyone agrees that the world of concepts shown above is inherent in human nature. We know that the world cannot be understood by scientific wisdom.

Kant's moral theory is propounded chiefly in *Grundlegung zur Metaphysik der Sitten* and *Kritik der practischen Vernunft*.

Reason orders human actions as an *a priori* mental faculty. Reason offers the subjective standard for actions (maxim). Kant called reason employed thus "practical reason."

Kant affirmed that the moral code within the human being is "one's inner moral code" which shines like a twinkling constellation arranged in beautiful order. In other words, he thought that humans are equipped with the moral code *a priori*, that this moral code is inherent in all persons as expressed by the categorical imperative (the absolute ethical standard established unconditionally); therefore, he believed that the categorical imperative is a rule which applies to all persons universally and that the moral world has a moral law (moral code) as the natural world has a natural law. The categorical imperative of Kant contains the following three ideas. Each of these is called a "formula."

①The formula of universal law (FUL).

Act only on that maxim which you can at the same time will that it should become a universal law. –Thomas E. Hill Jr. and Arnulf Zweig

Act only in accordance with a maxim through which you can at the same time will that it be a universal law. – Paul Guyer.

This is the first formula of the categorical imperative, or the formula of universal law.

This requires the universal application of conduct. It is natural that the principle engraved in the minds of many people as a moral code like so many stars in the night sky should be accepted universally. Kant thought that this principle applies to any person irrespective of nation, race, skin color or gender. This is the most basic moral provision.

②The formula of humanity (FH).

Act in such a way that you treat humanity, whether in your own person or in any other person, always at the same time as an end, never merely as a means. – Thomas E. Hill Jr. and Arnulf Zweig –

So act that you use humanity, whether in your own person or in the person of any other, always at the same time as an end, never merely as a means. – Mary Gregor–

This is the second formula of the categorical imperative, or the formula of humanity.

Kant maintained that the humanity in personhood should be esteemed in oneself and in others. Personhood should be regarded as a purpose of all human conduct, never only as a means.

This is closely related to the principle of human autonomy, which is becoming very influential in current ethical theories. Autonomy means to think freely without constraints, make decisions independently and act freely based on those decisions. Treating a person only as a means is a violation of that person's autonomy. The dignity of a human being consists in the respect shown for his or her autonomy, nothing else. Kant stated that the humanity in others and in oneself should be treated as a purpose. This means that a person can make decisions independently and act freely, under certain constraints. No one can live alone. Each person lives together with others in a community. In modern life, people are likely to treat others as objects or means. Under such circumstances, the second formula is very important.

③ The formula of autonomy (FA).

(the idea of) the will of every rational being as a will that legislates universal law.
– Thomas E. Hill Jr. and Arnulf Zweig –

(the idea of) the will of every rational being as a will giving universal law.
-Allen W. Wood-

This is the third formula of the categorical imperative, or the formula of autonomy. This is a constraint on the will to conform to reason. Human beings (rational persons) are legislative. When an intention is legislative, it is free. In other words, a pure intention is free. Autonomy is an important concept in Kantianism.
Thus, Kant expressed the universality of morality in the manner of formal logic in the first formula. He affirmed the dignity and freedom of human beings in the second formula. He proposed the autonomy of intentions and legislation in true rational existence in the third formula. These three ways of expressing the categorical imperative overlap one another. Or, they say the same thing from different standpoints. One of the most important themes of Kantianism is human autonomy or freedom. All concepts in ethics, such as dignity, justice, morality and the good, are based on this.

A human being, as a rational being (a being belonging to the world that can be imagined), thinks that the cause of his intention is based solely on the idea of freedom. This is because he or she is always independent, irrespective of the specific causes active in the world of sensibility (reason must think that this independence is its own characteristic), which means that he or she is originally free. The concept of autonomy is closely connected to the concept of freedom. The universal principle of morality is also closely connected to the concept of autonomy. The universal principle of morality underlies all conduct of a rational being in completely the same way as a natural law underlies all experience. (Kant: *Grundlegung zur Metaphysik der Sitten*, translated into Japanese by Hideo Shinoda, Iwanamibunko p. 156)

The theory of morality proposed by Kant exerted a strong influence on moral thinking in Japan from the Meiji Restoration to the end of World War II. During this period, the philosophical community in Japan learned a lot from Western philosophy, especially from German Idealism. The influence of Kantianism remained strong in post-war moral thought in Japan, when many ideas were imported from the U.S. and the UK.

In contrast, English-speaking countries such as the U.S. and the U.K. generated empiricism, utilitarianism and pragmatism. We should note that the proponents of these three approaches have comparatively little knowledge of Kantianism.

However, John Rawls (1921-2002), who died recently (November 2002), attracted attention. He investigated the theory of Kant in the U.S., causing controversy. One of his major works is *A Theory of Justice*, published in 1971. In that book, he discussed the expedient suppression of individual rights by the majority, and discussed this in the light of Kant's concept of freedom and justice. He is credited as the revealer of the modern significance of Kant.

5-2. Utilitarianism

Utilitarianism is a theory which judges the quality of the ethical norms underlying actions by evaluating the results of those actions.

The quality of moral rules is weighed in individuals as well as in communities (families, societies and nations). When the total quantity of good consequences is larger than the total quantity of bad consequences, the ethical standard which is the principle of the conduct that caused the result is judged to be rational. As people say, "The end justifies the means," and utilitarianism is a consequence-based theory. The famous expression, "the greatest happiness of the greatest number," encapsulates the idea that the quantity of good consequences of a given action is counted and different quantities are compared objectively. The greatest happiness of the greatest number of people refers to the total happiness (pleasure) of the constituent members of the relevant group. It is a principle that can be easily understood, because ambiguous concepts such as those of ethics, morality and law can be easily brought into the world of rational thinking and into society. In other words, it has the advantage that it can be used politically. It is a practical method for policy makers to glean the tendencies of the popular will when making political decisions.

Utilitarianism is apt to turn into populism, which enables individuals to pursue immoral actions; it is also said to be arbitrary. However, utilitarianism has clarity, simplicity and practicability, which are essential factors in ethical thought. Utilitarianism as a comprehensible ethical theory (moral theory) was generated in Great Britain under the influence of empiricism. The central figures of this development are Jeremy Bentham (1748-1832) and John Stuart Mill (1806-1873). Bentham thought of pleasure and pain instead of "reason" as the direct motive of human behavior. Pleasure is good and pain is evil. The standard of good and evil is reduced to utility. Pleasure obtained is happiness. He believed that the amount of pleasure can be calculated scientifically. Therefore, he used the expression "the greatest happiness." This was largely influenced by British empiricism.

Happiness is pursued at the individual level (act utilitarianism) and the public or community level (rule utilitarianism). Bentham focused on the latter, since he was interested in creating rules to manage civil life. In this sense, his method was like that of communalism. Bentham believed that humans can be controlled by imposing legal, religious, moral and physical sanctions (pain) on them. He believed that laws and regulations are indispensable for human beings. When a person is strictly subjected to criminal punishment, the pursuit of happiness at the individual level does not take precedence over the pursuit of happiness at the public level. Morality in civil life is meant to function based on common sense.

Mill took over the ideas of Bentham, but he relied on quantitative as well as qualitative factors to calculate pleasure. Mill modified and developed Bentham's theory because the relative importance of different types of pleasure was not always taken into account by Bentham. It is better to be a dissatisfied human being than a satisfied pig, better to be a dissatisfied Socrates than a satisfied fool. We often use the expression "What you don't know can't hurt you." A person who knows all things and behaves seriously enjoys a higher type of pleasure than a person who is satisfied without knowing all things. Controlling information in such a way that those with evil intent are abetted would be an ethical vice. The thoughts of Mill about qualitative pleasure are very important. The original draft will be cited as follows:

Whoever supposes that this preference takes place at a sacrifice of happiness — that the superior being, in anything like equal circumstances, is not happier than the inferior — confounds the two very different ideas, of happiness, and content. It is indisputable that the being whose capacities of enjoyment are low, has the greatest chance of having them fully satisfied; and a highly endowed being will always feel that any happiness which he can look for, as the world is constituted, is imperfect. But he can learn to bear its imperfections, if they are at all bearable; and they will not make him envy the being who is indeed unconscious of the imperfections, but only because he feels not at all the good which those imperfections qualify. **It is better to be a human being dissatisfied than a pig satisfied; better to be Socrates dissatisfied than a fool satisfied. And if the fool, or the pig, is of a different opinion, it is because they only know their own side of the question. The other party to the comparison knows both sides.**

— John Stuart Mill, Utilitarianism —

Mill added the internal sanction to the external sanction suggested by Bentham. This is the conscience formed in the human mind, and its sanction is remorse. Thus, he thought that humans can create and develop a society or a community with inherently universal values even if no external sanctions are imposed upon them. Furthermore, Mill asserted that humans are not only selfish and self-centered but also inherently altruistic. This characterizes the utilitarianism of Mill, in which personal ethical views are omnipresent in society. The basic assumption of Mill's theory is that a person is free and unique. Mill published *On Liberty* in 1859, in which he stated the importance of individual freedom and individuality as a precondition for "the greatest happiness" from the viewpoint of utilitarianism. This concept of individualism, as well as Kant's concept of autonomy, became the foundation of later liberalist theories.

Utilitarianism can also be called "consequentialism," and it had an influence on the birth of pragmatism in the U.S. (pragmatism is also a type of consequentialism because only laws or theories that can be put into practice are assumed to be true). Seen from the viewpoint of pragmatism, modern science and the capitalism that promoted modern science are valuable and useful because they function effectively to make human life convenient. Modern people, chiefly in the U.K. and the U.S., approve of the limitless development and utility of natural science. The reality of the modern world is that these nations lead the scientific community at present. Utilitarianism and pragmatism represent an important source of support for today's ethical mindset.

Pragmatism is a philosophical current originating from the U.S. It is comparatively new because it appeared in the 1880s, after the Civil War. At that time, Americans started to develop a truly specific American mentality, independent of Europe. New ideas (Marxism, existentialism, etc.) were emerging all over the world in reaction to the distortions of capitalism in the wake of the Industrial Revolution. American pragmatism accelerated the evolution of scientism. Pragmatism was transformed into optimism; a human-centered mentality focused exclusively on the modernization of life was eagerly adopted. Charles Sanders Peirce (1839-1914) and William James (1842-1910) founded the pragmatist movement, and John Dewey brought it to its peak. "*Pragma*" is a Greek word which means "behavior" or "practice." In pragmatism, ethical truth cannot be reached by the logic or reason found in the rigorism of Kant. Pragmatists believe that ethical truth can only be reached through the real experience of actual human behavior. In this respect, pragmatism was strongly influenced by British empiricism and adopted a stance contrary to German Idealism. The ethical theories of pragmatism belonged to social psychology. Moral rules that can improve social values were supposed to be better, and pragmatists took great interest in matters related to education. For them, the goal of education was to teach the student to solve problems through cooperation with others, and to expose the student to experiences in actual society in a practical setting ("leaning by doing"). Dewey is known for his instrumentalism, in which concepts and thoughts are viewed simply as tools to help humans adjust to their environment. Humans adjust to their environment as animals do. In addition, humans control their environment and nature in general. However, humans have a greater ability to adapt than animals, because humans use tools more frequently than animals. The utility of tools is evaluated based on the results. If a tool (a concept or thought) is not useful, it is modified to be useful. Throughout history, mankind has proceeded in that way with regard to tools in general. Instrumentalists typically believe that concepts and thoughts can change with the changes in society. Thus, instrumentalism is in sharp contrast to the theories of Plato and Kant. Dewey's theories of education did not focus on individual improvement, but on the improvement of society as a whole. The purpose of education was to transform individuals into useful members of society. This current had a large influence on the educational reform carried out in Japan after the war.

Pragmatism enabled American culture, which is based on the frontier spirit and the belief in the freedom of the people who developed the new continent, to leave behind traditional European culture. This departure was realized with the aid of considerable physical resources, such as the vast lands of the U.S., as well as assiduous scientific research and experimentation which allowed the development of science, the ensuing rapid spread of modernization, and the free development and synergistic effects of modern industries. We should remember that the special historical conditions which made this rise possible existed only in the U.S., a new continent, a *tabula rasa*. Pragmatism is based on British empiricism, especially on utilitarianism. Therefore, it recognizes the value of experimentation and first-hand experience. The truth does not issue from reason as in intellectualism; rather, it is established through actual experience. In pragmatism, there is no fixed, eternal truth; truth is a thing empirically proven to be useful for human society. Therefore, there are many truths. As shown above, pragmatism is a behavioral theory in which the truth is sought in reality, and so it is easy to understand for common people. Pragmatists believe that those things which are useful for humans are truth. It is an optimistic standpoint, because the modernized life, which is the result of the application of science, is assumed to be right, and it became the basis of the current American mentality. If empiricism and utilitarianism are the stem and the thick bough, pragmatism is the twig.

All ethical theories have advantages and weak points. The weak points of utilitarianism and its related ideas are as follows:

① The greatest number and the greatest happiness are those of specific communities (the Americans, the white people, the advanced countries, etc.).

This is an age when we should take into consideration human beings all over the world, as well as all environments around the globe. We cannot reverse the crisis facing the global ecosystem if we give in to national interests in matters of industrial regulation. The U.S. has adopted an evasive attitude in the international efforts to reduce carbon dioxide gas emissions. This amply illustrates the defects of the ethical theory on which American society is based. Things are the same with the grave problem of ozone layer destruction by artificial gases. We need a holy leader who will think of the whole earth, not just the interests of one nation. The greatest number should include at least all the people in the world. We should also include the global ecosystem.

② It lacks an impartial way to distribute happiness to less fortunate communities.

③ It cares about mobocracy.

④ There is a danger that happiness and pleasure of a community are pursued excessively. Negative feedback and sanctions are absolutely required for keeping a community in particular a nation from going crazy in promoting the national interest.

Utilitarianism is an ethical theory that underlies the development of the current scientific civilization and modernized life. It is felt that utilitarianism is intrinsically responsible for various contradictions of the present age, such as the North-South problems, the starvation in Africa, poverty, AIDS, public nuisances, ecocide, etc. The largest advantage of utilitarianism is that it can offer answers to any ethical question.

The major principle of judgment is to ensure the greatest happiness of the greatest number.

5-3. Virtue-based theories

Virtue is the behavior of a person in society, or a subjective propensity (a state of the soul), which is the foundation of spontaneous personal moral choice. It stresses independence, because it rejects the influence of strong external factors causing an internal regulation with a higher binding force, such as that seen in objective utilitarian decisions and in Kantian duty. Virtue is a complex of multiple ethical values expressed in many ways, and is a basic internal factor of the formation of the integrated human personality.

Japanese people have evolved in the midst of East Asian thought, from the establishment of the Japanese nation in the Asuka and Nara periods to the end of World War II. We resonate with virtue-based theories. Inazo Nitobe (1862-1933), who was an internationally recognized thinker and an Undersecretary General at the League of Nations, wrote *Bushido: The Soul of Japan* in English. In this book, he proudly introduced *bushido*, a complex mindset developed in the tradition of Japanese culture (tea, Zen, Shinto, poetry, art and martial arts), as well as the special theory of virtue related to it. The virtues he was especially fond of in *bushido* were wisdom, benevolence and courage. Wisdom is the excellence of intellectual resources, not scientific knowledge used to form moral character. The art of calligraphy, morality and literature were indispensable for the *bushido* way. Benevolence is the *samurai*-style mercy shown by the strong toward the weak; it is mild and tender, like that of a protective mother. Nitobe cited the historical example, from the Battle of Sumanoura (1184), of Kumagai Naozane, who felt sorry for Tairano Atsumori, a boy *samurai* whom he had wrestled to the ground. Courage is bravery. Intrinsically, a *samurai* is a man of action. Other virtues emphasized in *bushido* include justice, courtesy, loyalty and temperance. These virtues are still strong in today's Japanese culture and spirituality; this situation is apparent even in TV dramas broadcast by the national channel. In *Bushido*, published in 1899, Inazo Nitobe, who was a Quaker, mentioned that the spirit of the *samurai* would perish in history, but that it would exist forever as the core of Japanese culture. Japanese people should be proud of it and recognize it as the core of their identity. Daisetsu Suzuki (1870-1966), a Buddhist philosopher, actively introduced Japanese culture (the spirit of the *samurai*) to Europe and the U.S. from the viewpoint of Zen. The Japanese virtues and Zen thought emphasized by these two men of culture were imported from China in the earliest of times and blossomed in a way unique to Japan, becoming the axis of Japanese culture.

In Confucianism (Confucius: 551-479 B.C.), 仁 or benevolence (the perfect virtue) is placed at the summit of the hierarchy of virtues. Confucian benevolence is the virtue of humaneness originating from the Yin dynasty (the 16th to the 11th centuries B.C.) of ancient China. This virtue is to see things from other people's viewpoints or to experience empathy for others. It is a fundamental sympathy which arises when two persons meet. Other than benevolence at the individual level, Confucius emphasized the benevolence manifested by policy makers or persons of exalted rank toward their subjects or attendants. Mencius (372-289 B.C.) was a successor of Confucius. He believed that humans are naturally good, i.e. inherently benevolent and just. According to Mencius, the virtue of benevolence is expressed as feelings of compassion or pity towards others. The virtues of Confucianism other than benevolence and justice include courtesy (social benevolence in view of conserving the social order), wisdom (making sound moral judgments), belief (faith), cordiality (sincere kindness), and filial piety (filial devotion to parents). Society is stabilized, i.e. the order of the society (an artificial structure) is maintained, by introducing individuals into the common ethical framework via these virtues, allowing them to function as integrated members of society.

In Taoism (established by Lao Tzu), the first principle of all things is called the "*tao*." Taoists believe that various virtues, such as benevolence and justice, were generated when the *tao* passed away. In other words, the natural state is the original state of the *tao*. Virtues are necessary in the artificial state, when the natural state is lost. That is because the virtues are related to the *tao*.

These Chinese thoughts are being applied in leading educational doctrines since nearly 400 years ago. They have had a large impact on the formation of Japanese spirituality, and their influences remain to this day.

At almost the same time as Confucius and Lao Tzu, Socrates (470-399 B.C.), Plato (427-347 B.C.) and Aristotle (384-322 B.C.) were discussing *areté* and *agathon* in ancient Greece.

It is said that Socrates invented the method of induction. He tried to extract principles and approach truth using *logos* dialectically. He had little interest in physics and the human body. His life's work was to investigate the ethical question, "What is the Good?", or the relationship between the human being and the spiritual world. According to Socrates, the Good (*agathon*) can be reached through right knowledge and insight. The Idea of the Good is the principle unifying all Ideas, and is also the origin of wisdom (the observer) and the world of phenomena (the observed). Plato, who was a student of Socrates, thought in almost the same way. To discuss the nature of the Good meant to reach the source of the world of Ideas. Knowledge, as understood by Socrates, was ultimately this ideal knowledge (*sophia*), not merely scientific knowledge. Wisdom for Socrates was *areté* (virtue). Moral rules were generated from *areté* deductively.

Plato followed Socrates in his doctrine of Ideas. He discussed the three components of the soul and their respective virtues: wisdom (*psyché*, the rational part of the soul), temperance (the appetitive part of the soul) and courage (the willful part of the soul); he also discussed the virtue of justice, which is the order generated when wisdom, temperance and courage are in mutual harmony. In the *Republic*, Plato stated that an ideal society realizes these four virtues. At the same time, the leader of such a society understands the real nature of these four virtues. In this sense, an ideal state is a larger version of the philosopher; a philosopher's politics are ideal.

Aristotle expanded on Socrates' and Plato's doctrine of Ideas and their idealism about virtue. However, Aristotle was different in that he did not think that the Ideas, which cannot be reached by humans, are the good. He thought that the pleasure and happiness actually pursued by people are the good (the proper purpose of all human activity). Thus, he influenced later ethical thinking such as utilitarianism. Aristotle defined *agathon* (the good), or the purpose of human activity, in various contexts; for example, the good for doctors is the patient's health, the good for carpenters is the finished house. Thus, there are various things which are the good, depending on the context. However, there is a chain of dependency linking the various instances of the good, and the highest good is happiness. He made ethics understandable to ordinary people by transforming it into an artificial and practical humanistic method and making happiness, not God or the Ideas, the purpose of human activity. This Aristotelian ethic is a potent vein in present ethical, especially bioethical, discussions.

Every art and every inquiry, and similarly every action and pursuit, is thought to aim at some good; and for this reason the good has rightly been declared to be that at which all things aim.
(*Nicomachean Ethics*, Vol.1, Section 1, p. 15, translated into Japanese by Saburo Takada, Iwanamibunko)

What then is the good of each? Surely that for whose sake everything else is done. In medicine this is health, in strategy victory, in architecture a house, in any other sphere something else, and in every action and pursuit the end; for it is for the sake of this that all men do whatever else they do...
Now such a thing happiness (*eudaimonia*), above all else, is held to be; for this we choose always for

itself and never for the sake of something else, but honor, pleasure, reason, and every virtue we choose indeed for themselves (for if nothing resulted from them we should still choose each of them), but we choose them also for the sake of happiness, judging that by means of them we shall be happy. Happiness, on the other hand, no one chooses for the sake of these, or, in general, for anything other than itself.

(*Nicomachean Ethics*, Vol.1, Section 7, p. 29-31, translated into Japanese by Saburo Takada, Iwanamibunko)

Virtue (*areté*) is the state (*hexis*) of the soul required for humans to reach the Good, or the Ultimate End. Aristotle is well known for his notion that every ethical or moral virtue generally occupies an intermediate position between two extremes; each one is, in other words, a mean (the Golden Mean) between two extremes of behavior. Virtues are neither excess nor deficiency. As examples of such middle-path virtues, he mentioned courage as the mean between foolhardiness (excess) and cowardice (deficiency), temperance between abstinence (excess) and self-indulgence (deficiency), liberality between extravagance (excess) and meanness (deficiency); in the same fashion, he spoke about loftiness, self-respect, friendship, gentleness, justice, and so on, all of which, he believed, were cultivated in a community as habits (*ethos*). Of these virtues, justice is perfect and therefore the highest. He thought that justice has two meanings. In the wider sense, justice is to obey the law (regulating one's relationships with others) and perform right actions. In the narrow sense, justice is related to equality, or fairness, which is one of the principal concepts in contemporary ethics.

As a man who dedicated himself to the study of logic and developed the first well known theory of syllogisms, classified the 10 categories, and accumulated a broad background covering natural science, ethics and metaphysics as a partial successor of Plato, Aristotle divided the virtues (excellences) into two groups. One is the group of moral or ethical virtues, those discussed above. They are internalized as habits and customs, and, accordingly, are mainly formed in individuals through habituation within the social environment, although some parts subsist inherently in humans as potentialities; repeated virtuous acts in a community develop into habits which eventually take root in the individual as ethical virtues. Ordinarily, the term "virtue" is used in a narrow sense to refer to such ethical virtues. The other group of virtues, according to Aristotle's division, comprises the intellectual virtues, which are the fundamental requirement for the soul to reach the truth through the process of affirmation and negation. Intellectual virtues are therefore a part of the soul, or the soul itself. They include ①*techné* (technical expertise or art contributing to *genesis*), ② *episteme* (systematic or scientific knowledge based on reasoning), ③*nous* (intelligence or intellect, the possession of which distinguishes humans from other creatures and is at the same time concerned with divinity and therefore superhuman), ④*phronesis* (practical wisdom or practical judgment closely connected to practice or the choice of actions), and ⑤ *sophia* (philosophical wisdom as a combination of *nous* and *episteme*). Of these five intellectual virtues, the most important one for current or postmodern bioethics would be *phronesis*. It is discretion or prudence connected to *praxis* (moral practice). While ethical virtues are formed in the individual through habituation, intellectual virtues are cultivated mainly through education or learning for long periods of time. Such two groups of virtues are not clearly separated; ethical virtues are guided by *phronesis* on the one hand and closely affect the choice or *praxis* of *phronesis* on the other.

"*Phronesis*" is a difficult term to understand, because the virtue to which it refers is very individual and hard to generalize, unlike the first three intellectual virtues; *phronesis* can be said to lay the correct course towards the Good, the final aim, which is happiness, in a dynamic process of confliction of various virtues in each specific action; this confliction occurs whenever the appropriate *episteme* (transmissible scientific wisdom), *techné* and theoretical wisdom through *nous*, as well as all sorts of ethical virtues, are implemented together. Practical wisdom, or *phronesis*, generalizes various virtues in the actual moral behavior of every individual. So, it is like a conductor in the performance of an orchestra; it establishes the order and strength of each virtue in considering the overall situation, to bring about the best realization of Beauty or the Good. This virtue is directly responsible for the human being's attainment of the ideal objective in behavior or practice. *Phronesis,* a skill requiring mentorship and experience, has come back to the modern age in medical ethics as casuistry, which is individual and not at all theoretical or logical, and is acquired only through practical experience, apart from logical acumen.

As an actual example arising in bioethics, *phronesis* is becoming an important part of genetic counseling, because science will soon reveal almost all the genetic information about each disease. Here, the most sensitive and reproducible DNA analysis methods are always designed to pinpoint mutations, repeat numbers of bases, polymorphisms, and so forth. These methods represent "*techné,*" in Aristotle's terms. Tied to these, scientific or systematic interpretations of the abundant genetic data will be carried out, yielding exciting discoveries and novel theories which may necessitate further experiments. Further development of analytical techniques may also be promoted. These are all "*episteme*". Up to this point, things are rather easy for a scientist to do, because every scientist can perform such analytical processes automatically based on manuals. In order to succeed, he or she can simply be a clever person with plenty of static and scientific knowledge. However, genetic counseling deals with the complex problem of people living in communities who have been scientifically or objectively diagnosed as having genetic abnormalities. Here, it is *"phronesis"* that is needed. *Phronesis* is not science, but something far higher, and thus a genetic counselor has to be a practically wise person instead of a merely clever one. This is why *phronesis*, as practical or moral wisdom, is required for bioethics in general, including the ethics involved in genetic counseling.

As shown above, virtue is a voluntary propensity which determines human action at the level of personal ethics (individual morals) and social ethics. Therefore, some virtues have been lost over time and others have been generated, as reflections of the specific characteristics of the age and place.

The virtues which are often mentioned in bioethics are as follows:
① The intent not to perform actions harmful to others (non-malevolence)
② Mercy, good wishes, good deeds (benevolence)
③ Treating others with respect (respectfulness)
④ Impartiality (fairness)
⑤ Confidentiality (discretion)
⑥ Sympathy

① and ⑤ are mentioned by Hippocrates in ancient Greece. ② is mentioned by Confucius and the Buddha. The principle of treating others with respect (respectfulness) as shown by ③ has generated the principle of respect for human autonomy, which is the foundation of modern ethics (Kant and Mill). It is rooted in modern society as the right of procedural self-determination (informed consent). In modern bioethics, ④, ⑤ and ⑥ are linked to justice, privacy and humanity, respectively. They are expectations of human nature based on a common attitude called "humanity" (it is already mentioned by Confucius and Mencius).

Virtue is the value that should be targeted by human activity. It is the basis of good public order, customs and social conventions. There are virtues that change with time, ones that do not change with time, ones that are learned through education and custom, ones that are inherent, ones that accompany feelings, ones that do not accompany feelings, ones that control individuals internally, ones that regulate society, etc. They are not independent but interdependent. We should select the virtue with the highest priority whenever the relevant virtues compete with each other. Virtue-based theories do not have an internal mechanism of virtue prioritization. Other ethical theories must be used to determine which virtue should be enacted in each case. This is the weak point of virtue-based theories.

Another weak point is the individualistic consciousness and conservativeness. In general, ethical principles should evolve and abandon their old shells in this age of science. In this respect, virtue-based theories, which are individualistic, lack sociability, a characteristic appropriate for this new age. They are a strong type of doctrine that prospered in the political circles of ancient China and still supports the ethical fiber of modern East Asian countries. This important strain of thought should evolve with the help of outside inspiration.

Meanwhile, the usability of virtue-based theories consists in their flexibility; they tend to survive in any ethical theory. They link personal virtue to public or social virtue. When social decision as well as individual decisions (freedom and autonomy) may be made based on any theory, the virtue of reaching out to others and to society in general must remain. Bioethical decisions which disregard this opening toward others are not right. In this respect, virtue-based theories will play a more important role in the future.

In bioethics which has prospered in these last thirty years in the U.S., we could see that virtue-based theories were given a typically American face or, that of pragmatism (e.g., principlism).

The U.S. is a nation of liberalism and capitalism. It is also known as a nation of individualism and litigiousness, where individuals insist on their rights. In addition, bioethics and medical technologies have developed significantly in the U.S. in the latter half of the 20th century. Against this background, bioethics in the U.S. has developed primarily in the field of human medicine. Briefly speaking, it is largely a result of healthcare practitioners needing to defend themselves against malpractice lawsuits. This is a phenomenon unique to the U.S., a country of pragmatism. Bioethics should not be an abstract theory but a practical theory which addresses real issues. In this case, three or four of the virtues of common morality shown in the above discussion of virtue-based theories are actually considered practical skills in modern American bioethics. Suppose that a new drug or an artificial blood vessel is tried on a patient. We judge the ethical appropriateness of the action, which is assumed to be a bioethics problem, based on whether the action (judgment) is appropriate for the multiple virtues adopted in accordance with a specific method. The four practical virtues (medical acts and medical research) extracted by Beauchamp and Childress are shown below. They are all understood in their relationship with others (patients and research objects).

① Respect for autonomy
② Benefit
③ Harmlessness
④ Justice

③ is a reversal of ②. Therefore, ③ is included in ② (②: positive, ③: negative). In ethical judgments which target humans, specific checking as to whether an action is harmful or not for a patient is direct and effective. In other words, it is easily performed.

The judgment of the bioethical appropriateness of studies and medical procedures intended for human use based on these three or four virtues is called principlism. The minimally required principles mentioned in principlism should clearly reflect the respect for the individual rights emphasized in free nations. In other words, people should not win medical lawsuits generated by medical procedures (judgment). Principlism supports American medical ethics and is rapidly being imported to Japan, which is being affected significantly by American medical practice. Principlism has rendered bioethics more practical and easy to handle as a praxeology, which is one of its advantages. On the other hand, some people object to it on the grounds that it is merely a technique. Principlism is highly valued by pragmatists and utilitarians because it is useful in the praxis. However, we should discuss the utility of principlism further on other global cultures and ethical theories.

5-4. Communitarianism

In communitarianism, the interests of the community are more important than the happiness (autonomy, freedom and rights) of its individuals. This is an old concept put into practice since ancient times (ancient China, the Greek city states, etc.). This concept has had a large influence on socialist countries and nations with strong religious leadership.

All societies, including families, clans, villages, nations, races, etc., are communities.

Confucius (*Analects*) and Plato (*Republic*) believed that individual rights are to be sacrificed for the benefit of the community. Socrates killed himself by swallowing poison, saying, "Evil laws are also laws." He believed in the community or civil society bound by *nomos* (law). He thought that a person should ultimately obey the public order (civil society) even if his or her spirit is free to inquire and develop ideas. The public should be responsible for designing good laws through due consideration. In order to succeed, people should pursue the common virtues (*arete*). Socrates believed in the public, because he believed in the natural goodness of human nature.

Communitarianism is based on commonly observed moral rules and retains very much of humanity. It respects traditions, conventions and history, and is likely to generate conservative governance by elders. Communitarianism is set against liberalism and individualism, which value individual freedom and rights. Recently, liberalism is prospering on a global scale. Under such circumstances, communitarianism is now being revisited as a potential source of revitalization, especially with regard to morality. For example, the principle of respecting individual freedom and rights is a significant trait of American and European liberalism. People prioritize individual rights highly when making any ethical decision. When people demand that these rights be respected, they become self-absorbed and isolated. People forget sociability (emphasized by communitarianism); they forget to share in the common virtues with their neighbors. The warmth of sociability cannot be generated by people who lock themselves up in their homes pursuing their individuality. People have no feeling of togetherness, nor a commonly shared trend of life. The communitarianism through which families, homes, villages and towns supported each other before the war in Japan is vanishing rapidly because liberalism and individualism are blooming. For example, the concept of sexual freedom has spread even among junior-high-school students. This is because the awareness of individual rights has become excessive due to the imported liberalism; people are now requiring individual freedom at any cost.

Apart from the issue of the transformation of morality, the family system persists all over Japan in spite of legal amendments after the war. We still experience major traffic jams caused by passengers who go back to their home towns on the Bon holiday or the New Year holidays, which include ceremonies to ensure the peacefulness of one's ancestors, prayers for the welfare of the household, as well as attendance at ceremonies carried out at shrines and temples. The spirituality of Japanese people has survived throughout its long history and is not likely to change very rapidly even if the laws change. This is the situation in Japan today.

As shown in Japan's militarism before the war, communitarianism always risks sliding into fanatical faith. In communitarianism, individuals are sacrificed to the public, which is something like presentism, from the material viewpoint. For example, in some presentist communities, when a person dies, his or her skin is stored and recycled for reuse by the public. In the case of organ transplants, the dying person with communal beliefs benefits living persons. There is also the concept of eugenics, which seeks to eliminate disease-causing genes that human beings have lived with for a long period of time. These practices are directly connected to the bioethical problems of today. It is clear that communitarianism is opposed to liberalism. We should find a new way of life which conforms to new ages and cultures by combining communitarianism and liberalism.

5-5. Liberal individualism

Individual freedom and autonomy are the natural state of humans. A person can think, intend and behave freely. Today, a person is independent as an individual. He has a self-identity that does not depend on others. As stated during the French Revolution and in the American Declaration of Independence, freedom is a basic concept, and it underpins Western-style democracy, free-for-all capitalism, and Japanese postwar democracy and economic development. Freedom of conscience, religion, expression and economic activity are mentioned in the current Constitution of Japan, which was prepared under the guidance of the U.S. Liberal individualism and related ideas have been widely adopted throughout history except in ancient Greece, where slavery was approved of, feudal China, Middle-Age countries with strong religious leadership, Japan in its militaristic era, and some autocratic or socialist states today. In other words, the ethical theories in liberalist states are closely related to the concept of individual freedom. This is applicable to Kantianism, utilitarianism and pragmatism, as described above.

In accordance with the ideals of liberalism, American bioethics developed with an emphasis on individual rights. In bioethics, rights are used as a framework to protect human freedom. Many skills which play a role in the practical knowledge called bioethics have been developed. This is the attitude which allows the right to abortion, right to discontinue medical procedures aimed at prolonging life, the right to die, etc., based on the free will and the free decision-making capacity of human beings. This is the direction taken in bioethics in the U.S., where capitalism, modern science, modern industry, liberalism and individualism have been developed most acutely and the number of trials is the largest.

From the philosophical point of view, Leibniz, Kant, Fichte and Schelling in Germany remarked on the meaning of human freedom. Mill (utilitarianism) and Dewey (pragmatism) remarked on the essential importance of freedom. The present version of liberalism was developed based on the unification of Kantianism, utilitarianism, pragmatism, liberal individualism and capitalism, in a manner specific to the modern scientific civilization.

In liberal individualism, individual freedom and rights are maximal unless they violate those of others.

The point of autonomy is to protect free thinking, free will and free activity. In the U.S., there are specific ways to ensure this freedom, including informed consent and advance directives. In order to obtain informed consent, a doctor discloses to a patient sufficient information for him or her to make a free decision regarding any medical intervention to be performed. Advance directives are a way for the patient to stipulate the details of his or her end-of-life care in document form while he or she still has the ability to make free and rational decisions. Thus, the development of rights theories in the U.S. has contributed to the practical development of a new type of ethics called bioethics.

The Declaration of Helsinki was published in 1964 by the World Medical Association as a statement of ethical principles providing guidance to physicians and other participants in medical research involving human subjects. It is revised once every few years at the General Assembly of the World Medical Association. The latest version (2001) includes a list of items related to bioethical standards for medical research on humans. The ethical appropriateness of using placebos is also mentioned. This declaration refers to the practical activities encouraged by rights theories, including the observance of human rights, disclosure of sufficient information, confidentiality, non-maleficence, beneficence, justice, respect for autonomy, preservation of human dignity and practical methods for ensuring informed consent.

As shown above, liberal individualism (rights theory) is a major ethical current in today's capitalistic countries.

As a result of the rapid import of this current into Japan, even children say, "Crows are free to do as they please" or "I have the right." These have become household phrases. The tendency to value individual identity is spreading, especially among young people. On the other hand, communitarianism, with its virtues and its long history in Japan, continues to manifest itself in the common attitudes towards parents, family and hometown. We still have these traditional values, and the rights theories imported rapidly after the war are in conflict with them. In this sense, the Japanese people have lost their identity. We should reestablish an identity specific to the Japanese, by fusing modernism with Japan's racial history, culture, religion and ethos.

5-6. Relativity of ethical theories.

I have explained the major ethical theories above. In the present age where information is exchanged on a global scale, these ethical theories are not independent, nor far from those of ancient times. We should note that they are interdependent and relative, in an age where populations are increasing and exchanges are deepening among nations, and this is true for bioethical theories as well.

For example, the problem of autonomy and freedom is discussed in utilitarianism,

Kantianism, virtue-based theories and liberal individualism. It is also indirectly linked to the concept of individual freedom in communalism.

We can confirm that virtue-based theories were developed earliest in history, and they have seeped into all ethical theories, including those of today. Therefore, these theories can be said to find the basis of humanity in the human mind, not in a system of principles. We should understand that humanity is generated inevitably between two persons.

Rights theories were developed out of necessity, to protect individual rights in liberal countries. They are similar to communalism in the sense that human rights accompany duty in human relations. Rights and duties are inextricably linked to each other. A right is imposed by an individual on the outside, whereas a duty is imposed on the individual by the outside. In virtue-driven bioethics, it is preferable to emphasize duty above right. However, rights are emphasized in modern ethics because this is the more practicable approach. Rights-driven bioethics includes the equal right to medical treatment, the right to die, the right to refuse medical treatment, the right to abortion, as well as the right to life (natural right). The right to die of terminally ill cancer patients has been approved in Holland, which is one of the countries where the implementation of rights-driven bioethics is the most advanced (euthanasia).

Ethics is largely based on ethos (habits and customs). It is natural that differences in regional and historical characteristics generate differences in ethical theories. Under the present circumstances, Western ethics has been rapidly imported to morally incompatible regions in recent years. It is spreading across borders via the Western vectors of science and modern industry. Discontinuities and frictions between the old and the new ethics are being generated in East Asian countries.

Ethics is a part of culture. Ethics forms culture, and culture forms ethics. We should note that a superficial culture cannot change cultures and ethics that have a long history, such as those in East Asian countries.

It is no wonder that the spirit described in *Bushido* (1899) by Inazo Nitobe was not replaced by the ethics of Western liberalism, even if Japan has been Westernized to a point (maybe in 100 years it will be more replaced). In a similar manner, Japanese people do not accept individualistic decision-making in matters related to organ transplants, and sexual freedom and feminism are not rampantly spreading in Japan.

This may be mysterious for Western people with their monism. However, slowness and arbitrary codes are rather natural for Japanese people, considering their 2000-year history. This is an identity unique to Japanese people in a good sense. Ethical theories are relative. Various theories have been adopted by different nations and races, and the emphasis is always different, depending on the culture. We should adopt the principle of diversity in order to understand foreign cultures and races.

References
1) Yoshishige Abe and Tadashi Fujiwara: Kant Dotokutetsugaku Genron (Kant's Groundworks for the Metaphysics of Morals). Iwanami Shoten, Tokyo, 1921
2) Masaaki Kohsaka: Kant. Kobundo Shobo, Tokyo, 1939
3) Karl Jaspers: Von der Wahrheit. Piper, Munchen,1958
4) Karl Jaspers: Der Philosophish Glaube angesichts der Offenbarung, Piper, Munchen, 1962
5) Daisetsu Suzuki: Zen and Japanese Culture Revised Edition. Iwanami Shoten, Tokyo, 1964
6) Tetsuro Watsuji: Rinrigaku(Ethics) Vol 1. Iwanami Shoten, Tokyo, 1965
7) Karl Jaspers: Descartes und die Philosophie. Walter de Gruyter & Co., Berlin, 1966
8) Hayao Kawai: Jung Shinrigaku Nyumonm (an Introduction to Jungian Psychology). Baifukan, Tokyo, 1967
9) Karl Jaspers; translated into Japanese by H. Shigeta: Vom Ursprung und Ziel der Geschichte. Kawadeshoboshinsha, Tokyo, 1968
10) Karl Jaspers; translated into Japanese by S. Matsunami: Kleine Schule Des Philosophischen Denkens. Kawadeshoboshinsha, Tokyo, 1968
11) Charles F. Wallraff: Karl Jaspers. Princeton University Press, Princeton, 1970
12) Tatsuo Hayashi, Matao Noda, Osamu Kuno, Syoiti Yamazaki, Magoiti Kushida (Editors): Tetsugaku Jiten(Dictionary of Philosophy). Heibonsha, Tokyo, 1971
13) W.K.C. Guthrie: Socrates. Cambridge University Press, Cambridge, 1971
14) Descartes; translated into Japanese by Matao Noda: Discours de la methode. Tyuokoronsya, Tokyo, 1974
15) C.G. Jung; translated into English by R.F.C. Hull: Psychology and the East. Princeton University Press, Princeton, 1978
16) M. William: The Freud/Jung Letters. Princeton University Press, Princeton, 1979
17) Hayao Kawai: Tyukukozo Nihon No Shinso (A Hollow Structure as Deep Layer of Japanese). Tyuokoronsha, Tokyo, 1982
18) S. John: Minds, Brains and Science. Harvard University Press, Boston, 1984
19) Karl Jaspers; translated into Japanese by S. Hayashida: Was ist Philosophie? Hakusuisha, Tokyo, 1986
20) C.G. Jung; translated into Japanese by M. Hayashi: On Types. Misuzu Shobo,

Tokyo, 1987

21) Nagy Marilyn: Philosophycal Issues in the Psychology of C.G. Jung. State University of New York Press, New York, 1991

22) Tom L. Beauchamp, James F. Childress: Principles of Biomedical Ethics Fourth Edition. Oxford University Press, Oxford, 1994

23) Imanuel Kant; translated into English by T. K. Abobott: Kritik der Praktischen Vernunft, Prometheus Books, New York, 1996

24) Mary Gregor: Immanuel Kant Goundwork of the Metraphysics of Morals. Cambridge University Press, Cambridge, 1998

25) C.G. Jung; translated into Japanese by M. Hayashi: On Archetypes. Kinokuniya Shoten, Tokyo, 1999

26) Allen W. Wood: Kant's Ethical Thought. Cambridge University Press, Cambridge, 1999

27) Mark G. Kuczewski, Ronald Polansky: Bioethics- Ancient Themes in Contemporary Issues-. The MIT Press, Cambridge, 2000

28) Imanuel Kant; translated into Japanese by S. Hatano: Kritik der Praktischen Vernunft. Iwanami Shoten, 2001

29) Allen W. Wood: Kant's Ethical Thought. Cambridge University Press, Cambridge, 1999

30) Tom L. Beauchamp, James F. Childress: Principles of Biomedical Ethics Fifth Edition. Oxford University Press, Oxford, 2001

31) Aristotle; translated into Japanese by S. Takeda: Nicomachean Ethics Vol 1. 2001

32) Aristotle; translated into Japanese by S. Takeda: Nicomachean Ethics Vol 2. 2001

33) Aristotle; translated into English by Christopher Rowe; Nicomachean Ethics. Oxford University Press, Oxford, 2002

34) Thomas E. Hill, Arnulf Zweig: Kant Groundwork for the Metaphysics of Morals. Oxford University Press, oxford,2002

35) Imanuel Kant; translated into Japanese by H. Shinoda; Kritik der Reinen Vernunft. Iwanami Shoten, 2002

36) Inazo Nitobe; translated into Japanese by T. Yanaihara: Bushido. Iwanami Shoten, Tokyo, 2002

37) S. Matsueda, Y. Takeutsi: Lao Tsu and Lieh Zsu, Chinese Thoughts IV. Tokuma Shoten, Tokyo, 2002

38) J.J. Rousseau; translated into Japanese by K. Imano: Emile, Iwanami Shoten, Tokyo, 2002

39) Imanuel Kant; translated into Japanese by H. Shinoda: Prolegomena. Iwanami

Shoten, Tokyo, 2003
40) Imanuel Kant; translated into English by Norman Kemp Smith: Kritik der Reinen Vernunft. Palgrave Macmillan, New York, 2003
41) Stephan Holland: Bioethics A Philosophical Introduction. Polity Press, Cambridge, 2003
42) Glenn McGee: Pragmatic Bioethics. Vanderbilt University Press, Nashville, 2003
43) Mary Warnock: Utilitarianism and On Liberty. Blackwell Publishing, Malden, 2003
44) Stephen G. Post: Encyclopedia of Bioethics Third Edition. The Gale Group, New York, 2004
45) Aristotle; translated into Japanese by K. Boku: Nicomachean Ethics. Kyoto University Press, Kyoto, 2005
46) Paul Guyer: Kant's Groundwork for the Metaphysics of Morals. Continuum, London, 2007

Chapter VII: *Environmental ethics, environmental hormones and various current problems*

I will mention a number of major ethical problems that are important for us. They are past issues, but we will likely pass them on to the next generation.

1. *Silent Spring* and environmental ethics

On the planet called "Earth," organic matter was first generated. Then, single-celled organisms, plants, animals and humans came into being successively. Humans, as part of the wide-ranging biological ecosystem of Earth, have evolved into various races and nations and developed specific religions and cultures according to their adaptation to different geographical, meteorological and social conditions on Earth. The same mechanism of evolution holds for every plant and animal species.

When one looks at the minutely developed and finely balanced diversity of Earth's global ecosystem, one realizes rather solemnly there is a universal evolutionary process which all living organisms that have passed through the very long history of Earth, from long-lost generations to today, undergo. Or, if we adopt a teleological viewpoint, we can observe the vital flow of various biological systems towards an ultimate aim. However, this natural flow of global history is, since very recently, in a state of crisis brought on by the explosive and uncontrollable development of modern science, even if the crisis is as yet partial. Humans are on the verge of destroying their own environment all over Earth, as evidenced by anthropogenic global warming, atmospheric pollution and chemically induced misery.

When the population was not as large as it is today, and the industrialization process which leads to the destruction of nature was not so wide-spread as it is today, human beings remained an integral part of a healthy bio-diverse ecosystem by participating in it through coexistence and compartmentalization. This thought of coexistence is what we East Asian people, or Buddhists in general, have since long ago kept in mind as a basic worldview. Notably, there is the Buddhist precept against taking the life of other living things, such as worms, fish, birds, deer and of course humans since the days of the Buddha in India. Today, Buddhists never kill needlessly, and usually comport themselves in a compassionate way toward other living organisms because these are also members of the common ecosystem. They realize that all living things, be they humans or worms, depend on one another for survival. To use the vocabulary of a Buddhist, we and other organisms are all "made alive in the great light of the Buddha." For example, there is a famous painting depicting the *nirvana* of the

Buddha, in which birds, a snake, a cow, and even beasts such as a lion and a tiger, are present together with the many monks surrounding the lying Buddha, shedding tears in grief over his death. The concept of coexistence is eloquently captured in one of Issa's *haiku* poems, which can be loosely translated as follows: "Look, don't kill that fly! It is praying to you by rubbing its hands and feet." Yet another example would be Dogen's experience during his Zen meditation, described in Chapter V.

However, after the Industrial Revolution began in England, various world-wide processes were unleashed, including modernization, industrialization, colonization, wars, pursuit of national interests, the ruin of socialism, the unipolar domination of the capitalist ideology, globalization, the excessive control of nature, the exhaustion of fossil fuels and deep-sea mineral exploitation. In these processes, the original state of the global ecosystem is being unidirectionally destroyed. Finally, humans have realized that industrial waste is harmful to themselves, and humankind is now suffering the consequences of their modern science, which has developed excessively. Humans, who are part of the ecosystem and share the Earth with other living beings, cannot survive without self-regulation.

Artificial chemical agents that have not existed in the natural world are now being used as insecticides and herbicides, as part of the logic of trying to control nature. These killing agents have accumulated in the living matter of the natural world and have affected the ecosystem in a way opposite to what was expected. Some chemical agents are affecting generations of living organisms, just like radiation. Other chemical agents seriously disrupt the endocrine system, having effects similar to those of female hormones. In *Silent Spring*, published in 1962, Ms. Rachel Carson (1907-1964) mentioned that we should reflect on the fact that artificial chemical agents are causing the destruction of the environment. She was a major pioneer of the mass movement for environmental conservation that became popular 40 years ago and is still strong today.

The insecticides she mentioned in her book include DDT (dichloro-diphenyl-trichloro-ethane), DDD (dichloro-diphenyl-dichloro-ethane) and BHC (benzene hexachloride). She persuasively explained the effects of DDT over a large number of pages. DDD (dichloro-diphenyl-dichloro-ethane) is an insecticide which has one chlorine less than DDT (dichloro-diphenyl-trichloro-ethane).

DDT had been synthesized many years earlier by a chemist in Switzerland in 1874. However, its efficiency as an insecticide, unparalleled in previous history, did not become apparent until 1939.

World War II started in 1939.

Atomic bombs were dropped over the Japanese cities of Hiroshima and Nagasaki in

1945. DDT was referred to as the atomic bomb of the world of insects. The American military ordered chemical corporations in the U.S. to manufacture DDT in large quantities to kill fleas, lice and mosquitoes in the occupied areas of foreign countries. They stockpiled a large amount of inventory after the war.

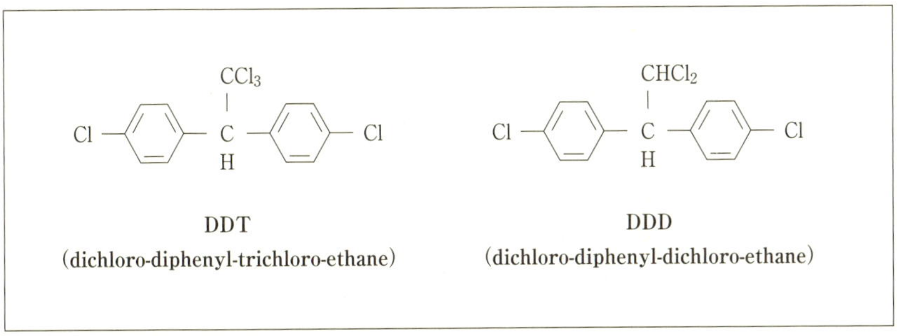

DDT
(dichloro-diphenyl-trichloro-ethane)

DDD
(dichloro-diphenyl-dichloro-ethane)

Fig.14 Organic chlorine insecticides

Modern weapons are demonic products whose purpose is to kill as many living beings as possible, to destroy nature as effectively as possible (atomic bombs, chemical defoliants, missiles, cluster bombs, etc). Western nations have developed these weapons in cooperation with the industry and the academic community, i.e. by unifying science and politics. In this sense, DDT is also a weapon. The ammunition industry developed rapidly and thrived during the war, motivated by it, of course, but also by the fierce competition among nations. However, they had trouble in disposing of these products after the war. Capitalist countries foster their core industries in cooperation with science. It is natural that they open markets for their stored stocks after the transition from war to peace.

Also in Japan, the Allied occupation forces gathered the Japanese people in schools and public halls just after the end of the war and sprinkled their entire bodies with DDT to exterminate the lice. This is still fresh in the minds of Japanese people. The same thing was done in Italy and Korea. DDT is still used in countries with frequent malaria cases (e.g., Africa, South America, Mexico, etc.). People thought that DDT is a safe agent because it is not absorbed through the skin. However, if it is absorbed by the body in some other way (and some studies show that it can also be absorbed through the skin), it accumulates in the fatty tissue and is never eliminated (biological accumulation).

DDD has a structure much like DDT, as shown in Figure 14. DDD is less effective than DDT, and has only one chlorine less than DDT. They are both organic chlorine insecticides. DDT started to be used in about 1950 in the U.S. to exterminate *Simulium* flies in woods, rivers and lakes.

As a result, *Simulium* flies were exterminated from the human environment. However, DDD was transferred to plankton and fish. Grebes which ate them died.

DDD has another effect, that of a cell poison. It destroys the adrenal cortex, which excretes the adrenal cortex hormones. It causes adrenocortical insufficiencies in dogs and Addison's disease in humans. This effect was discovered in 1948. DDD is now used as a drug (Mitotane) for treating Cushing's syndrome (in which the adrenal produces too much of the hormone called "cortisol"), which cannot be treated surgically and causes carcinoma of the adrenal cortex.

The significant insecticidal efficiency of DDT became clear in 1939. Since then, DDT has been used for exterminating lice, fleas and mosquitoes that transmit contagious diseases to humans.

Carson wrote *Silent Spring* in 1962 from the macro perspective, taking into consideration the entire ecosystem; she cited that DDT kills not only insects but also the birds and fish that eat the contaminated insects. This book got a lot of media exposure and provoked a mass protest against the deterioration of the environment. As a result, the production of DDT was stopped in 1972 in the U.S. However, DDT is still being used in malarial zones to exterminate mosquitoes which transmit contagious diseases. DDT is still accumulating in our bodies, although the amount of DDT being absorbed is decreasing.

With regard to the health condition of Carson herself, she was afflicted with breast cancer and died young as a result of metastasis to her entire body. People's awareness of that kind of fate was raised. She noticed two lumps in her left breast in the spring of 1960 and underwent a mastectomy of the left breast. The attending surgeon apparently overlooked the seriousness of her condition at that time, and performed the mastectomy only as a preventive measure. No radical surgery or radiation therapy, which was already common at that time, was performed. The lymph nodes along her right ribs became enlarged soon after the operation. No radiation was applied until then. After that, the cancer spread to her right breast and other lymph nodes and she could not endure the chest pain. The disease progressed unfavorably, spreading to her bony pelvis, and she developed a dysfunctional gait. She had anemia and was in pain due to the metastasis to her spine. Finally, the metastasis pervaded her entire body, including the liver. She had her pituitary removed at the Cleveland Clinic one month before her death. This operation was performed to suppress the secretion of female hormones. However, it had little effect and she died, 56 years old, in April 1964.

She prepared herself for this fate. While she was undergoing radiation therapy, she completed her life's work, *Silent Spring*, two years after the initial breast cancer operation. DDT is now believed to be an environmental hormone. Many environmental hormones have been correlated not only with the feminization of male organisms, but also with breast cancer. It has become clear that female hormones, generically called "estrogen" (one typical female hormone is estradiol), play a prominent role in the feminization of male organisms and in the development of breast cancer. Carson contended with pain in her entire body and the mental anguish caused by the breast cancer recurrences and the bone metastases throughout her entire body for four years, until her death in 1964.

She gazed out benevolently at all living creatures and human beings in *Silent Spring* and expressed her sorrow for them. This scientific book was published at the end of September 1962. It lingered on the best-seller list until December. It was a huge sensation all over the U.S., and President Kennedy ordered the Special Committee on Science and Technology to investigate the effects of agricultural chemicals. The report took due notice of the assertions made by Carson. People were pursuing efficient agriculture based on utilitarian, pragmatist and capitalist considerations, which were part of the prevalent American mentality at that time. People utilized the available scientific techniques of agriculture without doubting their safety and effectiveness. A wide range of woodlands and farms were sprayed with organic chlorinated agents, including DDT and DDD, using planes. Chemical companies became extremely wealthy by manufacturing insecticides. This was capitalism, and people took it for granted that companies had the right to pursue their capitalistic interests. As a result, a large amount of the agricultural chemicals produced not only killed insects but also accumulated in the fatty tissue of aquatic animals as a result of river contamination. DDT was detected in the larger fish caught in the outer seas; it was creeping up the food chain.

The general American consensus about the environment at that time was that it should profit humans. People wanted to exterminate insects from the human environment. They completely lacked the concept of the food chain, which includes the birds that eat the insects, the chemical substances that flow into the water and are absorbed by algae and plankton, the small aquatic animals that eat the plankton, the larger aquatic animals that eat the small aquatic animals, the even larger animals that eat those aquatic animals, and the humans fishing from a lake.

As a scientist and an excellent writer, Carson pointed out for the first time the facts of environmental pollution and the uncertainty of the future. However, she died too young, at 56. She got a master's degree at Johns Hopkins University and got a job at the

Fish and Wildlife Service. She researched and handled the publicity for aquatic organisms in seas and rivers. Not surprisingly, considering her career as a scientist, *Silent Spring* is rich in scientific observations, documentation and speculations. She took a global, not an anthropocentric, stance in her book. She mounted a critical attack on the risks of artificial chemical substances produced at a time when the government had no relevant regulations in place, adducing substantial proofs for her arguments.

Environmental problems have now mushroomed into a global ecological crisis. No one disputes that Carson, 40 years ago, was one of the pioneers in this field. She had several advantages which secured her position and achievements in the area of environmental awareness, as follows:

① She made clinical observations and organized her facts logically as a scientist, ② she had firm intent, ③ her writing was skillful, ④ she had an Asian attitude toward the ecosystem, ⑤ she had a sense of responsibility as a living human being preparing for death and ⑥ her mother, a deeply religious person, assisted her in her work.

The modern wisdom of Descartes, the greatest happiness principle proposed by Bentham and the moral theory of Kant are human-centered perspectives. Modern-day people need a new perspective in matters of morality, a perspective not covered by these ethical theories. Environmental ethics, which is an eco-philosophy that considers humans as part of the global ecosystem, has this new perspective. In this sense, Carson played an important role.

When reading *Silent Spring* again, a book written about 40 years ago, we notice that she predicted several issues being discussed in the 21st century. In this sense, she is really a pioneer of the now popular environmental ethics.

This book was written by a sincere scientist, not a journalist. This testifies to the truth and justice of her endeavor. The scientific analysis of facts generated scientific insights, and she refrained from making highly inflammatory remarks, unlike the common practice of journalism, allowing the scientific truth to speak eloquently and unfettered. This shows her confidence and strong intent as a scientist. Her attitude was that of a gentle illuminator whose goal was to help save people from the serious crisis facing the global ecosystem by informing them of the facts. She was a cool-headed scientist who tried to make politicians understand the scientific data.

We should clarify the present significance of this monumental work. The major chemical substance mentioned in this book is DDT. She raised the issue of environmental ethics, focusing her attention on DDT. Her perspective was innovative because she considered the use of DDT as very dangerous to human beings and the global biosphere in terms of the food chain. She stated that DDT (an artificial insecticide) is absorbed by biosystems and is accumulated over a long period of time. This pollution of the food chain extends to plants, birds, animals and humans, as DDT accumulates in the fatty tissue of animals. There were in particular high levels of DDT in the adrenal glands, testes and ovaries, where steroids generated from cholesterol in the fatty tissue, according to the scientific data. Based on these scientific and objective bases, she described the environmental phenomena she observed, such as the massive death of fish in rivers, the death of small birds such as robins, and the decrease in the eagle population after DDT spraying.

As early as 1962, she pointed out that DDT has the effects of an "environmental hormone," which is exactly what it is called today. She showed data proving that DDT was accumulating in the testes of robins, green pheasants, mice and deer. She predicted that the accumulation of DDT in the testes would reduce the masculine functions, leading to the feminization of the male organism in the form of testicular shrinkage and oligospermia. She also pointed out that the sex of mosquitoes which survive DDT spraying is not clear. These examples indicate that many of the environmental hormones were showing estrogenic effects through the activation of the estrogen (female hormone) receptor. Therefore, these environmental hormones are called endocrine-disrupting chemicals. As shown later, "environmental hormone" is a collective term for chemical agents such as dioxins, bisphenol A (BPA) and polychlorinated biphenyl (PCB). The existence of environmental hormones now prompts serious discussions about the feminization of the male organism in the natural world, abnormal female functions and carcinogenesis. Carson raised the issue of environmental hormones 40 years ago. The temperature dependence of the feminization of reptiles was revealed later. However, the significance of environmental hormones which Carson called to people's attention has not been lost, even today.

The third prediction made by Carson is that synthetic drugs damage the DNA in cells just as nuclear radiation does, and that the damage is carried over to the next generation. These chemicals, which are akin to nuclear radiation in their effects, appear to be carcinogenic. Typical cases are observed in nitrogen mustard contamination. Carson showed that DNA or genes damaged by chemicals leave an imprint on the next generation. In other words, environmental pollution is a problem of intergenerational ethics.

2. Environmental hormones

The term "environmental hormone" has become established at the social level.

However, experts often use the term "endocrine disruptor."

Hormones are normally synthesized by living bodies. They do not come from the environment. People use the term "environmental hormones" to describe certain artificial chemicals because, when these are discharged into the environment, they have effects on living organisms similar to the hormones generated naturally.

The study of hormones is called "endocrinology." Here, I will explain the basic characteristics of hormones, the mechanism through which environmental hormones act as natural hormones and the actual status of endocrine disruptors.

① General facts about hormones

Hormones are generated in the living body, in contrast to vitamins. Hormones play a role in humoral transmission in the living body. If nerves are comparable to electric wires with respect to the way they communicate information, the endocrine system is comparable to a system of water pipes: hormones, the informational substances of the endocrine system, flow through the "water pipes" of the living organism, ensuring humoral transmission.

For example, in stress situations such as hypoglycemia (low blood concentration of glucose) and intense fright, hormones such as CRH (corticotropin-releasing hormone) are excreted from the hypothalamus into the bloodstream. This stimulates the pituitary, inducing it to excrete adrenocorticotropic hormone (ACTH). ACTH or corticotropin flows into the bloodstream and reaches the adrenal glands locating above the kidneys. The adrenal glands excrete cortisol, an adrenal cortex hormone. This stress hormone, cortisol, corrects the low blood glucose that brought the body to the crisis level (recovery of blood glucose). The body is brought into a state of readiness to fight against the object of intense fright (blood pressure elevation, alertness and concentrated attention). Three hormones, CRH, ACTH and cortisol, are active here. They are excreted in conjunction with the biological reactions to crisis (low blood glucose, intense fright, etc). In other words, they function as information transmitters. Soluble substances called hormones flow within the living body, helping it to maintain a stable state (homeostasis) and thus, life. Therefore, an individual organism can keep on living by overcoming outer disruptions with the help of hormones.

There are many types of hormones. The classical hormones found long ago include the thyroid hormones, the adrenal cortex hormones, the gastrointestinal hormones, adrenalin and the pituitary hormones. In general, before they can have an effect, they must be transported to regions far away from the region where they were first excreted. Several other hormones were found more recently. Hormones with paracrine effects

Chapter VII : *Environmental ethics, environmental hormones and various current problems*   227

exert their actions chiefly in regions near the regions from which they were first excreted (vascular hormones, brain hormones and the Langerhans hormones in the pancreas). Some vitamins are taken in and modified to become hormones (activated vitamin D). Physiologically active arachic acids such as prostaglandin are also hormones. Nitric oxide, with its simple structure, is also a physiologically active substance that satisfies the definition of a hormone.

Now, I will explain the basic principles of endocrinology, the study of hormones.

② Control and feedback mechanism of upper hormones and lower hormones

Hormones are the behind-the-scenes errand boys who maintain the homeostasis of the living body. When the lower hormones are insufficient, a large amount of upper hormones is excreted to correct the deficiency. On the contrary, when the lower hormones are excessive, they hinder the excretion of the higher hormones (negative feedback).

For example, TSH is elevated in chronic thyroiditis (the state where the thyroid hormones are insufficient, also known as Hashimoto's thyroiditis). Patients take thyroid hormones orally as their treatment. The appropriate doses are determined based on the blood TSH levels.

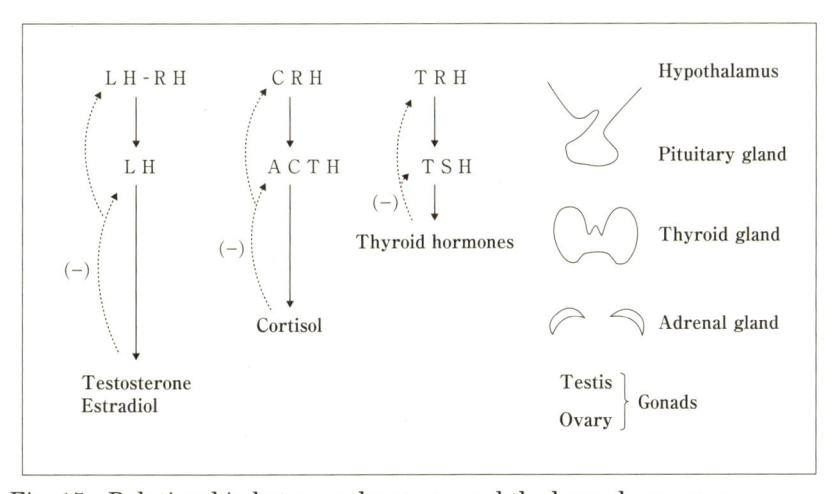

Fig. 15 Relationship between the upper and the lower hormones

In hypogonadism, where testosterone (the main male hormone) or estradiol (the main female hormone) is insufficient, sex-hormone drugs are administered to compensate for the insufficient hormone. The appropriate doses are judged by the reduction of the elevated blood LH (luteinizing hormone) values to normal values.

In Figure 15, the arrows along the dotted line indicate the negative feedback launched by the lower hormones to maintain homeostasis. When the thyroid hormones are insufficient, the excretion of TRH (thyrotropin-releasing hormone) and TSH (thyroid-stimulating hormone) increases. If cortisol is insufficient, the excretion of CRH and ACTH in the brain increases. In the same way, if the excretion of testosterone (testicular shrinkage in males) and estradiol (climacterium in females) is insufficient, the excretion of LH-RH (LH-releasing hormone) and LH increases.

③ Hormones act by way of receptors

This is an important rule. In general, a cell is composed of a nucleus (where the DNA is located), the cytoplasm surrounding the nucleus and the cell membrane surrounding the cytoplasm. Hormones are categorized into two main groups, depending on whether their receptors are situated in the cell membrane or in the nucleus/cytoplasm.

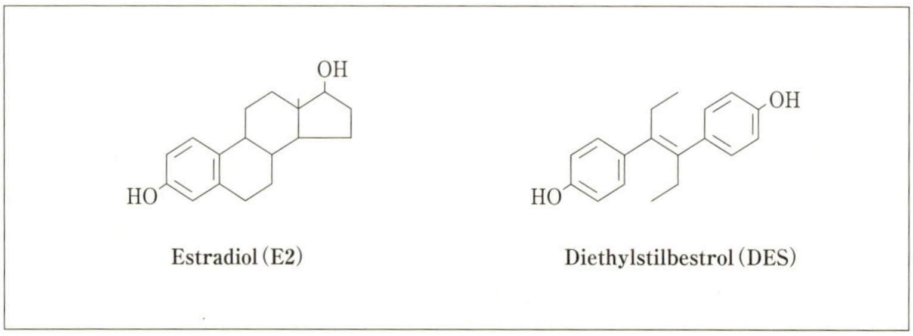

Fig. 16 DES of synthesized estrogen

The overwhelming majority of hormones have their receptors in the cell membrane. For example, peptide hormones (hypothalamic hormones, pituitary hormones, and parathyroid hormones) and adrenaline are of this type. Meanwhile, hormones with receptors in the nucleus or cytoplasm are the steroid hormones (testosterone, estradiol, cortisol, aldosterone, etc.) and the thyroid hormones. The locations of hormone receptors are different, but the hormones have common in these features: ① no hormonal action occurs in the cells without the action of the receptors, ② the hormones combine with those receptors for which they have higher affinity, and ③ chemical substances combining with receptors for which they have high affinity will have the same effect as the original hormones. One example of such a chemical substance is diethylstilbestrol (DES), which is an artificial chemical substance that combines with estrogen receptors.

Estrogen is the collective term for female hormones. "Estrus" means "mating season." The three natural estrogens generated in the living animal body are estradiol (E2), estrone (E1) and estriol (E3). Estradiol is the strongest and most important for female function and behavior. All estrogens chiefly combine with the estrogen receptors existing in the cellular nucleus and exert their effects within the cell.

　DES was synthesized as an artificial estrogen in England in 1938. The skeleton of DES is like that of estradiol (Fig. 16). To be precise, it has no steroid skeleton. Therefore, it is a non-steroid estrogen. As DES has an estrogenic effect, the Food and Drug Administration (FDA) in the U.S. approved DES for the treatment of menopausal symptoms and for use in hormone replacement therapies in 1941. Since 1943, a large amount of DES has been used as a wonder drug in the U.S. to prevent spontaneous abortion. DES has been used for various other purposes as well, for instance, to promote the growth of poultry, cattle and sheep. It has been used all over the world, and was sold in Japan at one time under the name of "Oibestine." Japanese women did not use DES because they had a different attitude toward the womanhood and the value of breasts from those of European and American women. As a result, the global DES drug disaster resulted in less damage in Japan.

　It has become apparent that DES exerts its estrogenic effect by combining with estrogen receptors. In the 1960s, side effects such as carcinogenicity, virilization, and fetal defects (when administered to pregnant women) became apparent. Because it is able to pass through the placenta, DES is easily transferred to the fetus and exerts its estrogenic effects there. As a result, girls were born with impaired reproductive functions and developed cancers in the vagina and the womb (clear-cell carcinoma) in their teens. Hypospadias and cryptorchidism (effects of excessive estrogen) were observed in boys. As a result of these side effects becoming apparent, the administration of DES to animals and pregnant women was prohibited in 1971 in the U.S. Also in Japan, the administration of DES to pregnant women was prohibited in 1972. DES so strongly combines with estrogen receptors that it has almost the same effect as the natural hormones E2, E1 and E3. The affinity of DES to estrogen receptors is far stronger than that of other environmental hormones (DDT, PCB, dioxin, BPA). Actually, DES is the strongest environment hormone that has ever existed.

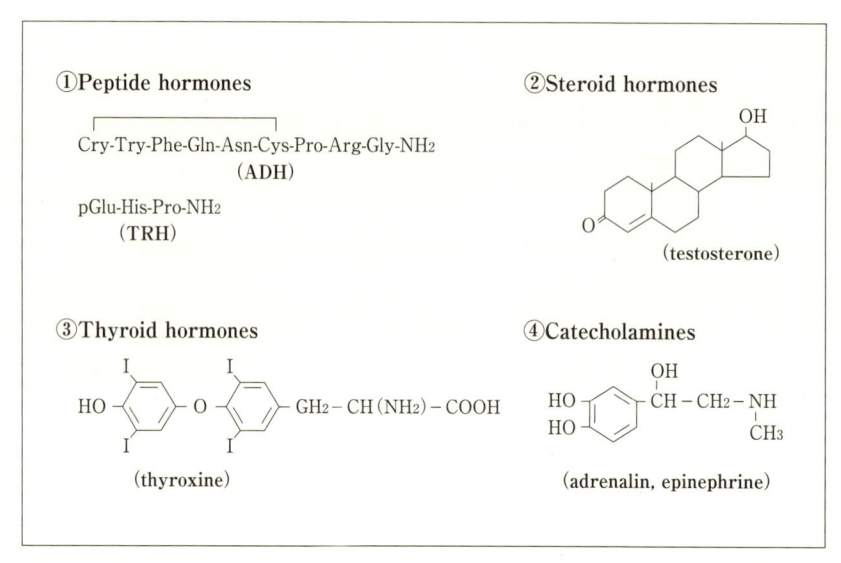

Fig. 17 Basic structure of hormones (*An Introduction to Endocrinology and Metabolism*, Norihiko Aoki)

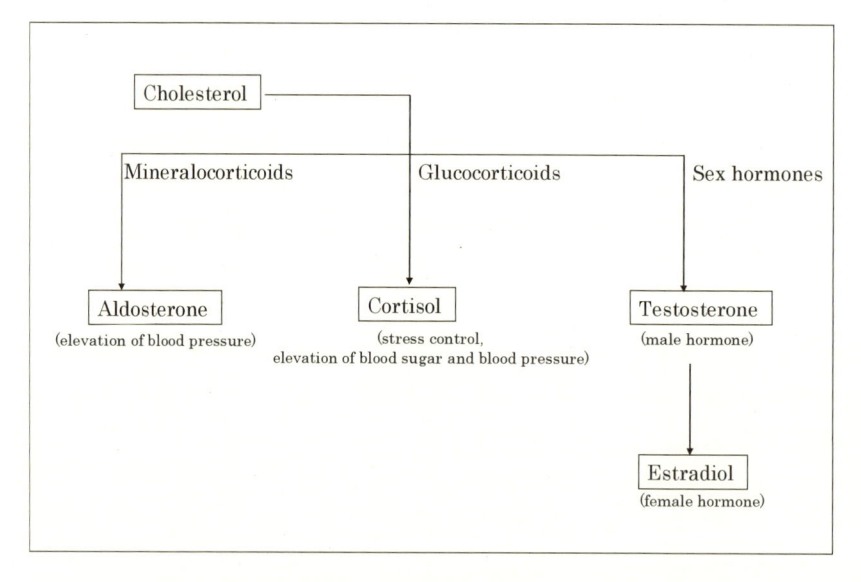

Fig. 18 Route of the generation of steroid hormones (modified from *An Introduction to Endocrinology and Metabolism*, Norihiko Aoki)

④ Structural classification of hormones

As shown in Figure 17, hormones are classified into five categories according to their structures: ① peptide hormones (largest group), ② catecholamine (adrenalin, noradrenalin), ③ thyroid hormones, ④ steroid hormones and ⑤ others.

Thyroid hormones and steroid hormones exert their effects by combining with receptors existing in the cell nuclei or in certain regions of the cytoplasm. In this case, the hormones pass through the cell membrane freely and transmit information directly to the nuclei. The receptors that combine with steroids, such as estrogen and glucocorticoids, exist not only in the nuclei, but also in the cytoplasm. They combine with specific hormones or ligands and such complexes move into the nuclei to activate the DNA. The basic mechanism by which these types of hormones send information to the nuclei is that two hormone-receptor complexes combine with each other to form a dimer. The dimer reaches the DNA (genes) of the nucleus and combines with the hormone response elements (HRE) to activate the genes specific to the hormone in question. Thus, increased amounts of messenger RNA cause various biological responses in cells, such as the synthesis of hormones and proteins. This chain reaction has been established as a general rule. In this case, the important point is that receptors form dimers. Even if a dimer is generated by an estrogen receptor that is activated by molecules other than estrogen, the estrogenic effect is still exerted.

Steroid hormones are called "steroid" because they have a steroid skeleton. As shown in Figure 18, the components of steroid hormones are lipids and cholesterol. Steroid hormones are categorized into three groups: ① pressor hormones, such as aldosterone (mineralocorticoids), ② stress hormones, such as cortisol (glucocorticoids) and ③ sex hormones (testosterone and estradiol). In this case, we should note that, in the system of sex hormones, the main male hormone (testosterone) is the precursor to the main female hormone (estradiol). The number of carbons in testosterone and estradiol is 19 and 18, respectively. Estradiol is formed by detaching one carbon from testosterone.

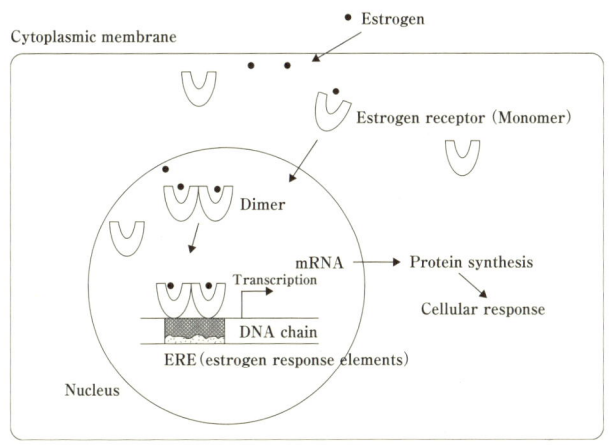

Fig. 19 Activation of estrogen receptors

⑤ Effects of estrogen

Estrogens are the collective term for female hormones. Meanwhile, male hormones are collectively referred to as "androgens." They are all collectively called "sex hormones." The major sex hormones in females and males are estrogen and androgen, respectively. Males have female sex hormones and females have male sex hormones, and each type of hormones has its own significance in the development and functions of the living animal organism.

All steroid hormones (estrogen, androgen, cortisol, aldosterone, etc.) have a common mechanism by which they combine with each specific receptors in the nucleus. Namely, natural estrogen (estradiol, estrone, and estriol) and synthetic estrogen (DES, diethylstilbestrol) activate genes specific to estrogen after combining with the estrogen receptors (acceleration of transcription). During transcription, the information carried by estrogen is sent to the messenger RNA. The nuclear receptor of estrogen is the transcription factor of estrogen. Nuclear receptors exist in the cell nuclei and the cytoplasm. If estrogen combines with the nuclear receptor, the receptor is activated. A dimer (two receptors combined) combines with the DNA in the nucleus (Fig. 19). This generation of dimers is important for unleashing the estrogenic effects. Combined artificial chemical substances (DES and other environmental hormones) or phytoestrogens, which are similar to estrogen, cause the receptors to form dimers. Based on the latest data, if a dioxin combines with the dioxin receptor, the dioxin receptor combines with the estrogen receptor. This process induces the estrogen receptor to become one half of a dimer. It is a bypass mechanism which explains why dioxin has an estrogenic effect.

Environmental epidemiologists are now demonstrating that the feminization of the environment is caused by artificial chemical substances (environmental hormones). Meanwhile, estrogen receptors are activated (dimer formation) by many estrogen-like substances for which living organisms have a certain degree of tolerance. It has become apparent that this mechanism diverges slightly from the precise definition of the relationship between general hormones (ligands) and receptors.

Steroid hormones and thyroid hormones combine with their respective receptors and the nuclear DNA in the form of dimers. The binding sites are called the "HREs" (hormone response elements). In the case of estrogen, they are called the "EREs" (estrogen response elements).

Estrogen affects the organs and tissues where the estrogen receptors exist.

We know that estrogens are the hormones which cause female rut and feminine traits. Affected organs include the internal genitalia, such as the ovaries, the ovarian ducts, the uterus and the vagina, and the external genitaria; also affected are the breasts, bones, skin, blood cells, pituitary glands and brain.

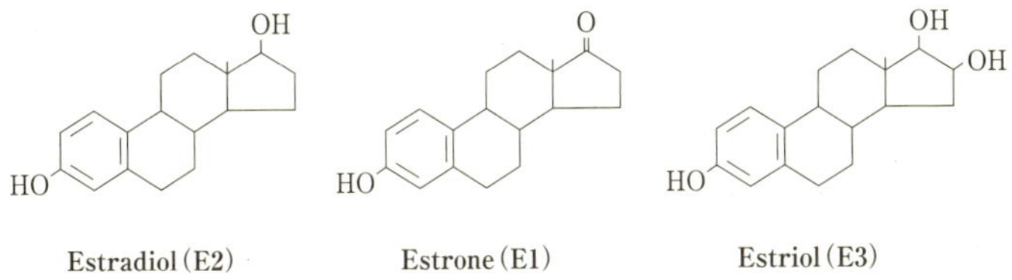

Fig.20 Steroid skeleton and the OH of estrogen

In 1996, it became clear that estrogen receptors are of the α or the β type. Type α has a stronger binding affinity to estrogen. The estrogen receptor which mainly exists in the genitals is type α. Type β mainly exists in the brain, affecting the growth and transformation of neurons and the development of cognitive functions. Females and males in whom α estrogen receptors have no effect are sterile, and the brain does not develop properly without the β estrogen receptors.

⑥ Environmental hormones (endocrine disruptors)

A chemical substance in the environment that disrupts a natural endocrine function by exerting a hormone-like effect in a living body is called an "environmental hormone." The technical term is "endocrine disruptor."

The worst environmental hormones with the highest abundance in the environment are artificial chemical substances that have the effects of female hormones (estrogen). Female hormones include estradiol (E2), which is the strongest, estrone (E1) and estriol (E3). The number after the "E" indicates the number of hydroxyl groups: E1 has one hydroxyl group, E2 has two hydroxyl groups and E3 has three hydroxyl groups (Fig. 20)

Estradiol (E2) is the major hormone of mature females. Most of the estradiol is excreted from the ovaries. Estrone (E1) is formed by enzymes from estradiol or androgen in blood and various tissues. The effects of E1 are weaker than those of E2. The effects of estriol (E3) are the weakest. Estriol (E3) is produced in the liver through estrone metabolism and is passed into the urine. All estrogens combine with their estrogen receptors in the cell nucleus. The hormone receptor complex then combines with the DNA in the nucleus to increase the amount of messenger RNA (mRNA) of the gene. As a result, protein synthesis is accelerated in the cytoplasm. Thus, the effects typical of female hormones become apparent (femininity, female functions and female secondary sexual characteristics). E2, E1 and E3 have similar structures. The A ring of the steroid structure has three double bonds (benzene ring) and is characterized by a phenolic hydroxyl group.

E1, E2 and E3 are physiological hormones (produced by the living body), not artificial environmental hormones. As shown above, the strong synthetic estrogen, diethylstilbestrol (DES), has no steroid structure. The benzene ring (phenolic ring) corresponding to the A ring of the steroid structure is the same as that in the estrogen structure. DES is a strong environmental hormone, and the endocrine disruptions caused by DES were very useful in research on environmental hormones such as bisphenol A (BPA) and polychlorinated biphenyls (PCBs), which later became the subject of discussion. The action mechanism of environmental hormones was less understood in Japan because, thankfully, few people in Japan used DES. A minor mistake can cause a major disaster.

We should understand the peculiar circumstances of DES use in the U.S. It is an artificial estrogen synthesized in 1938. As shown above, it in not a proper steroid. The FDA did not function as a responsible supervisor in this case and approved DES as a synthetic estrogen in 1941. DES became fanatically fashionable in the U.S., being used extensively by obstetricians and gynecologists who were convinced that DES prevents miscarriages.

Cancers of the vagina were not confirmed in children until 1971. The administration of DES to animals and humans was prohibited in the U.S. However, more than five million women had used DES during the nearly 30 years after its release. This is an example of a drug disaster that calls on administrations, companies, doctors and people to reflect on their past conduct. DES is an example of a synthetic substance having estrogenic activity. It is not a steroid like estrogen, but binds the estrogen receptors, thereby causing estrogenic activity. Accordingly, it is called a "nonsteroidal estrogen."

Phytoestrogens are also nonsteroidal estrogens, although their estrogenic activity is weak. Isoflavones, such as genistein and daidzein (Fig. 21), are naturally found in leguminous plants such as soybeans and foods derived from soybeans, including tofu and miso. These isoflavones bind the estrogen receptors in animals and humans through the aromatic ring structures which are similar to estradiol (E2), as shown in the figure, effecting estrogenic activity; they are thus collectively called "phytoestrogens" ("*phytó*" in Greek means "plant"). Equol, another isoflavone

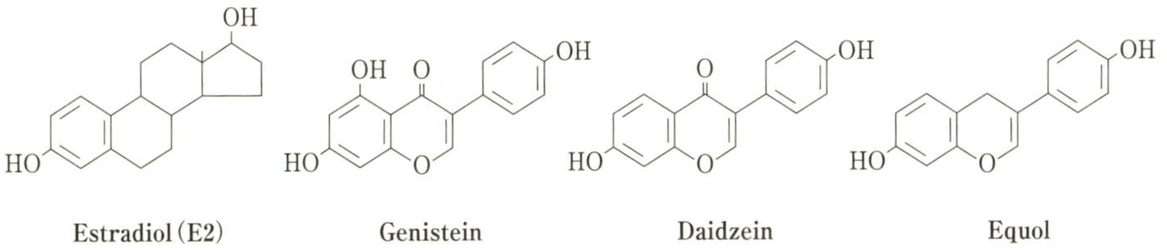

Chapter VII : *Environmental ethics, environmental hormones and various current problems* 235

Fig. 21 Phytoestrogens

(Fig. 21), is not a phytoestrogen and does not exist naturally, but is produced in the large intestine by the bacterial flora as a metabolite of daidzein. Besides showing estrogenic effects like genistein and daidzein, equol may be beneficial in the treatment of male baldness and acne, because it can act as an anti-androgen by binding 5-alpha-dihydrotestosterone (DHT), thereby preventing DHT from binding the androgen receptors.

Estradiol commonly has a phenolic hydroxyl at the position corresponding to the A ring of estrogen.

It is known that phytoestrogens combine with estrogen receptors. A chemical substance that combines with estrogen receptors is either activated to have estrogenic effects or occupies the receptor and prevents the original estrogen from combining (anti-estrogen effect). It depends on the structure and amount of the chemical substance involved (a ligand binding to a receptor). It has been reported that phytoestrogens have both types of effects (estrogenic and anti-estrogenic). The anti-estrogenic effect of phytoestrogens explains the epidemiological fact that breast cancers are less frequent among Japanese women, who eat tofu (soybean curd), miso (soybean paste), natto (fermented soybeans) and soy sauce. The estrogenic effect explains the statistical data that Japanese men have less prostate cancers. We do not clearly understand the action mechanism of phytoestrogens within the living body. But, it is known that phytoestrogens are also environmental estrogens (environmental hormones), like DES.

Meanwhile, more than a few chemical substances have been shown to be estrogen-like, other than DES and phytoestrogens.

They include DDT (dichloro-diphenyl-trichloro-ethane), dioxins, PCBs (polychlorinated biphenyl), bisphenol A, nonyl phenol, etc. Figure 22 shows the structures of dioxin, PCB and bisphenol A.

The mechanism through which the estrogenic effect is expressed is not uniform, but in the final phase, two estrogen receptors form a dimer which binds to the nuclear DNA at a specific site (ERE).

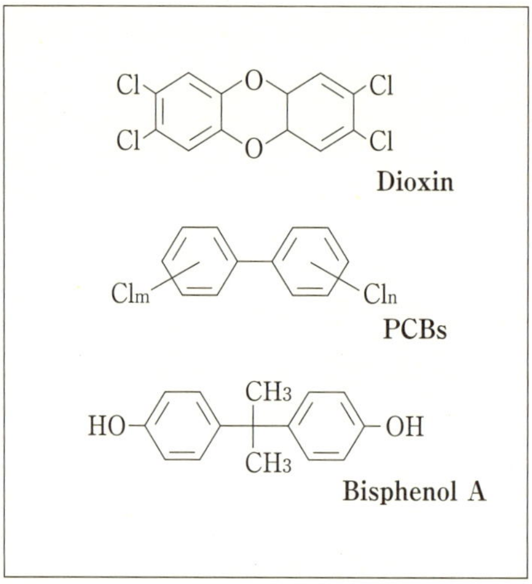

Fig. 22 Chemicals with estrogen-like activity

If estrogenic effects of chemical substances are generated when two receptors form a dimer; this leads to the feminization of the male organism. Some of these specific phenomena are now becoming issues of public concern and a major theme of environmental ethics.

For example, there are ecological and epidemiological studies on the reduced reproductive capacity of animals, including alligators. They have come to report abnormalities such as low sperm counts, developmental disorders of the male genitalia, and low sex drive in the males.

Low sperm count, endometriosis, infertility and increased incidence of breast cancer have also been reported in humans. There are no epidemiological data to establish a causal correlation; it is still just a hypothesis. But it can be speculated that such abnormalities are the result of the combination of pollutants pervading modern life. The environmental factors are too complicated for us to identify the specific factors responsible for these abnormalities.

Fortunately, we have succeeded in regulating the use of DDT. Now it is important for us to control and regulate the use of other chemical substances as well, such as dioxins (incinerators), PCBs (oil) and bisphenol A (dishes). The sources of dioxins are

Chapter VII : *Environmental ethics, environmental hormones and various current problems* 237

increasing in modern life, where many petrochemicals are used. We require regulations designed from a global bionomics perspective. Some substances disappear in the organic cycles of nature, in which case they pose no problems. The ones which do pose serious problems are those that do not enter the natural circulation and can only be eliminated through incineration.

We should also discuss hormones other than estrogen when talking about environmental hormones, because there are far fewer data on them than on estrogen.

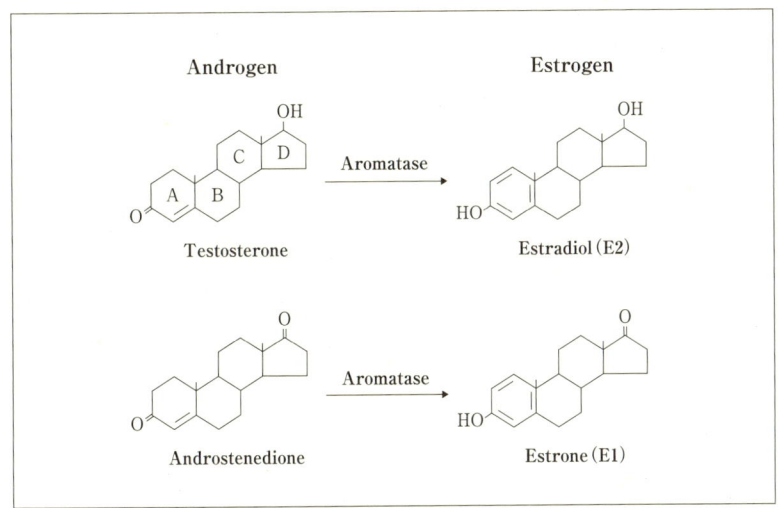

Fig. 23 Aromatization (modified from *An Introduction to Endocrinology and Metabolism*, Norihiko Aoki)

For example, the existence of a relationship between thyroid hormones and dioxin has been reported. But, again, the data are scant compared to those on estrogen, and so people pay less attention to dioxin when analyzing the ecosystem. People do not see other sex hormones, such as androgen, as a problem, even though the androgen receptors are independent of the estrogen receptors. One reason for this lack of proper interest in androgen is that, as shown in Figure 23, androgen is a precursor of estrogen; that is, androgen is changed into estrogen by aromatase (an enzyme) in the metabolic processes of the living animal body.

Estrogen has an aromatic ring (benzene ring) in place of the A ring of the steroid structure. Therefore, estrogen has an effect greatly different from that of androgen (its precursor). Aromatase (an enzyme) converts androgen into estrogen by changing the A ring into an aromatic ring. This enzyme changes testosterone (the strongest androgen) into estradiol (the strongest estrogen). Aromatase also changes another weak androgen, androstenedione, into estrone (a kind of estrogen). If an artificial chemical compound improves the effects of this enzyme, it strengthens the estrogenic effect, which can be another cause of feminization. Meanwhile, if there is a chemical substance that suppresses the enzymatic activity of aromatase, the female will become masculinized because female hormones cannot be formed in her body.

3. The thalidomide tragedy

Thalidomide brought to Japan a far more serious drug disaster than DES. When administered to pregnant women, thalidomide and DES cause drug-related defects in their children, not in themselves.

The number of reports of thalidomide-induced fetal malformation cases was largest in West Germany in the early 1960s, where the drug was produced. The U.K. and Japan ranked second. The frequency of reports was the same in the U.K. and Japan. In contrast, the U.S. experienced little of this drug disaster, and the thalidomide cases which did occur in the U.S. resulted from private imports by people who did not obey the regulations of the FDA (Food and Drug Administration). Human beings can learn many lessons from the thalidomide tragedy. Recently, there is a movement to begin reusing thalidomide, but it is a drug that has created and will create problems. Thalidomide has been legally rehabilitated. We cannot deny that there is still ambiguity in feelings of the Japanese public regarding the use of thalidomide. I will now explain the thalidomide incident in more detail.

In the 20th century, many chemicals were synthesized. They had unexpected side effects and caused wide-spread public nuisances and drug disasters. Indeed, we should call the 20th century "the century of public nuisances and drug disasters." A synthetic estrogen, DES, was synthesized in the U.S. in 1938 and was used as an over-the-counter drug. The significant insecticidal efficiency of DDT was discovered in 1939, and a large amount of DDT was used for spraying crops. However, the significant side effects of these two synthetic chemicals and their adverse effects on the global ecosystem become clear soon, and sales were stopped around 1970. Thalidomide, an analgesic and one of the most notorious drugs of the 20th century, inflicted its own serious damage on the Japanese population.

Thalidomide was first synthesized by a West German pharmaceutical company, Chemie Grünenthal, in 1953. It started to be sold in West Germany in 1957 as an analgesic and suppressor of nausea and vomiting during pregnancy (morning sickness), and it started to be sold in Japan as the sleeping drug Isomin in 1958. The production of thalidomide sky-rocketed in West Germany, from 30 kilograms in 1957 (the year of release) to 11 tons in 1961. Dr. Widukind Lenz (Hamburg) reported on the effects of thalidomide on children that same year, 1961, and the West German pharmaceutical company stopped selling it immediately. Sales in the U.S. were prohibited due to the cautious attitude of Dr. Frances Kelsey, a medical reviewer working for the FDA; this was extremely lucky for the Americans. She withheld permission to release thalidomide onto the American market because she believed that the results of the animal experiments were inconclusive. This historical decision helped save Americans from the thalidomide disaster. In 1962, President Kennedy gave her the Award for Distinguished Federal Civilian Service. The FDA has had recall events (DES), but it has also exercised good judgment, as shown in Dr. Kelsey's case. It is believed that she drew a lesson from the DES scandal.

Deformity of the arms and legs, collectively referred to as thalidomide embryopathy, was observed in newborn babies whose mothers had taken thalidomide during early pregnancy. The incidence was about 25%, a high rate. In this respect, thalidomide is a drug with a significantly high teratogenicity, causing specific abnormalities in the formation of limbs (brachymelia) and peripheral nerves (acoustic disturbances and facial palsy) of fetuses after passing through the placenta. Remarkably, thalidomide has no significant effects on the mothers.

In the beginning of the 1960s, several years after people started using thalidomide in 46 countries (though not in the U.S.), about 7000 cases of fetal deformity around the world, including 300 cases in Japan, were reported. In November 1961, a West German pediatrician named Widukind Lenz drew the public's attention to the relationship between limb deformity and the use of thalidomide. Based on this, the West German manufacturer of thalidomide quickly stopped selling the drug and recalled all of it on November 27 on its own initiative. In northern Europe and the U.K., it was decided to halt sales and recall unsold or unused stocks from November 30 to December 18. Thus, European countries immediately stopped selling and started recalling. But in Japan, thalidomide continued to be sold until August 1962. According to the records, thalidomide was recalled from the market in 1961. However, it continued to be seen on the market in Japan for eight months in 1962. The numbers of Japanese babies born with deformities caused by thalidomide were 12 (1959), 25 (1960), 58 (1961), 162 (1962), 47 (1963), 4 (1964) and 1 (1969); the peak was in 1962. As shown by the strict review of the FDA in the U.S. and the early response of European countries based on the reports of the side effects, appropriate administrative reviews, decisions and regulations during the early stages of drug disasters are important. Japanese people should learn much from this bitter experience. A drug disaster is never a thing of the past, and this particular disaster is fresh in the memories of many Japanese people because the victims are still living. The administration and the common people should not make the same type of mistake as in the thalidomide incident again. We should avoid drug disasters in the future.

People are likely to act fanatically and irresponsibly, driven by sensationalist journalism. Science and administration exist to increase the public's feeling of normality over a long period of time. Administrators should not be led by public opinion; instead, they should actively obtain scientific information and order the scientific investigation of unexplored issues. They should put restrictions on certain fields of research, and defy public opinion when necessary. Drug disasters should be prevented as much as possible, and administrators should not let themselves be influenced by politicians and big companies. Politics is a power game. However, drug disasters can be avoided through science. A drug disaster eventually comes to light sooner or later.

There are some reports that thalidomide is an effective suppressor of erythema nodosum in leprosy, myeloma, Behcet's syndrome, auto-immune diseases and the proliferation of blood vessels accompanying eye symptoms in diabetes, a disease which is now gaining momentum. Under these circumstances, people are likely to start reusing thalidomide under loose regulations. Younger patient groups and doctors who do not know of the thalidomide tragedy may begin to use it if its use is deregulated and private imports are allowed again. This is a serious ethical problem. We should feel responsible for the thalidomide disaster, and we should not allow the experience to fade from memory. The reuse of thalidomide should be allowed only under strict administrative guidance.

We should refer to a recent decision made by the FDA regarding the use of thalidomide. In 1998, the FDA, known for its strict regulations, approved the use of thalidomide only for treating erythema nodosum in cases of leprosy. They specified the strict conditions for its use as follows:

① Doctors and pharmacists who distribute thalidomide should register themselves in the System for Thalidomide Education and Prescribing Safety (STEPS). Only registered persons can administer thalidomide.

② Both male and female patients should agree with the STEPS to obtain the drug.

③ The administration of thalidomide to pregnant women is prohibited. Women who are capable of pregnancy should take several pregnancy tests before being allowed to take the drug, and they should report to the FDA if they become pregnant while taking the drug. They should also go to specialized institutions and receive counseling.

④ Male patients who take thalidomide should be controlled under STEPS just like the female patients, considering that there is no data on the safety of thalidomide in male ejaculate.

⑤ Scientific information on thalidomide should be conveyed to patients orally as well as in written form (the significantly high incidence rate of fetal malformation, the fact that administration at 35-50 days after the last menses yields the highest risk, that just one dose can cause fetal deformity, and that it has side effects such as nervous disorders, drowsiness, leucopenia and an increase in the HIV virus in the infected body).

These are strict FDA standards and administrative guidelines for using thalidomide based on the error of approving of DES and the foresight of Dr. Kelsey. The FDA has made this decision against the background of bitter experience.

These regulations are scientific and morally sound. It shows that ethics should not be affected by politics, economics or public opinion.

This decision of the FDA was also made based on pragmatist considerations.

The skin erythema which affects the limbs of people afflicted by Hansen's disease (leprosy) is very painful. Thalidomide, which the FDA never approved, is effective in alleviating the pain. No better painkiller for Hansen's disease exists at the present moment. Thus, the use of thalidomide is admitted only for this disease under strict administrative control. However, information on the thalidomide disaster is to be thoroughly disclosed to patients. Patients must always be placed under a doctors' supervision (prescriptions over restricted to one month at a time). This series of measures is pragmatic.

We should note that enough information has been disclosed and the disclosure has the purpose of controlling the use of the drug via scientists.

Another feature of the current thalidomide situation is that there are manuals for doctors, pharmacists and patients (both male and female) which enable its easy use. Practicability is the most important ethical condition.

As shown above, the standard for using thalidomide in Japan should not be looser than the FDA's. Furthermore, we should add the following important points, considering the narrow national territory, the population density and the prior experience of drug disasters:

① Personal imports and Internet sales should not be allowed. Every single tablet should be traceable.

② If this notorious drug, with such a high teratogenic rate of 25% as unprecedented in history may be discharged into the environment, epidemiological data should be collected for future generations.

③ Thalidomide was originally released as a sleeping pill and tranquilizer. We should investigate the diseases which respond significantly to thalidomide treatment and the mechanisms involved. We should not confirm the medicinal benefits of thalidomide based on ambiguous clinical evaluations. If we do, we will be the laughing stock of future generations.

④ It is becoming clear that thalidomide causes not only developmental anomalies in limbs, but also a wide range of nerve damage and blood circulation problems. If this notorious drug appears on the market again, it will be a tremendous social and biological experiment. Administrative control should strictly cover all research on thalidomide.

⑤ Regrettably, more than a few Japanese doctors eagerly adopt at the latest foreign medical trends. We should avoid the compulsion to be the first buffalo in a stampede. We should not restart the use of thalidomide in Japan in such a rapid frenzy. This is ungracious to the generation of victims. Strict clinical trials should be planned for targeted diseases (plasmacytoma, immunological diseases, etc.) under rigorous administrative guidance. It is imperative to enforce strict regulations according to which the use of thalidomide is only to be allowed in the treatment of thoroughly evaluated diseases.

As shown above, I have explained the real experience of the thalidomide disaster, and the latest movement to resume its use without strict regulations, which reveals the total lack of public moral sense in today's Japanese people. I have pointed out that thalidomide is a good symbolical test of future Japanese ethical and scientific attitudes. The U.S. has accelerated its research on environmental hormones based on the bitter experience of DES. Japanese people should always remember the bitter history of thalidomide and develop a sound environmental ethics and teratology with respect to thalidomide. In this sense, the thalidomide disaster is not a past affair but a current problem which challenges the Japanese mind to scrutinize its own motives.

Morality is generated in individuals.
Nations, governments and administrations establish rules.
Science and modern industries based on science are characterized by the principle of self-replication.

We should note the principle of the self-replication of science described above. If ethical rules do not function in an administration, science and industry expand without regard to principles. They do not take into consideration the whole picture. Humans should consider ethics if they want science and industry to develop in a healthy manner.

Deregulation is now being promoted all over the world to increase efficiency. However, regulations regarding the use of drugs, artificial chemical substances and industrial products should receive special treatment as they cover the global ecosystem and their deregulations should invade severely und in an unrecoverable way the earth. cover the global ecosystem. Therefore, the regulations should not be the same as the general deregulations.

I mentioned the pollution of the ecosystem and typical drug disasters in this chapter. Other examples include the ouch-ouch disease (1955), Minamata disease (1956) and Yokkaichi asthma (1968). They are results of unregulated industrial development and obsolete government regulations. History clearly shows that governmental regulations based on ethics are very important. Regulations should be the product of scientific insights and the ethical attitudes of humans. Meanwhile, common people are ignorant and sometimes turn into a mob. In this sense, people should be controlled by regulations based on science and ethics. Deregulation should not be confused with individual freedoms and rights.

References

1) Mitsushiro Kida: Sentenijyo no Igaku. Tyuokoronsya,Tokyo,1998
2) Alice L. Murkies, et al, Phytoestrogens, Journal of Clinical Endocrinology and Metabolism, Vol. 83, No 2, 297-303,1998
3) FDA Talk Paper. T98-44, July 16, 1998
4) T. Colborn, D.Dumanoski, and J.P. Myers; translated by Tikara Nagao: Our Stolen Future. Shueisya, Tokyo, 2001
5) Sheldon Krimsky; translated by Sanae Matsuzaki and Yoko Saito: Hormonal Chaos. Fujiwara Syoten, Tokyo, 2001
6) John Rawls: Justice as Fairness A Restatement. The Belknap Press of Harvard University Press, Cambridge, 2001
7) Tom L. Beauchamp, James F. Childress: Principles of Biomedical Ethics Fifth Edition. Oxford University Press, Oxford, 2001
8) Norihiko Aoki: Naibunpitsu Taisyagaku Nyumon (An Introduction to Endocrinology and Metabolism) Fourth Edition. Kinpodo, Kyoto, 2002
9) Rachel L. Carson: Silent Spring, 40th Anniversary Edition. Mariner Books/Houghton Mifflin Company, New York, 2002
10) Neurotoxicology and Teratology, Vol 24, 1-104, 2002
11) Judith Andre: Bioethics as Practice. The University of North Carolina Press, Chapel Hill, 2002

12) P. Reed Larsen, et al, Williams Textbook of Endocrinology 10th Edition, Saunders, 2003
13) Jan J. Brosens and Malcolm G. Parker, Oestrogen receptor hijacked, Nature, 423,487-489, 2003
14) Fumiaki Ohtake, et al, Modulation of oestrogen receptor signaling by association with the activated dioxin receptor, Nature, 423, 545-550, 2003
15) Dennis L. Kasper, Eugene Braunwald, Anthony S. Fauci, Stephan L. Hauser, Dan L. Longo (Editors): Harrison's Principle of Internal Medicine 16th Edition. McGraw-Hill, New York, 2005
16) Norihiko Aoki: Naibunpitsu Taisyagaku Nyumon (An Introduction to Endocrinology and Metabolism) Fifth Edition. Kinpodo, Kyoto, 2005

Afterword

The author believes that a book on bioethics evolved by a Japanese person should be written from the Japanese or Asian point of view. This is what induced him most to write this book.

Ethics is not science, but judgment regarding practice. Ethics is usually rooted deep in the culture, tradition and ethos of a community, at the core of which lies religion or the religious mind.

Even when only considering religion as a pillar of culture, there is a remarkable contrast between Christianity in the West and Asian religions, including Buddhism and Taoism, in the East. Further, the Islamic world exists as yet another presence. Historically speaking, religion has been essential or inevitable to human beings from the very beginning, while science has only been the late product of human intelligence. Now, scientific progress and the results thereof have become the common beacon which rallies human beings all over the Earth to promote further globalization. The rapid progress in the IT sector, space exploration and life science are good examples.

The author believes that the difference in the origin, as mentioned in this book, and the great disparity in the velocity of diffusion between ethics and science, are the deep pool which spews out today's ethical problems, many of which are so apparent in all parts of the world. When natural science and material civilization, both born and developed in the West, are introduced along with liberal individualism into an Asian country such as Japan, which has a long-standing and strong Buddhist culture and still enjoys a firm sense of communitarianism, it naturally takes time for them to be accepted by that culture, because ethnic or individual identity is nothing but strong self-affirmation based on religion and culture.

In this book, the author tries to demonstrate the basic structure of the distortion which has occurred in Japanese society, as evidenced by today's hot controversies in the life science fields regarding topics such as brain death, organ transplantation, embryonic stem cells, surrogate motherhood, gender identity disorder, sexual freedom and so on, all derived from the dissociation between the thoughts/facts introduced to Japan during the short period between the end of WW II and the present and the national character or ethical concepts formed throughout the long course of Japanese history, at least since the days of Prince Shotoku (who, as a member of Empress Suiko's dynasty, governed Japan at the end of the 6th century). The author hopes that Western ethics or logic will not be superficially accepted as if they are the sole and absolute forms of ethics and logic, despite the overwhelming achievement of basic and applied science; that is, the author hopes that tolerance will prevail in anticipation of a time when a novel ethical conclusion will be reached after science has been accepted and has matured in the deepness of culture or religion. This tolerance should be the general principle at any encounter between different cultures, and, in fact, tolerance, or *wa*, has been our tradition since the dawn of Japanese history.

This book was written based on a previous book on the same theme written by the author, which was published in Japanese about 4 years ago. The topics covered in the parts of this book entitled "Japanese religion" and "Culture and ethics" have been extensively researched after the publication of the previous book and consolidated here, it is hoped that this book will contribute to the international understanding of current Japanese mentality. The author is confident now, after the completion of this book, that Japan can accomplish a creative transformation of itself through the positive consciousness of its own tradition, as well as an active and alert attitude of perpetual scientific innovation.

The figures and tables in this book were prepared based on the author's own understanding of the cited references. However, the figure illustrating the structure of consciousness/unconsciousness in Chapter VII is simple and useful for understanding Jungian concepts, and it has been inserted after some modification upon obtaining permission from the original writer, Prof. Hayao Kawai, the Director General of the Agency for Cultural Affairs, who was an excellent introducer of the ideas of C. G. Jung to Japan and died much to the regret of all who know him a couple of months ago.

The publication of this book has become possible thanks to many dedicated people. The author expresses his special thanks to the late Prof. Yoshinori Takeuchi (Faculty of Literature, Kyoto University), his widow, Mitsu, and the late Dr. Masataka Sekoh (President of Kinki University). Also, the author expresses his thanks to his secretaries, Ms. Miho Hashimoto, Ms. Yoriko Uratake and Ms. Nobuko Sueyoshi, for their valuable work. Last but not least, the support graciously given to the author by his wife, Tomoko, and his three daughters, Mio, Aki and Sao, is greatly appreciated.

October 31, 2007

Author

Index

31-syllable verse, 149, 165
5-alpha-dihydrotestosterone (DHT), 235
Abe-no-Nakamaro, 111
Academeia, 64
ACTH, 226, 228
adrenal cortex, 222
adult T cell leukemia, 20
agathon, 204-205
Agent Orange, 1
AIDS, 7, 19-22, 24, 34
Akahiko Shimaki, 162, 169
Alcmaion, 50
Alexander the Great, 64
Amaterasu, 82
American bioethics, 212
Americanization, 120
Amida, 78
Amida-nyorai, 95
amino acid, 35
Amitabha, 78
Amitabha Buddha, 137
Anaxagoras, 51, 54
Anaximander, 48
Anaximenes, 48
androgen, 232, 237
androgen receptor, 235
androstenedione, 237
anima, 77
animism, 77, 130-131, 145
anti-androgen, 235
antisense strand, 29
arché, 47-52, 54, 56, 68, 168, 172
archetypes, 189
areté, 204, 206, 210
Aristotle, 55, 57-58, 63-66, 122, 172, 175, 179, 204-206
aromatase, 237
aromatic ring, 237
artificial insecticide, 225
Asanga, 88, 134
Asclepius, 62
Asia Minor, 47
Asuka, 78
Asuka period, 76, 84, 106, 126
Asuka-dera temple, 78
ATL, 7, 20-22, 24, 34
atmospheric pollution, 219
atomic bomb, 1, 6, 220-221
atomism, 52
atomos, 52
autonomy, 13, 197
Avatamasaka Sutra, 134
Avery, 27
Bacon, 176, 179, 190
Baekje, 100
Basho, 158
Beauchamp, 209
beneficence, 213
benevolence, 95, 127, 203-204, 208
Bentham, 199, 224
Benzaiten, 75
Berkeley, 190
Bewusstsein überhaupt, 181-182
BHC, 220
bio-diverse ecosystem, 219
bioethics, 1, 3, 12-13, 18, 24, 207, 209
biological accumulation, 221
Birusyana-butsu, 86
bisphenol A (BPA), 225, 234-236
Black Turtle-Snake, 116
blastocyst, 42, 44
Blue Dragon, 97, 116
Bodhidharma, 99
bodhisattva, 82, 95, 136
bosatsu, 95, 136

BPA, 229, 234
brachymelia, 239
Brahmanism, 90
breast cancer, 236
Buddha, 2, 51, 71, 75, 85, 112, 208
Buddha Rushana, 125
Buddhism, 75-76, 78, 84, 96, 108, 131, 169-170
Buddhism-Shintoism separation decree, 95
Buddhist precept, 219
bushi, 74, 92-93, 129, 137, 143-144
bushido, 74, 148, 203, 214
butsu, 95, 133
butsu-ga-ichinyo, 166
butsu-metsu, 145
by nature, 59
calcitonin, 37
calligraphic paintings, 138
calligraphy, 138, 159, 161-162
capitalism, 209
carbon dioxide, 15
Carson, 220, 222-223, 225
casuistry, 192
catecholamine, 37, 230
Categorical Imperative, 128, 191
causal mechanism, 188
causality, 175, 186, 189
CD4-positive T cells, 22
Cetaka, 75
Cha Chin, 104
cha-do, 145, 147, 157
Chaking, 104, 143
Chang' an, 111
cha-no-yu, 137, 147
chemical defoliants, 221
Chernobyl nuclear reactor accident, 18
Chi, 100
Childress, 209
Chinese Buddhism, 134

Chinese characters, 79, 106, 147
Chinese poems, 161-162
Chinese poetry, 159
Chinese thoughts, 121
Chinese-style poem, 159
cholesterol, 230
Chou, 71
chromatin, 28
Chronicles of Japan, 83, 132
Chu Hsi, 72, 127
Chu Hsi school, 72, 83, 94
Chuang-tzu, 72
clear-cell carcinoma, 229
clone, 41
cloned sheep, 7
codon, 34-35, 38
coexistence, 168, 219
cogito, 178
collective, 189
collective unconscious, 124, 189
common ecosystem, 219
communitarianism, 192, 210-211
compartmentalization, 219
complementary DNA, 29
complex, 188
confidentiality, 62, 213
Confucianism, 2, 71-73, 75-76, 95-96, 113-114, 126-127, 131, 139, 145
Confucius, 2, 71, 95, 127, 204, 208, 210
consciousness, 177, 188-189
consciousness in general, 181
consequence-based theory, 198
consequentialism, 200
Constitution of Seventeen Articles, 136
Corpus Hippocraticum, 58, 122
cortisol, 222, 226-228, 230-232
Cos, 62
CRH, 226, 228
crisis, 59

cryptorchidism, 229
cultura, 119
cultural transformation, 12
culture, 119
daidzein, 234-235
Dainichi-kyo, 86, 89-90, 135
Dainichi-nyorai, 86, 90, 95
Daisetsu Suzuki, 94, 203
Daruma-daishi, 99
Dasein, 181
DDD, 220-221, 223
DDT, 8, 220-225, 229, 235, 238
Declaration of Helsinki, 6, 213
Democritus, 52, 54, 58
DES, 228-229, 232, 238
Descartes, 15, 176-180, 186-187, 190-191, 224
Dewey, 201, 212
dharma, 79-80, 87
diabetes mellitus, 43
diethylstilbestrol (DES), 228, 234, 238
dioxin, 15, 225, 229, 235-236
diversity, 215
divinity, 57
DNA, 27-28, 32-34
DNA double helix model, 6
Dogen, 86, 92, 94, 104-105, 124, 136, 141-143, 159, 161-162
Dolly, 40
dopaminergic neurotransmission, 43
double-helix structure, 28
drug disaster, 239
dukkha, 133
duodenum, 65
E1, 229, 233, 237
E3, 229, 233
East Asian concept, 165
East Asian wisdom, 169
Eastern-style garden, 170
eco-philosophy, 224

ecosystem, 3, 13
Edo period, 127
ego, 188-189
eidos, 50, 56
Eihei-ji temple, 105
Eisai, 86, 92, 94, 104-105, 136, 140, 143, 157
eki, 145, 188, 190
Eleatic school, 52
emancipation, 88
Empedocles, 2, 51-54
Emperor Kanmu, 89
Emperor Okamoto, 153
Emperor Saga, 90, 93
Emperor Shomu, 87, 125, 136
empiricism, 176-177, 190-191, 194, 199, 202
Empress Suiko, 79, 84
emptiness, 134
encompassing, 180
endocrine disruptor, 226, 233
endocrine-disrupting chemicals, 225
endometriosis, 236
engi, 133, 169
enlightenment, 135
Enryaku-ji, 92, 140-141
environmental ethics, 1-3, 13-14, 18, 24, 224
environmental hormone, 18, 223, 225-226, 229, 232-233, 237
epidemic parotitis, 58
epilepsy, 60
epistemé, 58, 206
equol, 234-235
Erasistratus, 65-66
ES cells, 41-43
esoteric Buddhism, 86, 90, 135, 137, 141
estradiol, 223, 227-234, 237
estrogen, 223, 228-229, 232, 237

estrogen receptor, 229, 231-233, 235
estrogenic effect, 229, 232, 236
estrogen-like activity, 235
ethical theories, 202
ethics, 214
ethnicity, 120-121
ethos, 21, 58, 123, 206, 214
Existenz, 181-183, 186
Existenz-Transzendenz axis, 183
external nature, 167-168
extroversion, 190
fairness, 208
faith, 95
FDA, 229
Five Elements, 99, 102-103, 105, 145, 166
Five-Element philosophy, 116
flower arrangement, 101
food chain, 223
forms, 54
formula of autonomy (FA), 197
formula of humanity (FH), 196
Formula of Universal Law, 128
formula of universal law (FUL), 196
four bodily humors, 59
fragile X syndrome, 39
freedom, 212
freon gas, 3
Freud, 187-188
Friedreich's ataxia, 39
Fugen-bosatsu, 95
Fujiwara clan, 90-91
Fujiwara-no-Teika, 156
Fu-ryu-moji, 141
Galen, 66-67
Ganjin, 126
Geist, 181-182
General Shinto, 82
genetic counseling, 208
genetic information, 29

genistein, 234-235
Genji-monogatari, 147, 151
Genjo, 134
genome, 29
Genshin, 91-92
German Idealism, 191, 198
GHG, 17
Ginkaku-ji, 139
global ecosystem, 202, 220, 224, 243
global warming, 16, 219
globalization, 175
globalization of knowledge, 12
glucocorticoid, 230
gogyo, 105
gogyokaku, 102
Golden Mean, 58, 206
gongu-jodo, 91
Good, 204, 206
Gozan literature, 139, 143
Great Mother, 188
Great Sun Sutra, 86, 89-90, 135
Greek culture, 67
Greek natural philosophy, 47
green house gas, 17
Gyo, 88
Gyoki, 87
haiku, 74, 124, 150, 158, 162
Hannya-kyo, 85-86
happiness, 198
Harvey, 179
Hashimoto's thyroiditis, 227
Hayao Kawai, 188-189
Hegel, 177
Heian Buddhism, 94
Heian period, 90
Heike Monogatari, 154-155
hematopoietic stem cells, 43
Heraclitus, 50-51, 65
himorogi, 77
Hinayana Buddhism, 87, 93, 125
Hindu gods, 75

Hinduism, 90
Hippocrates, 2, 52, 58, 60-61, 63-64, 122, 146, 167, 176, 208
Hippocratic paternalism, 62
hiragana, 91
Historia Animalium, 57
HIV, 20-23
Hobbes, 176, 179, 190
hoen, 105
Hojo-ki, 154-155
Hokke-kyo, 86, 134
homeostasis, 228
Honen, 91-92, 138
honji, 82
honji-suijaku, 82-83
Horatius, 52
hormone receptor, 228
hormones, 226
Horyu-ji, 80, 96
hotoke, 78, 95
HTLV-1, 20-22
Hua-yen Sutra, 134
Hudo, 122
human dignity, 213
human ES cells, 42, 44
human existence, 190
human genome project, 29
human rights, 213
human science, 175
humanity, 208
Hume, 190
Huntington gene, 38
Huntington's disease, 38
hylé, 56
hypospadias, 229
I Ching, 188
Ideas, 50, 54, 56, 205
ikebana, 102, 145
Imperial Regime, 132
in vitro fertilization, 41, 44
Inazo Nitobe, 203, 214

Incan civilization, 120
Incan Empire, 120
Indian Buddhism, 140
Indra, 75
Industrial Revolution, 3, 220
industrial waste, 3
infertility, 236
informed consent, 213
initiator codon, 34
insecticide, 220-221
instrumentalism, 201
intellect, 186, 191, 194
internal nature, 167-168
introversion, 190
Ionia, 47, 49
Ionian school, 49
Ippen, 94, 138
isoflavone, 235
Issa, 124
IT revolution, 9-10, 12, 120, 176
IVF, 41, 44
Izanagi-no-mikoto, 132
James, 201
Japan Association for Bioethics, 1
Japanese culture, 129, 144
Japanese feelings in literature, 150
Japanese garden, 171
Japanese mythology, 98
Japanese poetry, 141
Japanese religion, 71
Japanese spirituality, 157
Japanese tea ceremony, 105
Jaspers, 5-6, 177, 180, 190
jichin-sai, 84
jin, 101
jinen, 167
jinen honi, 167
Jingu-ji, 81-82, 137
Ji-shu, 94, 138
Jizo-bosatsu, 95

Jodo, 138
Jodo-shin-shu, 92, 138
Jodo-shu, 92, 138
Jung, 2, 177, 187-188, 190
justice, 95, 208, 213
Kaga-go, 40
Kakinomoto-no-Hitomaro, 152
Kamakura Buddhism, 91-93
Kamakura Shogunate, 156
kami, 77, 132
kami-dana, 107, 132
kami-danomi, 132
Kamo-no-Chomei, 154
kana, 147, 151
Kanemi Yusho affair, 7
kanji, 72, 79, 106, 147-149, 151
Kan-jizai-Bosatsu, 136
Kan-non-Bosatsu, 136
Kanoe-saru, 98
Kanon-bosatsu, 95
kanshi, 149, 160
Kant, 177, 191-192, 194-195, 197-198, 201, 208, 224
Kantian ethics, 128
Kantianism, 192-193, 197-198, 212
Kan-ze-on-Bosatsu, 136
katatagae, 145
Kegon Sutra, 86, 126, 134, 137
Kegon-kyo, 86, 134
Keiji Nishitani, 94
Kenji Miyazawa, 16
kimon, 145
Kinkai-waka-shu, 155-157
Kinkaku-ji, 139
Kissa-yojoki, 104, 143
Kitaro Nishida, 6, 94
Kiyoshi Takatsuki, 20, 34
Klinefelter's syndrome, 28
koan, 104
Kofuku-ji temple, 134
Kofun (tumulus) period, 76

Koguryo, 78, 98
Koji Fukunaga, 80
Kojiki, 82-83, 100, 148, 165
Koke-dera, 125
Kokin-waka-shu, 151
Kongocho-kyo, 135
Ko-shin, 98
Kozen-gokoku-ron, 143
Kuan-ti, 99
Kublai Khan, 137
kuh, 85, 134
Kukai, 89-90, 93, 135, 147
Kumaarajiiva (Kumarajiva), 86, 134
Kyoto Conference, 17
Kyoto Protocol, 7, 17
lack of insulin, 43
Lao Tzu, 71-73, 96, 99, 204
Leibniz, 191
Lenz, 238
Leopold, 5-6
leprosy, 240
Leucippus, 52
LH, 227-228
LH-RH, 228
Li Bai, 135
liberal individualism, 212-213
liberalism, 13, 209, 212
life, 27, 192
Locke, 190
logos, 14
Lotus Sutra, 86, 90, 134, 140, 160
love and strife, 51
low sperm count, 236
Lu Wu, 104
Luwuh, 143
Lykeion, 64
macrocosmos, 135
Magna Graecia, 49, 54
Mahaparinirvana-sutra, 85
Mahavairocana, 86, 89, 137
Mahavairocana Sutra, 86, 89

Mahayana Buddhism, 71, 85, 87, 90, 93, 112-113, 125, 136
Mahayana sutras, 79
Makura-no-soshi, 98, 147, 151
mandala, 86, 188
mantra, 88
manyo-kana, 149
Manyo-shu, 147-151, 156, 165
mappo, 94, 137
material civilization, 3
maternal inheritance, 27
matsuri, 84, 132
matter, 56
Ma-tzu, 99
mechanicism, 14
mechanism, 186
meditative concentration, 135
medullary thyroid cancer, 37
Meiji Restoration, 106
MEN, 37
MEN2, 36
Mencius, 71, 204, 208
Mendel, 27
Mendel's law, 6
messenger RNA, 31-32, 233
metaphysics, 47
microcosmos, 135
middle-path virtues, 206
mikkyo, 135, 137
mikoshi, 84
Miletus, 47, 49, 52
Mill, 199-200, 208, 212
Minamata disease, 6, 18, 243
Minamoto-no-Sanetomo, 104, 144, 155-156
mind-body unity, 4
mineralocorticoid, 230
mitochondrial diseases, 27
Mitotane, 222
Mitsuji Fukunaga, 140
Miyoji Ueda, 164
modern bioethics, 208
modern science, 191
modern weapons, 221
modernization, 3, 220
Mokichi Saitoh, 163
monadism, 191
Mongolian invasions, 137, 146
monism of science, 175
Monju-bosatsu, 95
Mononobe clan, 79
monozygotic twins, 39
monsoon climate, 123
Montagnier, 20, 34
Mt. Etna, 52
Mt. Hiei, 89, 92, 142
Mt. Koya, 89
mu, 85
mujo, 94
multiple endocrine neoplasia, 2, 36-37
Murasaki Shikibu, 101
Muromachi period, 139
myeloma, 240
Naagaarjuna (Nagarjuna), 87, 134
namu Amida Butsu, 92
Nanpo (Southern) Zen, 104
Nara period, 81
national interests, 220
natura, 167
natural healing power, 59, 167
natural science, 175, 194
Nehan-kyo, 85
Neo-Confucianism, 72, 83
new millennium, 3
Nichiren, 92, 94
Nichiren-shu, 92, 94
Nicomachean Ethics, 58
Nihonshoki, 83, 132, 148
nirvana, 85, 88, 112, 219
nirvana pictures, 168
Nirvana sutra, 124

nomos, 210
non-maleficence, 213
non-malevolence, 208
nonsteroidal estrogen, 235
Norihiko Aoki, 169
Noto-go, 40
nous, 51, 58, 206
nucleic acids, 33
nucleotide, 28-29
nucleus, 228, 231, 233
nyorai, 86, 95, 133
Oath of Hippocrates, 62-63
Obaku Zen, 157
objectivism, 190
objectivity, 14
Ohjo-yoshu, 91-92
Ohno Yasumaro, 148
Okinawa, 96-97
Oku-no-Hosomichi, 158
Onmyodo, 101
onnade, 91
onozukara, 169
onri-edo, 91
On-yo-do, 100-101, 145
Orphism, 49, 52
Other Shore, 88
ouch-ouch disease, 6, 18, 243
Our Stolen Future, 7
Paekche, 78
pancreatic β-cells, 43
panta rhei, 50
parathyroid tumor, 37
Parkinson's disease, 43
Parmenides, 52
paternalism, 13
PCB, 8, 229, 235
Peirce, 201
Pergamum, 66
Peripatetics, 64
pheochromocytoma, 37
Phoenix, 116

phronesis, 58, 207-208
physics, 47
physis, 59, 167
phytoestrogens, 235
Pillow Book, 98, 101, 147
plasmacytoma, 242
Plato, 2, 5, 53-54, 57, 63, 172, 175, 179, 204-205, 210
Plato's astronomy, 54
pneuma, 66
poetic rhythm, 165
poiesis, 57
politeness, 95
polychlorinated biphenyl (PCB), 225, 234-236
polyglutamine disease, 38-39
pragmatism, 198, 200-202, 212
Prajna-sutra, 85-86, 133
praxis, 210
primary matter, 47, 49, 51
Prime Minister Shinzo Abe, 23
Prime Minister Yasuo Fukuda, 23
primitive Shinto, 76-77
Prince Shotoku, 23, 79-81, 83-84, 86, 88, 96, 106-107, 165
Principles of Biomedical Ethics, 193
principlism, 209-210
privacy, 208
psyche, 53-54, 77, 189-190, 205
psychological energy, 190
Pure Land, 137-138
Pythagoras, 49-50, 54, 63, 172, 179
Pythagorean community, 50
Pythagorean school, 52
rationalism, 177, 191
Rawls, 198
reasoning animals, 71
Record of Ancient Matters, 83, 100
religion in Vietnam, 112
religion of Vietnam, 108

replication, 29, 31
respect for autonomy, 213
respectfulness, 208
RET gene, 36-37
retroviral disease, 7
retrovirus, 20, 34
rights theories, 214
Rinzai Zen, 92, 94, 141, 157
Rinzai-shu, 92, 104
RNA, 32-34
Rushana-butsu, 125-126
Ryokan, 159, 161-162
Ryokan's waka, 165
Ryukyu, 96-97
Sacred Disease, 60
sacred rope, 107
Sagagoryu Ikebana School, 101
Saicho, 89, 104, 135
Saigyo, 153-154, 162
Saiho-ji, 125
Sakra devanam Indra, 75
samadhi, 135
Sami-Mansei, 152
samsara, 88
samurai, 74, 93, 95, 129, 137-138, 143, 203
sanganichi, 132
Sanka-shu, 153
sansaikaku, 101
Sanzo-hoshi, 134
Sarasvati, 75
satori, 88, 90, 135
scientific anarchism, 4
scientific experiments, 190
scientism, 4
Sei Shonagon, 101
Sein, 180
self, 189
self-help, 138
sense strand, 29
seppuku, 129

sex hormone, 230-232
Shaka-nyorai, 95
Shakuson, 85
Shakyamuni, 2, 71, 85, 138
shikantaza, 105, 142
shimenawa, 107
Shingon Buddhism, 93, 135
Shingon esoteric Buddhism, 90, 104
Shingon-shu, 89
Shinjin-datsuraku, 162
Shin-kokin-waka-shu, 141
Shinran, 91-92, 138, 167
Shinto, 75-79, 84, 106, 131, 140, 145
Shinto customs, 132
Shinto god shelf, 107
Shinto Shrines, 84
Shintoism, 83
Shinto-style festival, 132
Shinya Yamanaka, 44
Shitenno, 75
Shitenno-ji, 79-80, 96, 98
shizen, 167
Shobo-genzo, 105, 142, 162
Shofuku-ji, 93
shoin-zukuri, 139
shrine Shinto, 82
Sicilia, 49
Sicily, 49, 51
sickle cells, 36
Sikelia, 49, 51
Silent Spring, 8, 220, 222-224
Silla, 78
Sinnlichkeit, 194
six Nara Buddhism sects, 126
SNP, 30
social animals, 71
Socrates, 5, 53, 58, 175, 204, 210
Soga clan, 78
sokushin-jobutsu, 90, 137, 147, 166
sophia, 58, 205, 207

Soto Zen, 94, 142, 157, 161
Soto-shu, 92, 104, 138, 142
Southern Sung China, 157
southern Zen, 92, 99
Spanish flu, 6
spinocerebellar ataxia, 39
Spinoza, 191
spirit, 192
steroid hormone, 230-232
steroid skeleton, 233
stop codon, 34
Subjekt-Objekt-Spaltung, 183
sufficient information, 213
Sui, 76, 80, 112
suijaku, 82
Sung China, 104
sunya, 85
sunyata, 88, 134
supreme Buddha, 135
sutra, 80, 112
synchronicity, 189-190
syncretism, 131
syncretization, 78
syncretization of Buddhism and Taoism, 98
Syofuku-ji, 141
syogatsu, 132
T cells, 21
tai-an, 145
Tale of Genji, 101, 147
tamagaki fences, 84
Tang, 76, 112
Tang China, 104
tanka, 144, 149-151, 157, 160, 165
tantra, 86, 90
tao, 96-97, 204
Taoism, 72-73, 75-76, 96-99, 114, 127, 131, 139-140, 145, 204
tea ceremony, 74, 137, 143
tea plants, 104
techné, 58, 206-207

teleology, 67, 179
telos, 56
temae, 105
ten, 72, 101
ten-batsu, 72
Tendai-shu, 89, 92
ten-en tsi-ho, 101
ten-i, 73
ten-mei, 72, 101
ten-noh, 80, 101, 140
ten-sai, 72
teratogenicity, 239
testosterone, 227-228, 230-231, 237
Tetsuro Watsuji, 122, 146
Thales, 48, 52, 54
thalidomide, 238-240, 242
thalidomide disaster, 240-242
thalidomide embryopathy, 239
The Climate, 122-123
the unconscious, 189
Theravada Buddhism, 87, 112
thyroid hormone, 227, 230-232
Tibetan Book of the Dead, 188
Timaeus, 52, 54, 63
Todai-ji, 87, 125
tokonoma, 139
torii gates, 84
Tosa Nikki, 147, 150
total mind, 188
totality, 187, 190
traditional flower arrangement, 74
traditional verses, 165
transcendental, 138
transcription, 31-32, 34
transmigration of the soul, 88
Transzendenz, 180, 182-183
TRH, 230
triplet, 38
TSH, 228
tsi, 101
Turner's syndrome, 28

Tuskegee affair, 7
Tuskegee Syphilis Study, 12
Uji-cha, 104
uji-dera, 78
Umgreifende, 180-183, 186
unconscious, 177, 188-189
unmoving mover, 56
uranai, 145
utilitarianism, 198-199, 202, 212
Vairocana(Vairochana), 86, 125, 135
Vairochana
Vajrasekhara Sutra, 135
Vasubandhu, 88, 134
Vernunft, 182-183, 194
Verstand, 183, 191, 194
Vietnam, 96
vijnana, 88
Vimalakirti-nirdesa Sutra, 133
Vimalakirti-sutra, 86
vimukti, 88
virtue, 203, 205-206
virtue-based theories, 192, 203, 209, 214
vis medicatrix naturae, 59, 167
wa, 23, 79-81, 106-107
wabi, 94
wabi-cha, 105, 145, 147, 157
wa-fuku, 81
wa-jin, 80
waka, 74, 91, 111, 141, 144, 149-151, 157-162, 165
wa-koku, 80
wa-shiki, 81
wa-shitsu, 81
wa-shoku, 81
wa-shu, 81
Watson and Crick, 28
way of tea, 157
Welt, 180
Western concept, 166
Western wisdom, 170
Western-style garden, 170
White Tiger, 116
wisdom, 95
Wisdom Sutra, 85, 133
Wise Old Man, 188
Wissenschaftsaberglaube, 187
Wu Xing, 99-100, 143-144, 166
Wu-Xing theory, 100
X-chromosome, 28, 39
Xuan-zang, 134
Yakumo-tatsu, 149
Yakushi-nyorai, 95
Yamabe-no-Akahito, 152
Yamato, 81, 150
Yamato dynasty, 78-79
Yang, 97, 100
Yaoyorozu-no-kami, 146
Yayoi period, 76
Y-chromosome, 28
Yin, 71, 97, 100
Yin period, 73
Yin-Yang, 72, 99-100, 102, 105, 145, 166
Yin-Yang theory, 100
Yokkaichi asthma, 6, 18, 243
Yuima-kyo, 86, 134
zazen, 138, 142, 159, 161
Zen, 99, 141, 143-144, 157-158, 169, 203
Zen Buddhism, 74, 104, 138, 140
Zen meditation, 94
Zen practice, 146
Zhu Xi, 127
β-globin, 35

LIFE AND ETHICS IN JAPAN
- in consideration of history, religion and culture -

2008年3月28日　第1刷発行

著　者　Norihiko Aoki〔青木矩彦〕
発行者　柳原浩也
発行所　柳原出版株式会社
　　　　〒615-8107　京都市西京区川島北裏町74
　　　　電話　075 (381) 2319
　　　　FAX　075 (393) 0469
　　　　ホームページ　http://www.yanagihara-pub.com/

印刷・製本　大村印刷株式会社

Copyright © Norihiko Aoki2008　Printed in japan
ISBN 978-4-8409-7049-5